Public Policy and Health Care in China

W0234912

This book examines the introduction and ongoing development of public medical care insurance in contemporary China.

Based on extensive field investigations, residents' surveys and analyses by local policy experts and practitioners it provides a comparative analysis of the marketization of public policy in China in contrast to those in other countries, such as the United Kingdom and Germany. The book highlights system-specific issues of the centrally planned economy (CPE) during economic reform, such as alienation of entitlements from funding and historically rooted obligations in the realm of public policy, and as such fills the gap in research on the Chinese government's public financial management.

Public Policy and Health Care in China will appeal to students, academics and researchers interested in public policy and health care in China, as well as Chinese society and economics more broadly.

Peter Nan-shong Lee is Professor Emeritus at the Department of Political Science at the National Chung Cheng University, Taiwan.

Routledge Contemporary China Series

For more information about this series, please visit: https://www.routledge.com/Routledge-Contemporary-China-Series/book-series/SE0768

Public Policy and Health Care in China

The Case of Public Insurance

Peter Nan-shong Lee

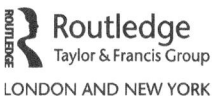
Routledge
Taylor & Francis Group

LONDON AND NEW YORK

First published 2024
by Routledge
4 Park Square, Milton Park, Abingdon, Oxon OX14 4RN

and by Routledge
605 Third Avenue, New York, NY 10158

Routledge is an imprint of the Taylor & Francis Group, an informa business

© 2024 Peter Nan-shong Lee

The right of Peter Nan-shong Lee to be identified as author of this work
has been asserted in accordance with sections 77 and 78 of the Copyright,
Designs and Patents Act 1988.

All rights reserved. No part of this book may be reprinted or reproduced or
utilized in any form or by any electronic, mechanical, or other means, now
known or hereafter invented, including photocopying and recording, or in
any information storage or retrieval system, without permission in writing
from the publishers.

Trademark notice: Product or corporate names may be trademarks or
registered trademarks, and are used only for identification and explanation
without intent to infringe.

British Library Cataloguing-in-Publication Data
A catalogue record for this book is available from the British Library

Library of Congress Cataloging-in-Publication Data
Names: Lee, Peter N. S., 1940– author.
Title: Public policy and health care in China : the case of public insurance /
Peter Nan-shong Lee.
Description: Abingdon, Oxon ; New York, NY : Routledge, 2024. |
Series: Routledge contemporary China series | Includes bibliographical
references and index.
Identifiers: LCCN 2023005218 (print) | LCCN 2023005219 (ebook) |
ISBN 9781032486192 (hardback) | ISBN 9781032486208 (paperback) |
ISBN 9781003389934 (ebook)
Subjects: LCSH: Medical policy—China. | Medical care—China.
Classification: LCC RA395.C53 L43 2024 (print) | LCC RA395.C53
(ebook) | DDC 362.10951—dc23/eng/20230502
LC record available at https://lccn.loc.gov/2023005218
LC ebook record available at https://lccn.loc.gov/2023005219

ISBN: 978-1-032-48619-2 (hbk)
ISBN: 978-1-032-48620-8 (pbk)
ISBN: 978-1-003-38993-4 (ebk)

DOI: 10.4324/9781003389934

Typeset in Times New Roman
by codeMantra

Contents

Acknowledgments

It has taken longer for the author to complete this research project, thankfully leading to the publication of the book entitled *Public Policy and Health Care in China.* The book could not have been completed without the assistance of numerous institutes and individuals, whom the author owes appreciation and gratitude. It would have been next to impossible to name them all, but in this limited space, the author wishes to register his sincere thanks to some most prominent ones.

One of the most notable institutes that the author feels grateful for is the Universities Services Center for China Studies (USCCS) where the author paid numerous visits and devoted considerably lengthy time through many years. The book would not have been possible without relying on the collection of USCCS. The documentary part of the research demonstrates how the public organization operates as it is based on written communication on an enormous scale featuring the attributes of impersonality (i.e., going beyond face-to-face relations) in the realm of public policy.

Two institutes in China to which the author is indebted greatly were the Guangzhou Academy of Social Science (GASS) and Shanghai Academy of Social Science (SASS) that were most helpful in scheduling and arranging interviews, about sixty interviewees (as individuals or panels of two or several), on policy actors and analysts in the arena of public policy in the two municipal jurisdictions. These interviews highlight the role of policy actors in real-life situations, enabling the author to articulate and observe public policy phenomenon at the local level from the interpretive frame of reference. Several colleagues deserve special thanks: Li Jiangtao, Cai Guoxuan, and Tong Xiapin in GASS and Wu Shusong in SASS.

The academic research on such a valuable subject-matter in China's public policy during economic reform gained additional strength due to funding by institutes concerned. The research project received generous financial assistance from the University Grants Committee of Hong Kong Government, SAR, making possible many field studies in China and the completion of two opinion surveys in Guangzhou and Shanghai respectively. The research project benefited from the grants from the National Science Commission in Taiwan, greatly facilitating a follow-up investigation in Xiamen, Fujian.

The research project benefits from guidance and inspirations on the subject-matter from several scholars in China, among whom are Professor Gu Xin of the Beijing University, Hu Shuyun from SASS, and Professor Du Lexun,

Harbin Medical University. The author repeatedly and continuously consulted their publications, journal articles, and books during the long process of research over years too.

For the write-up, the author received great help from Professor Timothy Guile who not only acted as a lay reader to push for clarity of text, but also, he alerted the author about the issues of academic writing from the perspective of a scholar. Also, thanks are owed to Dr. Crystine Lee (MD) whose help to solving the issues of computer greatly facilitated the editorial work. Finally, Dr. Chien Yuchin, spared her previous time and extraordinary skill to do all tables and figures with accuracy and excellent graphic designs within short notice.

Above all, credits ought to go to the acquisition editor Ms. Stephane Rogers and the entire editorial team of Routledge whose contributions to publishing a non-market-oriented academic book and promoting Social Science and China Studies are both unmeasurable and invaluable.

Preface

During the years of his graduate study, the author often heard about what the markets can do, but not often heard what the markets cannot. As the issue of marketization represented one of the most controversial topics among prominent economists such as Milton Friedman for decades during the turn of the century. To seek enlightenment, the author was eager to find an answer on the issue in the realm of public policy. After the beginning of his academic career, the author was very fortunate and found a rare opportunity to meet and listen to Professor Friedman and Mrs. Rose Friedman in their house at the Russian Hill at San Francisco during a worldwide study tour on the use of coupons and early childhood education in the USA, the UK, and other European countries back in 2002. The debate on the issue continued to occupy the author's mind for many years, providing stimuli to conduct serious research and finally produced this book volume. In connection with our memorable visit to the late Professor Friedman and Mrs. Friedman, the author would like to register much gratitude to the anonymous, enthusiastic, and intellectually stimulating sponsor who made the meaningful study tour possible.

This study's main intellectual and theoretical theme is concerned with "marketization," namely, introducing markets into the realm of public policy. And such an inspiring idea on marketization has been incorporated into public policy studies in the West, for instance, taken as a main theme in the so-called New Public Management since the late 1970s, remaining as an exciting theoretical vantage for several generations of students and scholars in the field. In view of acute shortage of empirical investigations on the subject-matter for years, it is always meaningful to make a close look at how markets have made it into the realm of public policy studies, so long a significant and fruitful breakthrough waits for interested and dedicated scholars. From a broad perspective, the study endeavors to initiate the intellectual and theoretical dialogs on the issue of marketization between Political Science and Economics as well as between Social Sciences of the West and China studies.

There were two market-oriented reforms in health care taking place in China during the era of reform: One regards revenue-generating endeavors through the introduction of user charges by the subsidized public providers, for example, in reforms centering on franchising of curative care services, drugs prescriptions, and medical devices at the public hospital level, and the other pertains to the introduction of public medical care insurance. Both are concerned with marketization with regard to public funding of medical care, as well as the use of markets in financial management in the public sector. However, they differ from each other with reference to problem area, major theoretical concern, and empirical research material and database. In the former, the representative works include *Re-engineering Affordable Care Policy in China* (by Peter Nan-shong Lee, first published by Routledge in 2019; paperback 2020). As an example of the latter, the current research monograph is concerned with the inauguration of public medical care insurance that relies on premium contribution and risk pooling mechanisms to help alleviate the financial burden of enrollees who seek cure from providers.

For more than three decades from the late 1980s to the 2020s, the making of public medical care insurance represents a landmark in the transformation from conventional funding mode of healthcare to the entirely new designs of public insurance, involving multiple layers of medical care demands, various sectors, and jurisdictions as well as inter-generational interactions in China. To examine this public policy change of historical significance, the study is focused on three packages of public medical care insurance, covering the entire population of 1.4 billion: The basic medical care insurance (BMCI) for the staff and workers in public enterprises and public personnel of the government and other public organizations, the urban resident medical care insurance (URMCI) for dependents of employees of public enterprises and public personnel of the government and other public organizations, and the new rural cooperative medical care insurance (NRCMCI) for the peasants. As soon as these three packages had been put into implementation, sovereign planners took a further step to promote the policy of integration at the municipal level, to initiate the combination between URMCI and NRCMCI at the municipal level by the late 2010s, promising a much long-term development of public medical care insurance in the foreseeable future.

In the Chinese context, healthcare policy was treated as an integral part of social security policy, and the study of healthcare is inseparable from an analysis of social security policy. It is meaningful to examine commonalities and differences between the two arenas. Nevertheless, it is worthwhile to go deeper and examine health care in greater details. As a public policy analysis on the Chinese case, furthermore, the study will work with two analytical foci that are interconnected in the inauguration of public medical care insurances. First, the study intends to address the issues of how policy actors make use of market mechanisms in both financing and spending functions of financial management of public insurance foundation. The study is focused on innovative forms of resource management, dealing with theoretical issues arising from the hybrid mode of governance in the realm of public policy. These issues include program specificity, product/service specificity, preference-mix, choice behavior in regulated market, behavioral adaptations in the markets, application of risk pooling mechanism, non-departmental public entity, and transaction-centered management, just to name a few. Second, the study will tackle the issues regarding how vested interests enter designing, packaging, and policy enforcement in the realm of public policy. For example, how the central policymakers interacted with their provincial/local counterparts in coping with the tension arising from the priority of HESI in the packaging of BMCI, URMCI, and NRCMCI?

Likely to be one of the most through and theoretically interesting analyses on the subject-matter for several recent decades, the study is solidly based on many trips of field investigations and extensive opinion surveys of residents, observations, and analyses by local policy experts, as well as policy guidelines, directives and regulations, and communication and analysis of practitioners who work on the first line of implementation. The volume heavily relies on several empirical case studies, such as Guangzhou, Shanghai, and Shenzhen, adding another empirical case study of policymaking that represents a rare commodity circulated in the circle of public policy studies.

It is next to impossible to handle the theme of public medical care insurance within a limited space in one book volume, given the lengthy time span, number and complexity, and multiplicity of analytical and theoretical dimensions. Accordingly, the study would be only able to answer parts of the questions so raised in this book volume, in so far as the empirical materials permit. Above all, the study has just mapped the theoretical and analytical perimeter for the investigation on public medical care insurance, one of the most innovative undertakings in public policy in China during economic reform.

Abbreviations

ACFLU	All-China Federation of Labor Unions
BLSS	Bureau of Labor and Social Security
BMCI	Basic medical care insurance
BMCIF	Basic medical care insurance foundation
CCP	The Chinese Communist Party
CCI	Comprehensive care insurance
CHCI	Commercial health care insurance
COE	Collective-owned enterprises
CPE	Centrally planned economy
CRSW	Congress of representatives of staff and workers
DRG	Diagnosis-related group
EAF	Enterprise adjustment fund
ESMCI	Enterprise supplementary medical care insurance
FUS	Financial undertaking system
HCI	Hospital care insurance
HESI	High expenditure serious illness
IRFS	Inward-resource-flow system
JFPURS	Joint family production undertaking responsibility system
LEMCI	Large expenditure medical care insurance
LIMC	Labor insurance medical care
LSMC	Local supplementary medical care
LSMCI	Local supplementary medical care insurance
MIF	Major illness fund
MII	Major illness insurance
MOA	Ministry of Agriculture
MOF	Ministry of Finance
MOH	Ministry of Health
NDPE	Non-departmental public entity
NHS	National Health Services
NHSA	National Health Security Administration
NIC	National health insurance contributions
NRCMCI	New rural cooperative medical care insurance
ORFS	Outward-resource-flow system

OPP	Out-of-pocket payment
OPMCI	Outside personnel medical care insurance
PA	Personal account
PAF	Personal account fund
PFMC	Public financed medical care
PRC	People's Republic of China
PPMCS	Public personnel medical care subsidy
PSC	Payment starting criterion
PSL	Payment starting line
RCMC	Rural cooperative medical care
RSS	Revene sharing system
SCI	Special care insurance
SP	Supplementary fund
SOE	State-owned enterprise
SMI	Subsidy for major illness
SMCI	Supplementary medical care insurance
SMCISW	Supplementary medical care insurance for staff and workers
SUF	Social unified funding
UIP	Urban insurance program
URS	Undertaking responsibility system
URMCI	Urban resident medical care insurance
URRMCI	Urban and rural resident medical care insurance
WUSMCI	Work unit supplementary medical care insurance

1   Introduction

With its massive size and largest population in the world, China is posed as a great intellectual and academic challenge for the observers and analysts alike to make sense out of the social security policy. In its early origin, there was a low degree of institutional differentiation within social security policy that embraced a broad range of entitlements and benefits, such retirement pension, health care, allowances and subsidies, welfare and relief, and facilities and amenities among others under the command economy. During economic reform, a separate program identity only took shape gradually in each functional area, coupled with expanding institutional, managerial, and financial autonomy. It is unavoidable for observers and analysts to engage in the constant trading between generality and particularity in a serious attempt to make sense of public policy, given a broad sphere including numerous functional components. From an epistemological perspective, one may find a metaphor of "forest and trees" illuminating in an intellectual endeavor to describe the relationship between social security and its components such as health care—the theme of the study.

Through the exercise of program specificity, for sure, the social security reform produced new programs that represented not only new types and standards of services, but also an upgrade and improvements in organizational, managerial, and financial terms. In the realm of public policy in China, for example, some entirely new programs of social security were introduced, as they were marked by new types of entitlements and benefits, funding sources, and funding levels, new approaches to provisions, spending control measures and new managerial tools during the reform era.

As a relatively new subject-matter in public policy and in China studies, it is by no means easy to find a handle to tackle public policy issues in general and health care in particular in China. So far a considerable number of authors and analysts have tried to conduct research on the subject-matter and produced some substantial research results (Dangdai Zhongguo congshu bianjibu 1988; Zhan, Yang & Zhang 1993; Yu & Song 1998; Wang 1998; Xu, Yin & Zheng 1999; Cheng 2000; Song 2001; Lee & Lo 2001; Zheng 2011; Qian 2021). The study represents a fresh attempt to analyze social security policy from the theoretical perspective of public management, making use of concepts and theories proposed and built in recent

DOI: 10.4324/9781003389934-1

decades. Meanwhile, it is an endeavor to bring Western concepts and theories into the field of China studies.

This introductory chapter will endeavor to provide mapping about the new funding system of social security, highlighting its key characteristics as well as some main conceptual and theoretical concerns. This study here will first examine the scope, types and characteristics of the three public medical care insurances (i.e., BMCI, URMCI, and NRCMCI). Next, this study here will deal with issues revolving around the application of a market-oriented approach to health care reforms, and the rise of the hybrid mode of governance in the public sector in light of the broad trend in public policy and management in China during recent decades. A chapter plan as well as highlights of the book volume will be given at the very end.

The Packages of Public Medical Care Funding

As sovereign planners endeavored to propel modernization and industrial growth, they began to establish the centrally planned economy in China from the 1950s onward. To accumulate financial surplus rapidly within a short time period, sovereign planners tried to enforce a tight budget of remuneration to the workforce. They needed to adopt a low wage policy to accumulate an enormous amount of revenue through paying the staff and workers less. Overall, not only were the employees insufficiently paid in form of wage compensation, but also non-wage compensation (such as social security) was inadequately funded under the low wage policy (Chapter 3). The government did promulgate a series of laws and regulations pertaining to types and standards about security, but the work units were given responsibility for funding and management in the situation where the government was not able to build a separate system of apparatus, funding, measure, and management (Chapter 4).

In building the centrally planned economy (CPE) during the early and middle 1950s, two public funding programs of medical care were made available to all personnel employed in the public sector. These two programs are: Public-Financed Medical Care (PFMC; *gongfei yiliao*; hereafter) and Labor Insurance Medical Care (LIMC; *laobao yiliao*). They offered comparable types and standards of medical care, but they remained institutionally and operationally separated from each other prior to the economic reform. The former catered to the medical care demands of civil servants and personnel of other public organizations (e.g., political parties, service units, educational establishments, and research institutes); the latter provided funding to medical care to the staff and workers of state-owned enterprises (SOEs), and subsequently collective-owned enterprises (COEs) (Dangdai Zhongguo congshu bianjibu 1988: 232–7). In the wake of the agricultural collectivization movements, rural cooperative medical care (RCMC; *nongchun hezou yiliao*) was first made available to the peasantry during the 1960s, and this continued to the 1980s and was then dismantled as the collective economy collapsed (see Chapter 10).

Against the background of conventional public funding packages, inaugurating public medical care insurances represents an endeavor to build new packages of funding to replace the pre-reform designs for the entire population, employed and unemployed (Gu 2010). Sovereign planners made attempts to introduce the first package of public insurance reform, namely, the so-called basic medical care insurance (BMCI) in anticipation of the transformation of CPE to a mixed economy, thereby accommodating employees in various ownership systems, covering multiple layers of medical care demands (Wang 2008). Facing a long period of transition after its commencement in 2001, BMCI had to include not only employees of the conventional CPE sector, but also fresh recruits from all sectors of the mixed economy. The second package pertained to urban resident medical care Insurance (URMCI), targeted at unemployed personnel in urban areas, for example, family members of employees in all public organizations, retirees, and students at all levels among others. The third package was concerned with a new rural cooperative medical care insurance (or NRCMCI) catering to demands for medical insurance for the peasants—the largest sector of the population in China (Gu 2010).

These three packages were not identical to one another in terms of their policy orientations, targeted enrollees, defined types of demands, funding modes and payment schemes, and managerial and institutional designs. And, each addressed various layers of medical care demands, and the level of benefits varied from one jurisdiction to another (Gu 2010: 60–8). The design of public medical care insurance covered the lowest level of benefits and was supposed to meet the requirements of essential medical care and ensure a floor of basic medical care available for all citizens throughout the country. From the very beginning, thus, the policymakers were inclined to recommend a thrifty version of basic medical care for all. Given the protection of medical care security at the essential level, meanwhile, residents were still given room to choose among alternative medical care insurances, so long as their financial ability and work unit's revenue conditions allow.

For comparison, it is germane here to examine each of all three packages of public medical care insurances systematically with regards to membership, types of services, funding modes, payment scheme, and organizational and managerial designs as given in Figure 1.1. In the case of BMCI, enrollees included both employees and retirees in the public sector, and their household registration was a basic requirement to join the package. Enrollees of BMCI enjoyed insurance benefits in terms of both clinical care and hospital care in addition to the benefits of HESI through supplementary medical care insurance (SMCI) as given in Chapter 8.

Overall, the entitlements of BMCI were intended to match what were offered by LIMC and PFMC addressing the alienation of entitlements from funding inherent in the program design under the considerations of compensation policy in the CPE developmental strategy. The funding mode features the design of co-insurance through which both the employer and employee have to contribute a share to the BMCI foundation, marking a distinct change from the conventional funding mode (i.e., PFMC and LIMC) where only the work unit (employer) shouldered all funding for entitlements. In addition, the BMCI registers an improvement by incorporating the spending control measures. The payment scheme embraced the standard elements of deductible, and co-payment and payment-ceiling. In terms of organizational and managerial designs, BMCI represents a new departure from LIMC and PFMC which operated with the budgetary and financial management of the work unit under the CPE. BMCI is run by a non-departmental public entity (NDPE) with the executive agency in charge, working with both transaction-centered and command-centered management. Besides, the government maintains "one-arm-length" in dealing with BMCI, allowing autonomy of decision-making in a market environment.

As shown in Figure 1.1, NRCMCI and URMCI each cater to the basic medical care demands of different sectors: The former addresses the medical care of the peasants while in the latter family members of the employees in the public sector, in addition to flexibly employed personnel who are holders of household registration in a respective municipal jurisdiction. By original design, both are targeted at the provision of large expenditure cases such as hospital care and HESI, but in the process of implementation both incorporated clinical care in adaptation to markets (to be elaborated in Chapters 9–11). The funding model for NRCMCI and URMCI is innovative in the sense that an insurance fund of considerable scale is built and sustained by premium contribution, operating with risk pooling mechanisms, in addition to the government's subsidies to the enrollee's premium contribution. In so far as the payment schemes, such procedures as deductible, co-payment and payment-ceiling are adopted, as what BMCI does. Moreover, both NRCMCI and URMCI adopt transaction-centered management tightly fused with command-centered management. In both cases, the executive agency oversees of the routine of financial management relating to premiums, payments and deposits. About the structure of command, the labor and social security bureau exercises supervisory functions over BMCI and URMCI in the urban setting. And the health bureau is given supervisory role over NRCMCI, coupled with its main responsibility over service delivery in the rural area.

Given their differences as given in Figure 1.1, the design of the said three packages lends recognition of inequality of medical care among various sectors of the population. As just noted, BMCI represents a relatively high level of medical care services, providing insurance funding to workers and staff of enterprises, public personnel of the government, political parties, service units, and other public organizations. It was originally intended to replace both LIMC and PFMC, but during the process of implementation, PFMC (mainly for the government officials and other public personnel) slowly merged with BMCI (Chapter 12). Compared with the other two insurance packages, the enhanced version of BMCI (its final drafts after 1998) was generous in covering both clinical and hospital care. Subsequently, it included cases of high expenditure and serious illness (HESI), as a supplementary medical care insurance (SMCI) was added from 1998 onward.

The institutional status of BMCI differs from that of LIMC, which is embedded in the conventional funding structure of the CPE and mainly relies on the retained revenue of public enterprises. The former is taken as a "quasi-foundation" remaining independent of the budgetary and accounting system within the party-state hierarchy, while the latter represents a separate "welfare fund" account jointly

Types / Features	Basic Medical Care Insurance (BMCI)	Urban Resident Medical Care Insurance (URMCI)	New Rural Cooperative Medical Care Insurance (NRCMCI)
Membership	Employees & retirees in the public sector; (household registration)	Family members of employees in the public sector; flexibly employed personnel (household registration)	Families & residents of rural community
Product/service-specificity	Clinical care, hospital care & HESI	Hospital care & part of HESI (clinical care only in some cases)	Hospital care & part of HESI (clinical care in some cases)
Funding design	Co-Insurance by the employer & employees	Insurance with the enrollee's premium partially subsidized by the government	Insurance with the enrollee's premium subsidized partially by the government
Payment schemes	1. Deductible, co-payment & payment-ceiling; 2. Lists and catalogs of services and drugs	1. Deductible, co-payment & payment-ceiling; 2. Lists and catalogs of services and drugs	1. Deductible, co-payment & payment-ceiling; 2. Lists and catalogs of services and drugs
Management & organization	1. Transaction-centered management & command-centered management; 2. Managed by NDPE and executive agency; and 3. Supervised by labor & social security bureau	1. Transaction-centered management & command-centered management 2. Managed by NDPE and executive agency; and 3. Supervised by labor & social security bureau	1. Transaction-centered management & command-centered management 2. Managed by NEPE and executive agency; and 3. Supervised by health bureau

Figure 1.1 Three Public Medical Care Insurances in China.

Source: Created by the author.

managed by enterprise management, the labor union, and the congress of representatives of staff and workers (CRSW) at the enterprise level (Lee 2019). The dissimilarities between BMCI and PFMC are considerable, too, as the latter relies on the state budget as its main source of funding. As a result of the reform, BMCI operates at the territorial level, and it is based upon a county/municipal jurisdiction, representing a viable scale of risk pooling, in addition to a better defined and more effective management apparatus. BMCI is a full-fledged medical care insurance program, the entitlements of which are mandated and defined operationally by laws and regulations, and it is indicative of the prominent role of the party-state hierarchy amid marketization.

Introduced in 2007, URMCI mainly financed hospital care plus some part of HESI for family members of staff and workers of public enterprises, unemployed residents and the marginalized sector of urban populations as indicated in Figure 1.1. Similarly, as shown in Figure 1.1, NRCMCI was inaugurated in 2003, originally intending to cover hospital care for peasants in addition to a part of HESI cases (Gu, Gao & Yao 2006; Lee 2019; Gu 2012). It took a relatively short time for NRCMCI and URMCI to incorporate targeted enrollees into the two respective packages considering the much smaller scale of funding, narrower scope of services, and lighter financial burden for various echelons of the government involved, coupled with budgetary surplus during the booming phase of economic reform.

Both URMCI and NRCMCI were focused on HESI (hospital care plus catastrophic illness), taken as the top policy priority of the government. The government carried weight in the designing of URMCI and NRCMCI, as it played a major role of subsidizing a large share of an enrollee's premium contribution as noted in Figure 1.1. However, HESI was considered as a higher-tier preference that covers the expensive and less frequent cases in both URMCI and NRCMCI. At variance with the central government's policy priority most enrollees were inclined to lend more weight to clinical care (representing lower-tier preference) that occurred more often in daily life, allowing to exercise a consumer's right of choice. It is therefore warranted to look closely into scenarios where policymakers in various echelons of the government—while working on the product/service specificity in the process of packaging—dealt with the tension between preference mixes in each enrollee (Chapters 8 and 10).

The network of three clusters of public medical care took shape in an evolutionary path over a long stretch of time for about three decades from the late 1980s to the late 2010s, as the two-step policy of program integration was entertained. The first step was concerned with merging PFMC and LIMC into BMCI as originally proposed in the 1998 Decision, and the second step pertained to combining NRCMCI and URMCI into urban and rural resident medical care insurance (URRMCI). It appears that the first step was less than successful as the PFMC has still maintained its separate program identity so far (Chapter 12).

Erecting yet another landmark in 2016, the government decided to take the second step to merge the URMCI and NRCMCI into an urban & rural resident medical care insurance (URRMCI). As promulgated by the State Council, the 2016 Opinion urged the provincial and prefectural/municipal jurisdictions to draft the plan and make preparation for the task of integration for URRIMC before June 2016, and made the concrete measures for implementation before December 2016.[1] And the National Healthcare Security Administration (NHSA), an entirely new ministerial ranking unit, was established in 2018. NHSA is supposed to oversee of all functions under both the BMCI and URRMCI, among others. However, the progress of implementation of URRMCI did not move as fast as expected. The 2020 Opinion by the Party Center, CCP and the State Council shifted to the priority on territorial integration with regards to building "unified funding" (namely, risk pooling mechanisms) at the municipal/prefectural level and strengthening vertical management at the provincial level (Zhonggong Zhongyang & Guowuyuan 2020). The 2020 Opinion remained silent on URRMCI. The study here has been focused only on the BMCI, NRCMCI, and URMCI, leaving URRMCI for further research till the dust is settled.

The foregoing analysis, in broad profile, provides a portrait of the inauguration of public medical care insurances on an exceedingly large scale, covering divergent sectors of the population (Lee 2019), and some statistical data attests the process of implementation up to the middle 2010s.[2] As the further progress of implementation was made under the leadership of the newly established National Health care Security Administration (NHSA) in 2018, the total enrollment in public medical care insurances reached 1,361,310,000 nominally as of the year of 2020, embracing 344,550,000 enrollees in BMCI and 1,016,776,000 enrollees in URRMCI. It is estimated that for one decade from the late 2010s to 2020, nearly 100,000,000 enrollees were added. However, considerably more effort is required to build URRMCI as an operational and managerial unit at the municipal level. Above all, the introduction of public medical care insurance entailed a process of marketization, that is, the application of markets in both financing and spending sides of financial management, an issue to be discussed in the following pages.

Policy Trend of Marketization

Marketization was introduced into the healthcare reforms in general and public medical care insurances in particular during the economic reform (Hu 2001; Gu, Gao & Yao 2006;Lee 2019). It represents an increasing tendency to use market transactions not only in the delivery of medical care, but also in the allocation of health care resources (Du et al. 2007, 2008, 2009). In conceptual terms, one may treat market activities here as transactions of equal value between two parties, normally the buyer and seller. The object of transactions is often taken as a commodity, involving either products/services or property rights or both in the health care sector (Li, Jiang & Chen 2008). Like elsewhere in the health care sector, marketization has pervaded all aspects of public medical care insurance throughout China.

Marketization refers to a process through which markets are adopted as public policy tools, and it assumes two forms. One pertains to the policy cases where markets are introduced to substitute for the role of the state in the delivery and allocation of health care resources, for instance, in case of expanding of market share of medical care through non-public sector: The legalization of private practices at the early phase of economic reform and the establishment of private hospitals according to the "classification" of hospitals in 2000. The other is concerned with the incorporation of market mechanisms in a managerial and functional sense into party-state hierarchies in connection with the use of user charges and inauguration of public medical care insurances at the micro level (Lee 2019).

Overall, the study argues that the inauguration of public medical insurance represents an unprecedented and innovative breakthrough in the evolution of public funding of healthcare in China, producing an entirely new system with the distinctive characteristics as follows: First, the creation of a risk pooling mechanisms sustained by premium contributions; second, its financial management operates with the inward-resource-flow (IRF) system in the markets; third, its scale of financial pool goes beyond the work unit, working with local jurisdiction promising further expansion; fourth, it relies on a new form of public organization, the non-departmental public entity (NDPE), and fifth, it is focused on the new package of medical care, lending priority to high expenditure and serious illness (HESI) and taking into consideration of positive externality of basic medical care in each local community.

Public medical care insurance is a kind of insurance with considerable state intervention not only in financial terms (e.g., tax exemption, subsidies to low-income brackets such as the vulnerable and marginalized social strata), but also in the granting of franchises and the exercising of other forms of regulatory governance. Overall, each of three public medical care insurances (i.e., the BMCI plus its enhanced version, URMCI and NRCMCI), is given franchise, namely, rights of entry into the market for some mandated and well-defined categories of medical care services. As the public insurance caters to the medical care demands of each enrollee personally, it also endeavors to provide positive externality to third parties, that is, the other residents in the community. Here "positive externality" is taken as quasi-collective goods in terms of effective control of common and frequent diseases, quick recovery from illness, and better overall health to the multitude of undifferentiated but needy people, coupled with productive workforce in each jurisdiction.

By definition, a health insurance refers to a design of risk-pooling mechanisms through which each enrollee contributes a premium to an accumulative funding pool, and meanwhile each enrollee can draw from the said funding pool and make payment for curative services rendered by the provider. Given an actuarial scheme, it is expected that each episode of sickness for a given patient would take place at a different time, resulting in a pattern distributed evenly over a longer time frame while building a funding pool to fulfill obligations for payment one case at a time (Sultz & Young 2006: 251–4; Porter & Guth 2012: 71–106). In other words, just as a particular enrollee helps everybody else, everybody else helps that enrollee.

The public medical care insurance programs represent marketization on both the funding and spending side of its financial management system. On the funding side, an insurer collects premium from enrollees (and often a share from their employers too in co-insurance) in an insurance plan, while the insurer undertakes contractual obligations to cover medical bills when enrollees become ill. In theoretical terms, enrollees and employers have choices among competing insurers, even though these choices might be restricted depending on local conditions. On the spending side, enrollees have to pay providers for curative care and other services in the form of deductibles and co-payments, together with the share of payment by the insurer. Also, spending control is necessary to maintain the budgetary balance of the on-going financial pool. Like any other health care insurance program, moreover, the insured (i.e., enrollees) are given the right to choose among several competing providers just as in the case of Germany, but the room of choices depends on the actual situation on a case-by-case basis (Chapter 2).

During inaugurating public medical care insurances, marketization took place in conjunction with the packaging of insurance benefits and entitlements (Chapter 2). The said packaging exercise represented an effort in the exercise of product/ service specificity, ensuring that the types of basic medical care were a part of the quasi-collective goods the externality of which was spread positively to the entire community, although each patient (i.e., enrollee) enjoys them as private goods. With regards to product/service specificity, basic medical care was identified, defined and mandated through two phases of packaging during the health care reform (Ge & Gong 2007; Lee 2019) to be discussed further in Chapter 2.

The BMCI represents a full-fledged public insurance program, indicative of a movement toward marketization. As a novel design, the BMCI differs from the conventional funding packages (i.e., PFMC and LIMC). The former works with an inward-resource-flow (IRF) system managed through market mechanisms (Chapter 2). In the latter the funding functions are handled as an integral part of the financial system of the party-state hierarchy, that is, as an outward-resource-flow (ORF) system in part or in full. For example, LMCI works with a financial system of public enterprises that does not require strict budgetary connectivity of spending with financing in view of soft budgetary constraints where the government might interfere with financial and accounting procedures at the work unit level for broad policy considerations. Also, PFMC relies on the public financial resources provided entirely through non-market channels, such as the state budget, as spending is not always accountable to funding (Chapter 4).

The inauguration of BMCI is concerned with the marketization of both the funding side and spending side of public financial management in the health care sector. On the funding side, co-insurance means that both the employer and employee shoulder a portion of premium contribution in transactions with the insurer for insurance payments for medical care, while in conventional funding programs, the employer's contribution was solely responsible for funding medical care. On the spending side, both the insurer and insured are responsible for a share of co-payment in transactions with the provider under BMCI. Whereas in the conventional funding system, public organizations, such as government units and public enterprises, act in the capacity of purchasers in transactions with providers to pay for basic medical care services on behalf of the patient. The patient's share of co-payment is relatively small.

As a new funding system, moreover, BMCI ceases to be a work-unit-centered system of funding and management. Both employer and employee work within a non-departmental public entity (NDPE) when coming to the risk pooling as indicated in Figure 1.1. Not only is the said NDPE independent from the government in an emerging mixed economy, but it also promises a viable funding source operating with a set of risk-pooling mechanisms with a scale of economy. Furthermore, BMCI (especially its enhanced version funded partly by SMCI) is comparable to the conventional public funding of PFMC and LIMC with regards to the types of basic medical care that each enrollee enjoys. In the cases of PFMC and LIMC, moreover, the work unit, be it a SOE or department/bureau, acted as the vehicle for public funding, but financial resources for BMCI are managed independently within an institutional framework. By and large, to finance LIMC, SOEs rely upon retained revenue from monopolized production at the enterprise level, while public organizations (including government units) depend financially on public finance, including taxation and revenue remittance from the SOEs.

In the two other cases, namely URMCI and NRCMCI, the coverage focuses on high expenditure and serious illness (HESI) cases, that is, hospital care plus catastrophic medical events as indicated in Figure 1.1. It is explicitly stated in policy papers that NRCMCI is intended mainly to prevent the impoverishment of the peasant family resulting from the unbearable costs of HESI (Gu, Gao & Yao 2006: 308–51). Meanwhile, URMCI was intended to fill the gaps within the public funding for the demands of basic medical care pertaining to families of employees, flexibly employed personnel, and other unemployed residents. It is noteworthy that the membership of LIMC and PFMC is employment-centered, not family-centered. That is to say, the eligibility of enrollees to LIMC and PFMC depends on their status of employment, but their family members (mostly dependents) are not employed in the same work unit. Nonetheless, family members of employees had been given some measures of medical care entitlements prior to the health care reforms, albeit in a scaled-down version (Chapter 4).

In funding URMCI, various echelons of the government covered a share of premium contributions as each enrollee was also responsible for his/her own portion (Chapter 8). In the case of NRCMCI, various echelons of the government subsidized for a large portion of the premium while a smaller portion was contributed by the peasant's family (Chapter 10). In the two insurance plans discussed above, the government adopted the "coupon method," that is, the government's subsidy to the user's premium contribution rather than the government's direct subsidy to the provider on behalf of the user. That is to say, the coupon method allows money to follow the user who deals with the provider directly through transactions in the health care markets, lending weight to the patient's choice in a quasi-market procedure (Gu 2010: 27–32).

The government had to deal with some issues arising from the application of market mechanisms in both URMCI and NRCMCI since markets operated unexpectedly and at variance with the government's original policy priority. To satisfy most enrollees, policymakers at the local level had to work with a mix of HESI and clinical care in packaging medical care services for an insurance plan. In fact, the enrollee's willingness and choice were crucial in order to maintain a sizable market share to sustain a healthy flow of funds from the enrollees into the financial reservoir of the insurance foundation of URMCI and NRCMCI, as a result, the insurance plan was accordingly modified in order to accommodate the enrollee's preference mix, meaning to bring clinical care in the respective programs (Chapters 8–10).

Regarding co-insurance in the case of BMCI as indicated in Figure 1.1, for example, both employer and enrollee (or employee) are required to shoulder a given share of the premium contribution in conjunction with the establishment of two accounts: A personal account (PA) and a unified social funding account (USFA) (Hu 2001: 205–94; Gu 2008). PA pays for clinical/minor illness, and its funding sources are derived from a share of contributions by employer and employee each, while the financial pool for USFA consists of a large portion of contribution from the employer and a smaller portion from the employee. In cases of NRCMCI and URMCI, in contrast, enrollees (often involving family membership) make their own premium contribution, but they are heavily subsidized by the government.

These three sub-types of service represent three different coverages, as shown in Figure 1.1. By far, BMCI (the enhanced version) is most generous in that it covers all three sub-types of curative care. In comparison with conventional funding packages such as LIMC and PFMC, the enhanced BMCI goes one step farther by explicitly addressing HESI through SMCI, on top of clinical services and hospital care. With a limited budget, priority is given to HESI cases in both URMCI and NRCMCI, allowing some room for discretion for local authorities to decide on the coverage of clinical/minor treatments according to their economic and financial conditions (Gu 2006).

The spending control measures stand out notably as one of the most salient features in designing public medical care insurances. And they were introduced to all packages throughout the jurisdictions involved. As a form of spending control, for example, a method of co-payment was incorporated into all three packages as well, to allow patients to make their own choice of services while transacting with the provider, coupled with deductibles and payment-ceiling (Hu 2001; Gu 2010; Liu 2012). Users were invariably required to shoulder a share of co-payment where both insurer and insured on the one side enter transactions with providers on the other side. Consistent with the policy of affordability, the user paid less progressively as the payment scale moved up to more expensive items. Theoretically speaking, moreover, that co-payment would result in better spending control as users tend to become more cost-conscious in view of payment obligations to be shouldered in seeking a cure. Also, it is argued that co-payment tends to curtail spending because the insurer is more knowledgeable and capable of striking better deals with the provider on behalf of the insured (Gu 2010: 123–47). The foregoing analysis has endeavored to highlight key dimensions and distinct characteristics of three public medical care insurances, and the study will outline the chapter plans next.

Highlights and the Chapter Plan

The book volume is devoted to an analysis of BMCI, URMCI, and NRCMCI that are evolved from the conventional fund programs under the CPE, and cater to the basic medical care to residents (both employed and unemployed) in the urban sector and the peasantry in the rural sector. The study chooses Guangzhou,

Shanghai and Shenzhen as an empirical database, partly because of availability and feasibility, and partly for its representativeness and desirability in the eyes of sovereign planners.

The issue of representativeness deserves discussion, given the study is only able to cover empirically a limited part of the universe under investigation. To begin with the three cases are focused on BMCI and to a lesser extent URCMI and other insurance plans working in the urban sector (Chapters 5–9). More likely than not, the three metropolitan-scale municipalities represent the "successful" cases, considering their leadership strengths, financial capability, administrative/managerial proficiency, economic resources, and size of population. It is arguable that the three empirical cases chosen can represent the true profile of implementation in more than 300 municipalities throughout China. Neither can the three municipalities demonstrate how public medical care insurances are introduced in some jurisdictions where the municipal leadership is weak and financial and managerial resources are in short supply. Nor the database of three municipalities chosen is adequate to illustrate how a package can operate smoothly, if not successfully, under an environment where market economy is underdeveloped, as marketization is taken as the core component for the insurance plan. Nonetheless the study makes use of the three empirical cases to show not only the process of policymaking and program packaging but also managerial and financial details. Besides, the study applies three empirical cases to illuminate the direction of policy development desired by sovereign planners.

Moreover, the book volume deals with NRCMCI in two chapters, covering the peasants, the largest, but rapidly shrinking sector of population in China (Chapters 10 and 11). To be examined in the study, the use of the empirical database centering on the county can better represent the true picture of implementation and policy outcomes, albeit this falls short of the original policy intent of sovereign planners to build NRCMCI at the municipal level, leaving the unfinished task of program integration for the future (Chapter 12).

Apart from the introduction given here, this book consists of four major parts in addition to the introduction (Chapter 1) and the concluding chapter (Chapter 12). Part I consists of three chapters that are devoted to an analysis of the policy and political dimensions of public medical care insurances. These three chapters (namely Chapters 2–4) cover the main issues, theoretical perspective, legacy, and vested interests, coupled with early origins and policy precedents that paved the way for public medical care insurances during economic reform.

In Chapter 2, this study endeavors to substantiate the claim that public medical care insurances (i.e., BMCI, NRCMCI, and URMCI) are unprecedented and innovative by demonstrating how these differ significantly from the conventional funding modes in PFMC, LIMC, and RCMC prior to economic reform. Chapter 2 will examine two dimensions of the subject-matter. From a conceptual and theoretical dimension, the chapter will examine the financial strategy of public medical care insurance considering an inward-resource-flow (IRF) system in contrast to an outward-resource-flow (ORF) system. Also, the study will compare Chinese public medical care insurance with the mandatory plan of Germany and the National Health Service (NHS) in the UK to highlight the salient characteristics of the Chinese case. From the disciplinary orientation of Political Science, furthermore, to focus on resource management, this study proposes an analytical framework consisting of three modes of governance: The market mode, the hybrid mode, and the hierarchy mode, as the hybrid mode is adopted in case of public medical care insurance in China.

On a policy and historical dimension, Chapter 3 is devoted to an analysis of the policy legacy of social security (including health care) and vested interests built in echelons of the government and various sectors of society during the forced modernization under CPE, and takes into consideration cultural, relational, and political aspects of social security. This study will examine three main approaches dealing with public policies, including basic medical care: The work unit approach, the corporatist approach, and the compensation approach. It is argued that in designing and implementation, sovereign planners needed to address the problems of program specificity, for instance, the spending/cost control measures and alienation of entitlements from funding, coupled with historically rooted obligations.

In Chapter 4, this study will try to examine the early origins of public funding and the policy precedents regarding basic medical care in conjunction with the introduction of PFMC and LIMC, two conventional public funding medical care packages made available to public personnel at an earlier stage of policy development through the CPE strategy. Furthermore, this study will analyze various remedial responses to spending control issues as well as new policy experiments and pilot programs dealing with the issues of funding HESI events across jurisdictions, which prepared the ground not only for launching BMCI reform starting in the mid-1990s, but also for the exercises of program specificity and product/service specificity in the designing of NRCMCI and URMCI during the 2000s.

Part II is concerned with the details of BMCI, the center of gravity of policy discussions regarding public medical care insurances which were being constructed for the first time throughout China. Consisting of four chapters (Chapters 5–8), Part II demonstrates how the early designs of BMCI were formulated and how new components were incorporated subsequently. Moreover, it will try to identify how pure policy concerns were fused with politics in the process of drafting and implementing BMCI.

Chapter 5 is concerned with an analysis of the dynamic interactions between the central government and provincial/local governments in the process of designing, building, and implementing BMCI programs. As this study argues, BMCI needed to address the funding issues by focusing on the senior cohorts of workforce to settle two sorts of "historical debt"—conceptually embracing alienation of entitlement from funding (i.e., unfunded, and under-funded PFMC and LIMC programs), and historically rooted obligations of social security to the workforce prior to economic reform. The study argues that the politics of social security is characteristic of tension, disputes and even conflicts on the issue of sharing of financial burden more than the strains, competitions and fights for revenue and economic interests.

The BMCI program intends to cover the workforce in the country, but its emphasis is placed on the issue of non-wage compensation of senior employees and retirees in the process of implementation. As illustrated in three empirical cases, Guangzhou, Shanghai and Shenzhen, the central government engaged in persuading local governments to find the ways and means to take care of the vested interests of the earlier cohorts of the workforce (i.e., senior enrollees and retirees) under PFMC and LIMC in the designing, packaging, and implementation of BMCI.

In Chapter 6, this study will discuss two salient issues arising from the exercises of program specificity in the process of packaging and introducing BMCI in China: Focusing on product/service specificity, first, what kinds of services ought to be included? And second, how are insurance services to be provided? Given that funding represents one of the many analytical dimensions of marketization, this study will endeavor to analyze how BMCI financially makes medical care services available and accessible to enrollees, covering such matters as the size of a jurisdiction, transaction-centered management, payment schemes, and spending control measures. Moreover, this study will examine selected empirical cases to illustrate how policy actors tackled issues surrounding the types and provisions of BMCI at the provincial/local level.

Chapter 7 is concerned with financial management (including especially the PA-USFA scheme)—one of the core features of the risk-pooling mechanisms and transaction-centered management characterizing BMCI. It is argued that the new public management of BMCI constitutes an integral part of the market oriented IRF system. In terms of institutional design, financial resources are held and handled by a non-departmental public entity (NDPE) operating independently of the government. From a political perspective, this study examines how, in the process of designing and building BMCI, sovereign planners tackled issues of non-funded or under-funded claims for social security entitlements—unsolved issues left during the pre-reform era. This study will also make use of two cases, Guangzhou and Shanghai, to illustrate how the provincial/local governments endeavored to find means and ways to ensure the medical care entitlements of all senior employees and retirees to be honored and funded properly through BMCI.

Chapter 8 represents an attempt to document the case of supplementary medical care insurance (SMCI), discussing how policymakers at the central and provincial/local levels dealt with the funding of basic medical care that exceeded the payment-ceiling in the early, thrifty version of BMCI packages. As the study argues, in essence, SCMI tries to bridge the funding gaps between the early, thrifty version of BMCI and the conventional funding programs (LIMC and PFMC). In addition, SCMI tackles the issue of HESI, which was not treated in the conventional funding of health care. This study also shows how policy actors dealt with the matters of SCMI in three empirical cases, Guangzhou, Shenzhen, and Shanghai, from both political and policy considerations, for instance, in the establishing risk pooling mechanisms in insurance funds and, meanwhile the handling of vested interests of various sectors and organizational units.

Part III consists of three chapters, mainly dealing with URMCI and NRCMCI, respectively, two public medical care insurances in the non-planned sector of the economy. Both will offer a narrower coverage largely centering on HESI cases with a smaller scale of funding than that of BMCI. In Chapter 9, this study is devoted to an analysis of URMCI, addressing issues relating to basic medical care insurance for family members of staff and workers of public enterprises. In this chapter, the study will begin with some discussion of the origin and background of URMCI, coupled with an analysis of the exercise of product/service specificity as it relates to HESI. In addition, the study will examine the insurance plans—to be illustrated in the cases of Guangzhou, Shanghai, and Shenzhen—that are made available to flexibly employed personnel, and the agricultural laborers (who are normally not holders of household registration) in urban areas. These two categories of workforce represent an expanding labor market that needs to be recognized considering rapid urbanization within several decades of economic reform.

Chapter 10 renders an account of the origin and legacy of RCMC, underscoring its differences from NRCMCI in terms of its funding model. NRCMCI represents a case of marketization under the sponsorship of the government, a move halfway from the party-state hierarchy to markets, as demonstrated in the separation of financial management (including the budgetary system) from that of the government. Also, NRCMCI is run by an autonomous NDPE managerially and financially independent of the government. Moreover, NRCMCI addresses the question of how to apply market mechanisms in funding certain categories of specific product/services to enrollees, together with the provision of positive spill-over effects onto an undifferentiated multitude of residents, who are not a party to NRCMCI, in each jurisdiction.

Chapter 11 is focused on the hybrid mode of governance, examining the operation and management of NRCMCI, including the key issues of financing and spending on the two sides of a given transaction. Two key aspects of marketization in the case of NRCMCI will also be addressed: How did policymakers apply the government subsidy to help peasants make premium contributions to the NRCMCI foundation, how product/service specificity pertaining to NRCMCI was made, and what packages of product/services were offered to enrollees under NRCMCI. In addition, the study will also analyze, in turn, the designs and management of funding, the funding role of the government, and, finally, the results of implementation.

In Part VI, Chapter 12 will first make an attempt to address the extent that public medical care insurances have covered as well as the gaps to be filled. Then, the study will examine some key functions that public medical care insurances perform, for instance, risk pooling mechanisms, enhancement of affordable care, and spending control measures among others. To be followed, the study will dwell on the government's changing position on HESI in the endeavors to work out the operational definition of HESI and to fine-tune the insurance plans for HESI. In addition, the study is devoted to an analysis of the policy agenda of integration of public medical care insurance at the municipality level. To focus on the evolutionary path, the study will try to monitor and analyze integration with regards to two pairs of public medical care insurances: First, incorporating LIMC and PFMC into BMCI, and second, combining NRCMCI and URMCI into URRCMI.

Concluding Analysis

To sum up, the making of public medical care insurances was focused on marketization in the health care sector during China's economic reform. Among various policy options, marketization represented a large-scale reform movement and an exceedingly complex phenomenon in China's health care sector starting in 1979 (Duckett 2004, 2013; Huang 2014, 2020; Lee 2019). In managerial and institutional terms, the inauguration of public medical care insurance represents a movement away from the framework of CPE but has gone only half way in the direction of marketization, producing a hybrid mode of governance suspended between markets and hierarchies in the realm of public policy. Although the national policy and institutional framework have been laid down, insurance plans are still separately managed by executive agencies at the municipal level in the case of BMCI and at the county level for URRCMI by the 2020s. Formally established in 2016, NHSA is in charge of public medical care insurances throughout the country, promising the long-term policy objective of program integration among insurance plans first at the municipal level, and eventually at the provincial and national level.

Notes

1 On January 1, 2016, the State Council promulgated "The opinion of integration of the resident basic medical care insurance systems of cities and towns" (abbreviated as the 2016 Opinion hereafter) (Guowuyuan 2016).

2 By the middle of the 2010s, enrollment in each new package of public medical care insurance was registering a steady expansion, reaching the total enrollments of 1,268,000,000 with a breakdown of 237,000,000 for enrollees in BMCI (including PFMC), 195,000,000 for urban residents in URMCI, and 836,000,000 for peasants in NRCMCI in 2010 (Ma & Gui 2012: 73–87). According to the 2008 National Resident Survey, percentages of various categories among interviewees (given some overlap) are: BMCI, 12.7 percent; PFMC, 1 percent; URMCI, 3.8 percent; NRCMCI, 68.7 percent; other insurances, 1 percent; and no social insurance, 12.9 percent (*China's Statistics Yearbook 2009*: 182). Almost all Chinese citizens were covered by one or another package of medical care insurance, albeit a portion of the population was not yet included, say, about a hundred million people such as agricultural laborers, "flexibly employed personnel," among others (Gu 2010).

References

Cheng, S. (Eds.) 2000. *Zhongguo shehui baozhang tixi de gaige yu wangshan (The Reform and Improvement of Social Security System in China)*. Beijing: Minzhy jianshe chubanshe.

National Bureau of Statistics of China 2009. *China Statistical Yearbook 2009*. Beijing: China Statistics Press: 182.

Dangdai Zhongguo congshu bianjibu 1988. *Dangdai zhongguo caizheng, Xia (Finance in Contemporary China, Volume II)*. Beijing: Zhongguo shehui kexue chubanshe.

Du, L., Zhang, W. et al. (Ed.). 2009. *Zhongguo yiliao weisheng fazhang baogao, No. 5 (The Development Report of China's Medical Care and Health Care, No. 5)*. Beijing: Shehui kexue chubanshe.

Du, L., Zhang, W., Huang, Z. et al. (Ed.). 2006. *Zhongguo yiliao weisheng fazhang baogao, No. 2 (The Development Report of China's Medical Care and Health Care, No. 2)*. Beijing: Shehui kexue chubanshe.

Du, L., Zhang, W., Wang, P. et al. 2008. *Zhongguo yiliao weisheng fazhan baogao, (The Development Report of China's Medical Care and Health Care, No. 4)*. Beijing: Shehui kexue wenxian chubanshe.

Duckett, J. 2004. State, collectivism and worker privilege: a study of urban health insurance in China. *China Quarterly* 177: 155–73.

Duckett, J. 2013. *The Chinese State's Retreat from Health*. London & New York: Routledge.

Ge, Y., & Gong, S. 2007. *Zhongguo yigai: wenti, genyuan, chulu (China's Medical Care Reform: Problem, Roots and Solution)*. Beijing: Zhongguo fazhan chubanshe.

Gu, X. 2008. *Zuoxian quanmin yibao: Zhongguo xinyigai de zhannu yu zhanxu (Towards Universal Coverage of Health Care Insurance: The Strategic Choices and Institutional Framework of China's New Medical Care Reform)*. Beijing: Zhongguo laodong baoxian chubanshe.

Gu, X. 2010. *Quanmin yibao de xin tansuo (New Exploration of National Medical Care Insurance)*. Beijing: Shehui kexue wenxian chubanshe.

Gu, X. 2012. Zouxian quanmin jiankang baoxian: lun Zhongguo yiliao baozhang zhidu zhuanxing (Towards national health insurance: On the transformation of medical care insurance in China). *Shehui baozhang zhidu (Social Security System)* 11: 48–52.

Gu, X., Gao, M., & Yao, Y. 2006. *Zhengduan yu chufang: zhimian zhongguo yiliao zhidu gaige (Diagnosis and Treatment: Facing the Reform of Medical Care System in China)*. Beijing: Shehui kexue chubanshe.

Guan, Z., Dong, C., & Cui, P. 2006. Zhongguo yiliao weisheng: Tiaozhan yu chulu (China's medical care and health care: Challenges and solutions). *Zhonguo weisheng jingji (China's Health Care Economics)* 25.10: 5–9.

Guowuyuan. 2016. Guowuyuan guanyu zhenghe chengxiang jumin jiben yiliao baoxian zhidu de yijian (The opinion of the state council regarding the integration of basic medical care insurance for urban and rural residents). Retrieved from http.//baike.baidu.com/reference/4277454/1873UrwzYuLMHXs…IGXsOc388e3krl_Ao2rhdf6MFcp65MFcp65Hs8woThXBrYgRSi1-PJjw

Hu, S. 2001. *Yiliao baoxian he fuwuzhidu (The Medical Care insurance and Delivery System)*. Chengdu: Sichuan renmin chubanshe.

Huang, Y. 2014. *Governing Health in Contemporary China*. London & New York: Routledge.

Huang, X. 2020. *Social Protection under Authoritarianism, Health Politics and Policy in China*. New York: Oxford University Press.

Jin, W. 1996. Laodong jiaohuan yu guoyou qiye zhigong de laodong jijixing (Labor exchange and incentives for staff and workers in state-owned enterprises). In Li, D. (Ed.), *Zhongguo de xiandai qiye zilu* (The Road to A Modern Enterprise System in China). Beijing: Guoji wenhua chubanshe gongsi. 75–85.

Lee, P. N. 2019. *Re-engineering Affordable Care Policy in China, Is Marketization A Solution?* London & New York: Routledge.

Lee, P. N., & Lo, C. W. (Eds.) 2001. *Remaking China's Public Management*. Westport, CT and London: Quorum Books.

Li, L., Jiang, Y., & Chen, Q. 2008. Gaige kaifang Beijing xiade woguo yigai 30 nian (Health care reform with the background of reform and opening in China for the last 30 years). *Zhongguo weisheng jingji (China's Healthcare Economics)* 27.2: 5–9.

Ma, L., & Gui, J. 2012. Wanshan jiben yiliao baozhang zhidu yanjiu (Research on the improvement of basice medical care security system). *Tizhi gaige (System Reform)* 4: 73–87.

Porter, M. E., & Guth, C. 2012. *Redefining German Health Care, Moving to a Value-based System*. Springer, London & New York: Springer.

Qian, J. 2021. *The Political Economy of Making and Implementing Social Policy in China*. Singapore: Palgrave Macmillian.

Song, X. 2001. *Zhongguo shehui baozhang tizhi gaige yu fazhan baogao (The Report concerning the Reform and Development of the Social Security System in China).* Beijing: Xinhua shudian.

Sultz, H. A., & Young, K. M. 2006. *Health care USA, Understanding Its Organization and Delivery.* Boston, MA, Toronto, London & Singapore: Jones and Bartlett Publishers.

Wang, D. (Eds.) 1998. *Zhongguo shehui baozhang zhidu (The Social Security System in China).* Beijing: Qiye guanli chubanshe.

Xu, D., Yin, Z., & Zheng, Y. 1999. *Zhongguo shehui baozhang tizhi gaige (The Reform of Social Security System in China).* Beijing: Jingji kexue chubanshe.

Yu, G., & Song, X. (Eds.) 1998. *Wei shichang jingji de lieche pugui (To Pave Railway for the Train of Economic Reform).* Beijing: Xueyuan chubanshe.

Zhan, H., Yang, Y., & Zhang, Q. 1993. *Zhongguo dalu shehui anquan zhidu (The Social Security System in Mainland China).* Taipei: Wunan tushu chuban gongsi.

Zheng, G. (Eds.) 2011. *Zhongguo shehui baozhang gaige yu fazhan zhanlue (The Strategy for the Reform and Development of Social Security in China).* Beijing: Remin chubanshe.

Zhonggong Zhongyang & Guowuyuan 2020. Guanyu Shenhua yiliao baozhang zhidu gaige de yijian (Opinion regarding the further reform of medical care insurance system) (abbreviated as the 2020 Opinion). Retrieved from http://www.gov.cn/zhengce/2020-03/05/content_5487407.htm 12/9/21, 11.23 AM. 1–5

Part I

Public Policy and Health Care

2 Main Issues and Theoretical Perspectives

From the early 1950s onward, the top policymakers began to follow the Stalinist style of CPE as the strategy for their ambitious modernization project, and command was taken as the major tool for policymaking and implementation. Upon the arrival of the era of economic reform, the top policymakers did make a comprehensive review of their policymaking system in the realm of economic development (Lee 1987: 213–5). In search of the direction of change, they talked about the markets more than hierarchies in the realm of economic policy. Evidence indicates, however, that they were inclined to apply administrative instruments in economic policy, if not public policy, suggesting that they remained cautious and conservative about the market approach (Naughton 1996).

In defiance of the imagination of China watchers and analysts, sovereign planners dared to adopt the markets and tried to propose something totally new in the realm of public policy during economic reform. It is difficult to suggest whether the use of market tools is of importation from abroad or derived from an indigenous experience. After all, the use of the markets in public policy is not entirely alien to policymakers in China. For instance, the centrally planned economy (CPE) is characterized for its reliance on monopoly production, that is, involving application of franchise in the markets. Nevertheless, it does not seem an easy task to find an answer to the issue of marketization in social security policy, as much as all other relevant policy issues during economic reform. Accordingly, the study intends to investigate marketization in the realm of public policy covering all important aspects, from the origin and evolution to policymaking and key designs, vested interests and politics, and programs and implementation, among others.

The main concern of the study is how the markets work in the realm of public policy, especially in social security, in China. Here public medical care insurance is chosen as a case study in social security policy for it marks an entirely new departure from conventional funding mode of social security under CPE in China. And it represents a novel style of public financial management that not only goes beyond the narrow revenue/profit orientation of the markets but also represents an endeavor to fulfill broad public policy goals.

This chapter will deal with the issues of marketization as manifested on various managerial and institutional dimensions pertaining to public medical care insurance. The study will first address the exercise of product/service specificity,

DOI: 10.4324/9781003389934-3

namely, choices of insurance entitlements, and then proceed to analyze the financial strategy adopted by the policymakers. To be followed, the study will examine resource management regarding funding, spending, and financial reservoir of public medical care insurances. On top of the discussion of key aspects of marketization, furthermore, the focus will shift to analyzing which mode of governance in the public medical care insurance is adopted by the government, as well as its key characteristics and functions. The last section will examine behavioral adaptations with reference to how policymakers tackle the gap between program design and actual performance, and between the policy goals and implementation.

Repackaging and Financing Public Insurances

Conceptually and theoretically speaking, health care covers a vast territory, part of which is penetrated either by the state hierarchy, or market or both. In other words, it is appropriate to address marketization in terms of varying extents (i.e., more or less) rather than as a whole (i.e., yes or no). One cannot treat all kinds of health care services indiscriminately as a singular form of commodity. To study marketization in the case of public medical care insurance, one needs to address several issues: What kinds of services the enrollee needs to get from the provider through market transactions? In what quantity? How to pay for an insurance plan from the insurer? And how much does it cost?

To begin with, one needs to tackle the issue regarding what kinds of services are chosen to be the object of transactions. In his celebrated article on medical care welfare economics, Kenneth J. Arrow is one of the earliest authors to initiate theoretical discussions of the marketability of health care. Arrow's analysis focuses on the effectiveness of market mechanisms whereby medical care services can be both offered and demanded upon payment of a price, and involve an action that is "identifiable, technologically possible, and capable of influencing others" (Arrow 1963). Arrow is fully aware that not all types of health care services are marketable as he addresses the issue of how to distinguish non-marketability from marketability. For example, he identifies non-marketable cases in public and preventive health care with reference to "social costs and benefits," for example, prevention of communicable diseases and immunization in the health care sector. According to Arrow, it would be necessary for the state to intervene in the form of a subsidy or tax or compulsion in non-marketable types of health care (Arrow 1963: 944–8).

To echo Arrow's view on the subject-matter, this study will first examine how practitioners and policy analysts dealt with the marketability of health care services, including health insurance. Amid policy experimentation on marketization of health care during the reform era, it took two phases for repackaging health care services that were in correspondence with two market-oriented reforms in health care in China. And each phase represents a form of marketization focusing on packaging of objects of transactions.

In the first phase, a classification scheme of health care was constructed and introduced in connection with the new policy of user charges and revenue-raising endeavors during the early 1980s. The classification scheme embraced four categories: Category 1 pure-public health care, Category II quasi-public health care, Category III basic medical care, and Category IV non-basic medical care (Lee 2019). Among these four categories of health care services, theoretically speaking, Category I pure-public health care is taken as collective goods to be financed with government funding, while Category IV non-basic medical care is treated as private goods, open to full-fledged marketization. Standing in between the hierarchy and market, Category II quasi-public health care and Category III basic medical care are subject to partial marketization, and often rely on a mix of funding sources (Lee 2019).

It is evident in the repackaging of health care that the above classification scheme reflects the theoretical and conceptual concerns of Western analysts, authors and practitioners (Ostrom & Ostrom 1977: 7–14; Savas 1978: 35–58). While Category I pure public health care pertains to a form of externality, namely benefits produced by the public organization and made available to all users undifferentiated in society, such as are clean water; fresh, unpolluted air; safety and quality of drugs; hygiene education and property protection, etc. Category IV non-basic medical care is treated as "private goods," that is, services that are attributable and retrievable, and thus subject to higher user charges, for instance, upgraded wards, appointments with senior doctors or consultants and imported medicine among others (Lee 2019). However, Category II quasi-public health care and Category III basic medical care are quasi-collective goods, representing a combination of collective goods and private goods. And they are the kind of benefits that patients can enjoy personally on an individual basis, and meanwhile are also benefits to the undifferentiated multitude of residents in a given community.

It is noteworthy that health care demands represent multiple levels of human existence, from the biological and personal level through the material/economic level to the cultural and abstract level. At the lower levels, for example, health insurance provides personal benefits related to control of illness, pain-relieving, wellbeing, longer work hours and income-earning ability as well as social benefits to foster a healthy, productive labor force, and thus bolsters the growth potential of an economy. At the higher levels, the risk-bearing notion of insurance deals with healthcare in terms of risk probability, a constructed and abstract category in an actuarial, financial, economic and policy sense. In fact, healthcare demands contain culturally constructed elements, often taken as ideational products beyond what is stipulated merely according to medical and biological criteria.

The second phase of the repackaging of health care services was largely focused on public medical care insurance in the early 1990s. Here the funding service from public insurance represents a kind of product/service in market transactions, and it can help pay for medical care in time of need. Overall, policymakers in various echelons were confronted with tensions between quests for funding economic growth on the one hand, and financial pressure for healthcare, welfare, and education on the other hand. In a number of a few local jurisdictions, insurance schemes of "large expenditure" were introduced on an experimental basis, focusing on so-called high expenditure and serious illness (HESI, including catastrophic medical events). As noted in PNS Lee's study, China's policy designers took one more step forward to making choices among three zones of healthcare services: Zone I clinical care, Zone II hospital care, and/or Zone III above payment-ceiling expenditure including HESI) during the healthcare reforms (Lee 2019). Clinical care in Zone I is taken as outpatient care whereas the last two zones belong to inpatient care, albeit the classification of zones is operationally difficult in view of a problematic operational definition as well as considerable tension inherent in the interpretative frame of reference of the actors in various echelons of the government involved.

Arising from the policy experimentations in the early 1990s, local jurisdictions' principal concern was on the HESI cases that might result in devastating effects of both medical and financial nature on the staff and workers themselves as well as the public enterprises with which they were affiliated. When the central policymakers were drafting the BMCI insurance policy, they were caught in between policymakers of local jurisdictions whose main concern was HESI events on the one hand (Chapters 5 and 8) and, on other hand, staff and workers in the public enterprises who were in favor of maintaining their vested interests (for instance, the then existing level of clinical care and hospital care) that were taken as non-wage compensation—an integral part of the remuneration package under the CPE legacy (Lee 2019).

When the drafts of the enhanced version of the basic medical care insurance (BMCI) were being worked up in 1998, supplementary medical care insurance (SMCI) was eventually incorporated to address the discrepancies in the early, thrift version of BMCI as well as the HESI events for both staff and workers and employees of the government and other public organizations (Lee 2019; Chapter 8). Furthermore, in the URMCI programs and NRCMCI programs, the priority was given to covering HESI cases too (Lee 2019; Chapters 8–11).

The classification of various types of healthcare demands is inseparable from the choice of financing strategy. For example, some types of healthcare services such as Category I pure public health tend to rely more on tax revenue, while it is feasible for Category IV non-basic medical care to tap the potential purchasing power of the high-income classes. Questions arise from choosing among the alternative financial strategies to finance different types of healthcare services during repackaging healthcare services. What are their merits and demerits? How do they each fare in designing an effective public insurance plan? The study will try to tackle the questions so raised in the next section.

The Choices of Financial Strategy

Since public medical care insurance plans are designed to meet selective categories of health care services, it is germane to dwell next on the issue of financing, namely, how to pay for the healthcare services. In public policy, the core issue of financing is concerned with resource management. By and large, one may consider two systems of financial strategy to characterize the relationship of resource flow between the organizational unit and its task environment. As just noted, the two systems are: An outward-resource-flow (ORF) system that is embedded in the party-state hierarchy and an inward-resource-flow (IRF) system that rests on the markets.

The ORF system represents a cluster of mechanisms and procedural tools that allocate resources externally to the environment by relying mainly on public funding for the implementation of public policy goals. Accordingly, revenue and spending are treated as separate streams, which are managed by the party-state hierarchy, making use of tax revenue and other forms of public finance, and relying on mandatory power rather than market transactions. Compatible with the tasks and functions of the territorial organization, furthermore, the ORF system is most suitable in the provision of collective goods that are non-marketable and often aimed at producing considerable positive externality for an undifferentiated multitude of people in each task environment.

The IRF system consists of a cluster of procedures and mechanisms, transferring resources (often in the form of revenue/profit) from the task environment as much as possible into the organizational unit concerned, often through market transactions. It invariably operates with simple, well-defined revenue/profit goals, working with financial accountability and ensuring profit/revenue earned through each transaction. As a rule, spending and revenue are closely tied together with each other in budgetary and accounting terms. Meanwhile it tends to internalize resources from and externalize costs to the task environment in view of its profit/revenue orientation. In most cases, it works with marketable goods and services. To work with the design of insurance plans in general, the study argues that the IRF system tends to be revenue-oriented and address the issue of resource management effectively to collect premiums and sustain a viable reservoir of risk pooling based on the scale of the economy.

To implement policy goals, the public organization is often financed through a basket of financial means including both non-market avenues (e.g., public finance, taxation) and market avenues (e.g., user charges, revenue from franchising, etc.). When working with an ORF system that is supported by tax revenue, the public organization performing various types of function/service is *not* expected to be tied proportionally to any amount of earning, for example, in the case of providing collective goods such as education, welfare, and public/preventive health. Although the public organization is not financially oriented in most cases, revenue could often be one of its important policy goals when the issue of resource management assumes some measure of priority. In some exceptions, for example, a public organization may adopt the IRF system in chosen services to raise revenue by making use of franchises or introducing user charges (e.g., wine and tobacco monopolies or user charges for certain types of services). During the early phase of health care reforms in the 1980s, the government did make use of franchise for revenue-raising purposes through introducing the undertaking responsibility system (URS) at the public hospital level as previously noted (Lee 2019). The making of public insurance also relies heavily on the IRF system, which is the study's main theoretical concern.

To finance healthcare, it is up to the government to opt for either the IRF system or the ORF system or both in China and elsewhere, recognizing different types of services and depending upon the purchasing power of various strata in the society. On the one hand, certain private insurances covering health care are a good illustration of the IRF system at work as an experience in the USA cited by Davidson (2010). By design, private health care insurances rely heavily on formal contracts as the funding vehicle, coupled with a judiciary system in the case of needed adjudication. Owing to its concern for profit, an insurance company tends to adopt an IRF system by enforcing resource-internalizing and cost-externalizing at the same time. For instance, the company concerned endeavors to maximize premiums contributed by enrollees and minimize costs through conventional financial management, featuring the IRF system (including the available budgetary and accounting tools) in conjunction with the obligation of payment in each medical care episode. Typical of the IRF system, for example, the cost-externalizing behavior includes screening out potential enrollees with pre-conditions, and lending preference to young, healthy, high income enrollees who are more affordable but make less use of medical resources (Davidson 2010: 18–23).

As a good illustration of an ORF system, on the other hand, the National Health Service (NHS) in the UK relies mainly on public expenditure that comes mostly from general taxation, coupled with a small amount from National Insurance Contributions (NICs). In general, taxes include income tax, VAT, corporation tax, and excise duties (fuel, alcohol, and tobacco). No general tax revenue is earmarked for the specific purpose. NICs are collected on earned income from all employers, employees, and self-employed people in the UK. The NHS is not contingent on NICs, albeit about 10 percent of NICs contribute to NHS funding. General taxes and NICs are collected at the UK level and then allocated to England and local authorities through the Department of Health, while block grants of all devolved services including a portion to healthcare are given to Northern Island, Scotland, and Wales respectively. Apart from the said two sources of the statutory financing, the remaining financing for healthcare comes mostly from a combination of out-of-pocket payment (OPP), private medical insurance, and other forms of private expenditure: 9.3 percent, 2.8 percent, and 5 percent of total healthcare expenditure respectively (Cylus et al. 2015: 41–62).

In the Chinese health care sector, both an ORF system and IRF system are employed too, depending on the types of services and functional areas chosen. For example, the ORF system is normally applied to public health care that is non-marketable, where public financing plays a principal role to handle externalities such as preventive health care, immunization programs, and defined benefits to women and children etc. In the case of non-basic medical care services that are marketable, the IRF system is often employed as the funding vehicle. For instance, user charges are introduced to non-basic medical care (i.e., special care services) where externality is not considered a main concern. However, it appears that public hospitals can adopt the IRF system partially to maintain a steady flow of revenue through URS in addition to the government's subsidies through the ORF system as previously mentioned (Lee 2019).

As the public insurance packages in China mainly adopt the IRF system as a financial strategy in all three programs (BMCI, URMCI and NRCMCI), the insurer endeavors to make full use of accounting and budgetary tools to collect premiums effectively, avoid and/or minimize a deficit, and thus maintain a funding reservoir to honor the financial obligations of insurance payments. This is supplemented by financial resources that stem from the ORF system to finance the provision of externality to residents in the community. Representing a defining feature in the ORF system, for instance, premiums of the peasants in case of NRCMCI and the enrollees of URMCI, such as minors, students, and those under welfare, are to be partially subsidized by the central government and provincial/local jurisdictions.

Resource Management of Healthcare Services

It is not unusual for modernizing countries to introduce marketization in the public sector in view of the evolution of public policy during the last two centuries, as the conventional state bureaucracy has gradually expanded its new functional territories into education, welfare, social security and healthcare among others (Shonfield 1965). Accordingly, the hybrid mode of governance that originally existed in the private sector (Williamson 1996), has made an inroad into public resource management. To study the resource management of healthcare services, it is useful to divide the hybrid mode of governance into the partial case and the full-fledged case. The former is concerned with introducing the market mechanism only to one link within resource management, for example, the spending link, while the latter includes both fund-raising and spending links. The partial case of the hybrid mode is illustrated by American Medicare and Medicaid whose revenue source stems from the government at both the federal and state levels, while the spending function is performed through purchasing exercises—characteristic of transactions—between the government and provider (Sultz & Kristina 2006: 241–91; Starr 2011: 41–50). Accompanying the waves of policy initiatives called "privatization," meaning the transfer of policy implementation from the public sector to the non-public sector, governments in the USA in various echelons have experimented with and introduced managerial reforms on a broad front, for example, purchasing or contracting out services in such functions as policing, public utilities, welfare and education (Savas 1978; Propper 1993; Lowery 1998: 137–72).

The partial case of the hybrid mode is also exemplified by the quasi-markets experiments in the British National Health Services (NHS) system, that was considered as the marketization of the spending link in public resource management for about two decades from 1980s to 2000s (Le Grand & Bartlett 1993; Ham 1994, 2009; Webster 1998; Grand, Mays & Mulligan Eds. 1998; Baggott 2004; Greener 2009). In essence, the "quasi-market" experiment was focused on the purchasing side of public financial management (Le Grand 1991). By introducing the so-called "quasi-market" institution, the government purchased healthcare services from the provider on behalf of the users. In operational terms, funding for the British NHS system relied upon tax revenue, in addition to a small amount from the National Insurance Contributions (NICs) as just noted. The system embraced four separate health services in the UK: NHS England, NHS Scotland, NHS Northern Ireland, and NHS Wales. Each of these was run by its respective home nation's ministry which assumed political responsibility to fulfill public policy goals, in operational terms, for example, health care demands for everyone, free services at the point of delivery, and the priority of clinical care rather than ability to pay, among others. Then healthcare resources were allocated, and services rendered through arms-length bodies rather than directly through government departments. The spending exercise involved the purchasers who were represented by hundreds of commissioning groups, working with their counterparts, namely, the providers who comprised a number of trusts, foundation trusts and private companies. The purchaser and provider were connected by a "service agreement." That is to say, the former "paid" the latter for health care services (quantity and quality of which were to be specified) on behalf of the patient, a third party pertaining to the "service agreement." In the process of implementation, the purchaser often dictated the terms of franchising of healthcare services in view of its monopoly status. Through the NHS policy experiments pertaining to the quasi-markets, by and large, the separation between the purchaser and provider meant that each stood equally in a market-like transactional relationship, albeit the so-called "service agreement" was much less than a legal contract.

Germany represents a full-fledged case of the hybrid mode of governance in the realm of resource management with regards to marketization of both the spending link and revenue link of public financial management (Porter & Guth 2012; Busse & Bumel 2014). Germany is credited for offering one of the earliest and largest national health insurance systems in the world, dating back to 1883 in the wake of Otto von Bismarck's policy initiatives in social legislation during the 1880s. The statutory (or public) plans today cover approximately 90 percent of the population in the country, the private plans take care of the remaining 10 percent or so.

Centering on the spending link, a package of medical care services is provided and paid for by statutory plans which rely on risk-pooling systems to satisfy essential demands of the insured as well as enhance positive externality in healthcare services for undifferentiated multitude of residents (e.g., a healthy and productive labor force) at the societal level. Each statutory plan offers a constructed category of services which is made available to each enrollee in time of need. Patients have considerable room for choice within a two-tier system of healthcare services in Germany: Choice of hospitals and outpatient care doctors. As the statutory plans managerially depend upon market mechanisms to provide the choices to the patient and encourage competition among providers, administrative measures characteristic of hierarchies are adopted for the purpose of cost control, such as the standard reimbursement catalog, deductible, and co-payment scheme (Porter & Guth 2012).

Operating through statutory plans, the revenue source is channeled through a funding system, featuring mandatory enrollment, co-insurance of employer and employee, income-dependent premiums, family coverage, equal access to care regardless of ability to pay, and an obligation to underwrite every enrollee, among others. The statuary plans are invariably managed by self-governing statutory corporate entities under the supervision of the governments at the federal and regional level. There exists intense competition among hundreds of corporations, often centering on costs, but not necessarily on measurable value. Since the opening of insurance markets in 1996, plans have shrunk from 476 in 1997 to 169 in 2010 (Porter & Guth 2012).

Like Germany, China's public medical care insurance plans also fall into the full-fledged case of the hybrid mode of governance, installing market mechanisms to both the revenue link and spending link of each insurance plan. As previously noted, for instance, the enhanced version of the basic medical care insurance (BMCI) plan, coupled with the SMCI, incorporates market mechanisms into both the revenue link and spending link of resource management, as is characteristic of mandatory enrollment, co-insurance of the employer and employees, income-dependence design, co-payment, deductible and ceiling payment-ceiling. The enhanced BMCI plan covers both outpatient services (i.e., clinical care) and in-patient services (i.e., hospital care) in addition to HESI cases. Clinical care covers routine cases that depend partially on the accumulated savings which come from personal contributions overtime, while hospital care and HESI cases rely heavily on a risk-pooling scheme. In the implementation, moreover, the enrollees are given almost no choice of insurer, but have limited choices of providers (e.g., often out of two designated providers in curative care and in dispensary services) as mentioned (Chapter 6). In the NRCMCI and URMCI plans (Chapters 9–11), the government units in various echelons assume the important role of funding by subsidizing a large share of premium contributions, together with the enrollee's smaller share. In relation to the provider, the insurer and the insured assume the role of purchaser to be responsible for medical bills in the forms of out of pocket payment (OPP), co-payment and deductible, indicative of market transactions in full swing (Lee 2019).

As mentioned previously, the medical care insurance plans adopt an IRF system as the financial strategy bearing close resemblance to what is adopted by the business sector. The core of managerial and financial activities of the said plans is revenue-centered, if not profit-oriented, working under budgetary, accounting and auditing procedures like their counterparts in the non-public sector. It is evident that market mechanisms are installed into all three basic medical care plans, namely, the enhanced BMCI, URMCI, and NRCMCI, but questions as to whether the patterns of transactions would remain stable after the inauguration have yet to be empirically assessed.

Toward the Hybrid Mode of Governance

Here the study will treat the case of public medical care insurance programs as a hybrid mode of governance that saddles in between the state and markets with reference to major institutional and managerial features.[1] From the disciplinary perspective of Political Science, which differs from its sister disciplines such as Economics and Sociology, the study is focused on resource management—a functional area which is most distinguished in the hybrid mode. It is pertinent to dwell on Williamson's early analysis on the mode of governance, and then proceed to demonstrate how the public organization differs from the economic organization in handling public policy issues.

To account for behavioral patterns of profit-seeking in market situations, Williamson proposes a theoretical scheme of three modes of governance in a kind of continuum: From the market mode to the hybrid mode, and the hierarchy mode (Williamson 1996: 93–119). Highlighting the differences between the public organization and economic organization, the study applies the three modes of governance here as well, while taking the disciplinary perspective of Policy Studies into full consideration. Through reformulating, the three modes will be treated here as three managerial and institutional alternatives for coordinating and organizing activities in the realm of public policy (including public medical care insurance) as given in Figure 2.1. The market mode and the state hierarchy mode each stand at one far end of the policy continuum while the hybrid mode is in the middle, and it is often taken as a mixture of the two. For analytical purposes, each mode has six dimensions: Goal orientation, actors involved, institutional form, funding vehicle, financial strategy, and decision-making style to be further elaborated below.

Overall, it is readily apparent that three modes of governance differ from one another regarding goal orientation, actors involved, and institutional forms as given in Figure 2.1. While the market mode is characteristic of profit/revenue pursuits, the state hierarchy mode is concerned with multiple, broad goals of public policy (often including financial goals). The hybrid mode represents a case where public financial management is an integral part of public policy, but tries to go beyond

Modes / Dimensions	Market	Hybrid	State-hierarchy
Goal orientation	Revenue/ profit	Policy goals (including revenue targets)	Policy goals (including citizens' demands)
Major actors	Buyers and sellers	Executives & clients	Officials & citizens
Decision-making style	Full autonomy & response to price signals	Limited autonomy & policy guidance (bilateral dependency)	Command & relational elements (e.g. unilateral dependency)
Institutional apparatus	Corporate entities & private enterprises	Public organizations (No-departmental public entities)	Bureaus & government units
Financial strategy	Inward-resource-flow system	Inward-resource-flow system (highly regulated)	Outward-resource-flow system (grants, subsidies & tax exemption etc.)
Funding vehicle	Transactions (contacts supplemented by judicial system)	Transactions under regulatory control (e.g., user charges, compensation & revenue franchise)	Taxation

Figure 2.1 Modes of Governance: Market, Hybrid, and State-hierarchy.

Source: Adapted and reformulated from Williamson, O.E. (1996). *The Mechanisms of Governance.* New York & Oxford University Press. 105.

the narrow horizon of profit/revenue orientation of the economic organization. Moreover, one needs to make differentiation among the three modes according to the key actors in each: For example, government officials serve as principal actors in the state hierarchy mode; in the market mode profit-seekers assume the roles of investors, sellers, buyers and owners; and in the hybrid mode, the key actors are often task-oriented personnel such as appointed managers/or property oriented directors, executives or administrative heads of the public organizations rather than civil servants. From an institutional perspective, the market mode often operates in the form of a corporate entity, enterprise, or investor/property owner; the state hierarchy is coordinated by government units such as bureaus; and the hybrid mode is managed by non-departmental public entities (NDPEs), keeping an arm's length from the government while handling the tasks and functions mandated and given to them.

As indicated in Figure 2.1, the market mode tends to rely upon transactions as the principal vehicle of funding by making full use of contracts in addition to the judicial system for the resolution of conflicts. Its financial strategy features resource-internalizing coupled with cost-externalizing as adopted by the IRF system previously noted. According to Williamsom, in the market mode, the decision-making style is taken as fully autonomous while relying on price signals with a strong propensity toward Adaptation (A), often price sensitive, consumer-oriented, and market-oriented. The attributes of managerial instruments are performance appraisals, differential incentives, and measurable and marketable results (Williamson 1996; 93–119).

Focusing on financial and managerial functions as shown in Figure 2.1, the state hierarchy mode tends to make public revenue, including taxation, its main funding vehicle, and adopt the resource-externalizing mechanisms as the principal financial strategy. While emphasis is placed on overall budgetary balance of the entire government, the state hierarchy mode does not require the matching of costs and benefits for each item of policy action. The decision-making style shifts from an emphasis on price signals to "relational" (including political) considerations in Adaptation (C), for example, mutual dependence between counterparts, suggesting that, given the costs of information, risk control and provision of collective and quasi-collective goods might often take precedence over profit-maximization. In the state hierarchy mode, moreover, the coordination of activities tends to depend heavily on command rather than market transactions. In the exercise of command, the managerial tools are largely procedure-centered, relying on rules and regulations, written communication, supervision, and control where performance and outcome are not often quantifiable, measurable and marketable. It is noteworthy that the state hierarchy mode is comparable to the market mode in that both have revenue concerns in the context of resource management; however, the former works for a broader goal mix while being oriented to both marketable and non-marketable results. Nonetheless, Williamson does not draw a conceptual distinction between command and reciprocal relations—the defining features of two entirely different disciplinary orientations, namely Political Science and Sociology, by treating both in an undifferentiated fashion as "relational."

As the main theoretical concern of this study, the hybrid mode of governance represents an amalgam of the market mode and the state hierarchy mode as indicated in Figure 2.1. As a funding vehicle, the hybrid mode relies heavily on transactions by maintaining a budgetary balance between financing and spending in the IRF system. For example, in public medical care insurance in China, premium contributions are closely tied to payments to cover expenses of an enrollee's illness based on financial calculation. In terms of financial strategy, the hybrid mode tends to adopt an IRF system with modifications, in connection with resource-internalizing mechanisms centering on transactions. For public policy considerations, meanwhile, the government does have an option to work through the ORF system by subsidizing, in part or in full, premium contribution of the needy and marginalized sector of the population in conjunction with the enrollment in public insurance of basic medical care.

Working in hybrid mode, the principal actors (e.g., the insurers of a public insurance plan) tend to maintain a bounded autonomy in their decision-making style in the sense that not only do they take price clues from the marketplace to make relevant decisions, but also they consider other relevant variables to guide their policy-making (e.g., collective or quasi-collective benefits as just noted). In the design of public medical care insurance, for example, insurers can lend greater weight for the fulfillment of externality and provision of collective and/or quasi-collective goods, while moving away from pure pursuit of revenue maximization and a decision-making style strictly guided by price signals, as in the market mode of governance.

The study proposes to adopt two different formulations in the analysis of the hybrid mode of governance, namely, the policy-oriented formulation and non-policy-oriented formulation. The two formulations here address the differences between the public organization and economic organization respectively at the conceptual and theoretical level. To begin with, questions arise on how the public organization performs its revenue-oriented functions in the public sector in comparison with its economic counterparts in the non-public (or private) sector, and whether the former acts in either a way like or different from the latter. The public organization and the economic organization are found comparable when both perform similar functions in resource management, for example, the government's role in purchasing functions, building infrastructure, managing public facilities, running public enterprises, and providing subsidies to the needy (Hughes 1998: 81–128). However, the former assumes a significant role in public policy, while the latter is mainly concerned with non-policy-oriented tasks. In some instances, the latter might produce externalities in the realm of public policy, in both positive and negative terms, but they are neither intended, nor controllable.

Applying the policy-oriented formulation, the study differs from Williamson's analysis of public policy, for example, in a case of public medical care insurance in China. The study treats the said hybrid mode as representing an attempt to examine how the markets and hierarchy are fused with each other in the realm of public policy. That is to say, public medical care insurance operates in close resemblance with the performance of the economic organization in Williamson's sense, for example, adopting the IRF system centering on funding/spending goals, placing emphasis on maintaining budgetary balance with regard to each item of service provided and exhibiting the cost externalizing tendency. The central gravity of the task here tends to lean on funding/spending and rely on resource management. The case of public insurance represents one among many types of public organization that mainly performs revenue-oriented functions.[2] In the policy-oriented formulation, the hybrid mode is concerned with the public organization that is confronted with externality going beyond narrow concern of revenue pursuit, and it needs to work with the ORF system, and to be involved in public funding and guided by broader policy goals.

In the policy-oriented formulation, moreover, the hybrid mode can address the policy concerns pertaining to a viable choice of public funding for the basic medical care demands. First, as a tool of public resource management, an independent funding source needs to be installed to face challenges arising from the alienation of basic medical care entitlements from institutionalized funding as found in conventional public funding modes such as LIMC and PFMC. Instead of relying on fragmented and diverse funding sources from various channels and the work units, it is effective to adopt an institutional form of funding, that is fully separate from other public organizations including the governments, to maintain the continuity, stability and reliability of funding requirements for basic medical care services in novel forms of public funding, such as BMCI, URMCI and NRCMCI.

Second, in public medical care insurances introduced during the reform era, the independent funding source so installed makes it possible to be insulated not only from fluctuations of the economic cycle, but also disturbances of policy and political changes. Public medical care insurance is designed to avoid the drawbacks of market-oriented alternatives to the funding system, and non-market-oriented options. On the one hand, it is intended to be immune from risks of profit pursuits and to ensure the reliability and security of funding sources. On the other hand, it needs to be separated from the government's revenue, in order to minimize and prevent diversion of insurance funding to answer other demands of changing and variegated revenue policy of the government.

Third, the public medical care insurance fund must address a preference mix with two policy concerns: As private goods in terms of personal demands of curative care (treatments, drugs and devices) and as collective and/or quasi-collective goods regarding a healthy and productive workforce for the economy. Fourth, the independent funding operates in adherence with the sound principles of financial management, in accordance with strict budgeting and auditing procedures and rules, as well as ex ante and ex post interventions by the party-state. Above all, the hybrid mode of governance represents an effective financial strategy to organize and manage the public funding for various types of public services, especially basic medical care insurance.

Patterns of Behavioral Adaptations

It is germane here to examine how Williamson's theoretical construct extends to an analysis on behavioral adaptations in the hybrid model of governance in public medical care insurances in China. In Williamson's theoretical formulation, any design of governance adopted (presumably positioned in between the markets and hierarchy) tends to make adaptations once again toward one or other direction (i.e., toward either the markets or hierarchy), as it is put into practice. Theoretically speaking, behavioral adaptation represents the endeavor of bridging the gaps between the design and implementation.

According to Williamson, the profit-oriented pursuit often leads to two patterns of behavioral adaptation in the context of markets: Adaptation (A) centering on responses to market signals (including price) in order to internalize resource-flow through transactions, often coupled with its byproduct such as cost-externalizing tendency, intended or unintended; and Adaptation (C) forging "relations" while facing uncertainty and uncontrollable risks arising from the economic environment (Williamson 1975, 1996). By and large, Adaptation (A) pertains to the patterns of decision-making behavior that is dictated by market signals, oriented toward revenue-concerns in transactions. Adaptation (C) is concerned with non-market information, and it is oriented toward "relational" variables other than revenue/profit-oriented pursuits.[3]

Theoretically speaking, Williamson needs to answer on three accounts as he addresses the issue of the linkage between transactions and "relations" that is taken as "mutual reciprocity," "cooperation," and forms of authoritative dominance, etc., in different contexts. First, why do there exist discrepancies between the ideal type (or design) and practices of transactions, and between formal contracts of transactions and actual market behavior in the first place? In other words, a rational profit-oriented actor tends to move away from the ideal type of market behavior, for example, only responding to price signals in the marketplace, and always in full compliance with a formal contract.[4] Second, how does behavioral adaptation take place? And in which form? In the case of profit seeking activities, for example, the rational actors need to make behavioral adaptations under a variety of circumstances where they might be found in shortage of information, limitation of competence, and divergent operational definitions of profit-seeking goals (Williamson 1975, 1996). Third, it is likely, as the study argues, that behavioral adaptations might simply result from the shifting commercial strategies as well as changing operational definitions of profit goals, for instance, profit maximization within a short time span, steady profit stream over a long time, or the maintenance of market share at a cost while waiting for an optimal profit-making opportunity in the future, etc.

This study works with the hybrid mode of governance in its policy-oriented formulation, based on a case study of public medical care insurance in China. And it represents an attempt to examine how the markets and hierarchy are fused with each other in the realm of public policy. From the disciplinary perspective, the study is concerned on how politics (including public policy) is "embedded" (or takes root) not only in market transactions but also in social networks respectively.[5] In the process of building the hybrid mode of governance in conjunction with public medical care insurances, there witnessed considerable tensions between Adaptation (A) and Adaptation (C) regarding decision-making on four key issues: The issue of program specificity (often including product/service specificity), the application of franchise, the network of regulatory control, and the relationship of asymmetric information among actors. The study will dwell on these issues in conceptual and theoretical terms here, saving empirical cases in the rest of the book.

First, Adaptation (C) takes place through the exercise of program specificity (including product/service specificity), attesting the growth of hierarchy in inaugurating public medical care insurance. In introducing public medical care insurance plans, product/service specificity is made in the process of packaging a specific product and/or rendering service—a category of insurance package constructed for chosen clients. The provision of a constructed category regarding basic medical care insurances is sustained by premium contributions and the risk pooling mechanisms based on a specially designed program. The exercise of program specificity entails considerable investment and costs of research, technology and professional expertise, exercise of command, and other non- market-oriented decisions. In conceptual terms, this bears close resemblance to the notion of "asset specificity" as noted by Williamson (Williamson 1996: 59–60).

Adaptation (C) tends to occur when policymakers are confronted with the exercise of product/service specificity, for instance, whether only hospital care and other expensive and serious cases (HESI) rather than clinical care ought to be incorporated into insurance plans in China? In packaging BMCI plans across jurisdictions, for instance, there witnessed the tensions about the relative weight between clinical care on the one hand and hospital care and HESI (i.e., more expensive, and serious illness beyond payment-ceiling) on the other hand. While the provincial/local jurisdictions that bear financial burden tend to support the incorporation of HESI only, the central government was inclined to include both, maintaining consistency with the compensation policy and in deference to vested interests of enrollees in BMCI. As a matter of official line of central policymakers, moreover, priority was given to hospital care and HESI and to absorb the risks of infrequent, but serious and unusually expensive illnesses, indicative of a movement toward Adaptation (C). Just opposite to the BMCI case, however, provincial/local policymakers tended to heed the enrollees' preference mix and underscore clinical care/common and frequent illnesses, representing Adaptation (A) to be dictated by market signals and concern for revenue in the marketplace in URMCI and NRCMCI.

Second, the use of franchise was concerned with both politics and policy in introducing public medical care insurances in China, often producing a salient tendency of moving away from Adaptation (A) to Adaption (C) as the government's intervention increased. Theoretically speaking, the policy of franchise/monopoly represents an endeavor to allocate market shares among competitors in the marketplace through exercise of mandatory power of the state. It often produces two kinds of outcomes: Adjudication among vested interests, and policy outcomes regarding economic and managerial dimensions. And politics and policy are often intertwined. In political terms, Gordon Tullock, for instance, is focused on highly politicized situations in the USA, where the plurality of interests often remain considerably active, and meanwhile pursuing rents through seizing the right of entry into the markets by political means (Rowley 2005). In a way, rent-seeking behaviors involve fighting for control of market opportunities through political manipulation within the institutional arena.

In the Chinese case, both policy and politics are found relevant in making public medical care insurances. Considering policy merits, franchise applied to all three public medical care insurance programs, that is, BMCI, URMCI and NRC-MCI. For example, the insurer's market shares were certified and franchised by local authorities. Moreover, patients enjoyed only a limited choice of providers—normally a few of them that are "designated" (meaning franchised). From a policy consideration, the impetus toward adaptation (C) was reinforced by policymakers' granting of market share, considering economies of scale, and making it more feasible to build viable risk pooling mechanisms to meet payment obligations in all public medical insurance plans. Moreover, sovereign planners introduced a brand of privatization in medical care during the health care reform but, in politicized situation, private providers, such as clinics and hospitals, were often denied a franchise to enjoy any market share in public insurance plans, even though private facilities were legitimized and licensed since 2000 to enter healthcare markets according to the "hospital classification" policy (Lee 2019).

Third, tendency toward adaptation (C) was manifested in the process of building a network of regulatory control in connection with public medical care insurance plans in China, where transactions among relevant parties were found nested in a network of regulatory controls—the main tools characteristic of an exercise of command within the state hierarchy. In other words, transactions of key actors (e.g., buyers and sellers) were not only dictated by price fluctuations, but were also required to adhere to public policy goals, for example, low-price policy of medical care services, safety and quality of drugs, externality in terms of good health and social security available to all, etc. To govern the actors as well as the transactions between them in the execution of public insurance plans, in fact, the government employed a variety of regulatory tools of an administrative nature and went beyond formal written contracts in private commercial settings.

The market mechanisms began to operate in two arenas which are under regulatory control in case of BMCI, for example: In the first arena where a co-insurance scheme was applied, an insurer assumed the role of seller of an insurance benefit package while the employer and employees (enrollees) acted as buyers in the transaction. In the second arena, largely focusing on purchasing functions, the insurer and enrollee acted as buyers by "paying" their respective shares for the services rendered by the providers according to the hurdles of deductible and co-payment scheme. Whereas in case of NRCMCI and URMCI, the government worked with the enrollee, subsidizing a substantial part of premium contribution in transactions with the insurer, and in turn, the insurer and enrollee worked together in the role of "buyer" of medical care services rendered by the providers who represented the selling side under the network of regulatory control.

Among many possibilities, fourth, adaptation (C) is likely to take place in conjunction with asymmetric information between the two sides of a transaction, namely, between the purchaser of public medical care insurance (i.e., the insurer and enrollees) and provider (Lee 2019). Some authors make observations about desirable policy outcomes of public medical care insurance with regards to the new role of the insurer in public management, in substitution for the bureaucratic control (Gu 2008: 117–21). In addition, Williamson raises theoretical issues about the scenario regarding Adaptation (C), where the contract holder might be able to gain advantage of asymmetric information once entering the contract. For example, when facing other competitors in the marketplace, as mentioned by Williamson, the contract holder might gain "idiosyncratic knowledge" to fend off potential competitors; make asset specificity of the supplying corporation to gain advantage in holding contracts; and grant franchise to public utility company to minimize the costs of unexpected changes (Williamson 1975: 20–40; 1996: 106–9).

In the situation of asymmetric information, the insurer's position is likely to be strengthened in two ways. One pertains to franchising that enables the insurer to assume predominance in the insurance market. In other words, the insurer can substitute for the bureau in undertaking the supervisory role overseeing the performance of the provider in accordance with the service agreement signed by the two parties as well as the laws and regulations of the state. In the other way, once the insurer finds its entry to the domain of insurance profession, it tends to accumulate knowledge and skills and act as a counterweight to other actors such as medical doctors in the same field. The discussion on behavioral adaptation has pointed to a cluster of exceedingly complex episodes of choice making so far, warranting some further empirical investigation into concrete cases in the remainder of the volume.

Concluding Remarks

In conceptual and theoretical terms, this study treats public medical care insurance in China as a hybrid mode of governance in the policy-oriented formulation. Public medical care insurance plans represent a case where transactions are encapsulated within the state hierarchy. On the one hand, the principal actors are revenue-oriented, if not profit-oriented, operating within the hybrid mode. By design, all three public insurance plans—BMCI, URMCI and NRCMCI each—work with an IRF system, armed with resource-internalizing mechanisms such as budgetary and accounting tools, to ensure that costs in each transaction will be matched by earnings. On the other hand, actors involved are guided by higher policy goals while conducting transactions in the marketplace. Operating through the ORF system, the government subsidizes the enrollee to pay for premium for insurance plans such as in NRCMCI and URMCI, and yet the government is not a party in the transactions concerning buying insurance within the IRF system that operates independently. Whereas the broad outline of the public medical care insurance plans has been depicted here, the remaining chapters will describe their origin, evolutions, key characteristics, and management, as well as the discrepancies between implementation of the plans and policy relating to such plans.

Notes

1 To risk over-simplification, one may study China's economic reform broadly as a process of marketization, that is, transformation from a state-centered system such as the CPE to a market-oriented system but falling short of a full-fledged free market system. Accordingly it is equally meaningful to focus on the intermediary mode, namely,

the hybrid mode, in addition to the state and markets. According to Charles Lindblom, standing on one extreme of a continuum of public policy alternatives, the market is taken as the strategic model centering on voluntarily coordinated interaction in the realm of public policy, while the state represents the synoptic model theoretically guided by and depending on command as the vehicle of coordination. Lindblom's analysis does theoretically anticipate the intermediary model of policymaking but it has yet to take on one step forward to map the major characteristics, institutional forms and managerial mechanisms, operational flow and outcomes (Lindblom 1977).

2 Like public medical care insurances, one finds that the revenue-earning monopolies in wine and tobacco. In China under the CPE, public enterprises work with franchises to squeeze enormous revenue sources from the society to the government and from the agricultural to industrial sector. In fact, much of marketization in the health care sector is concerned with the use of franchises as a revenue tool, for instance, in case of URS and the wholesale/retail ratio in drug sale at the public hospital level (Lee 2019).

3 Williamson leaves "relations" in Adaptation (C) operationally undefined, without addressing the distinction between "relations" in Sociological sense and authoritative relations in Political Science. In Ferlie's discussion the "relational" dimension of "quasi-markets" in social and "institutional" terms, he tries to work out an operational definition for the concept of "relations" with regards to "social embeddedness" and "institutional embeddedness," each of which can theoretically be analyzed as an independent domain (Ferlie 1992). As an alternative, overall, it is appropriate and more fruitful to draw conceptual distinctions among three arenas, namely, market transactions, social network and power relations, and to examine the key features, the process, operation and mechanisms pertaining to each (Ferlie et al. 1996). Arguing in terms of restoration of politics in public policy analysis, this study is focused on political behaviors that are taken, in part, as "relations" with reference to Adaptation (C) in Williamson's formulation. Also, the study argues that an important part of so-called "relations" are actually political relations that operate within a state hierarchy, while the other part is concerned with social networks. It is argued that neither political relations nor social networks are reducible to market transactions.

4 The concept of transaction needs to account for a dynamic and changeable relationship subject to behavioral adaptations over a long stretch of time. In light of Gunnar Mydral's conceptualization, the contract embodies a demand or expectation "before event" (ex-ante), while bilateral dependence represents part of an actual economic result "after event" (ex-post) (Mydral 1939: 46). That is to say, the contract represents what is originally intended by the two contracting parties, but in the process of implementation, the actual result of the transaction differs from what was originally contracted, leading to behavioral adaptations in two directions, either Adaptation (A) more in response to price signals in the marketplace or Adaption (C) more cooperation in a non-market sphere (Williamson 1996). Williamson uses the notion of "incomplete contracting" to point to the discrepancy between ex-ante and ex-post, and resonates with Herbert Simon's formulation of "bounded rationality" in the sense that the contract is intended as rational, but its outcome is "satisficing," that is, less than originally expected. In Simon's view, the cost of information cannot be equated to zero, and as decision-makers, contracting actors cannot ensure a completely satisfactory result of the contract in question.

5 By the same token, it is theoretically meaningful for authors to work further on the connectivity of any pairing of other two variables, for example, market transactions with either social networks or power structure. Also, Williamson makes an effort to explore how economic decisions are made in conjunction with the variable conceptualized as "relations" that includes other two variables, namely social networks and hierarchy (power structure). Parallel to Williamson, Ferlie proposes the concept of "embeddedness" pertaining to "quasi-markets," suggesting to look into "relational" variables in connection with both social networks and "institutional" (or political) variables (Ferlie 1992: 79–97).

References

Arrow, K. 1963. Uncertainty and the welfare economics of medical care. *American Economic Review* 53.3: 941–73.

Baggott, R. 2004. *Health and Health Care in Britain.* Houndmills, Basingstoke, Hampshire & New York.

Bendix, R. 1962. Max Weber, *An Intellectual Portrait.* New York: Anchor Books, Doubleday & Company.

Busse, R., & Blumel, M. 2014. Germany: *Health System Review. Health Systems in Transition* 16.2: 1–296.

Cylus, J., Richardson, E., Findley, L., Longley, M., O'Neill, C. & Steel, D. 2015. United Kingdom: Health system review. *Health Systems in Transition* 17.5: 1–125.

Davidson, S. M. 2010. *Still Broken, Understanding the U.S. Health Care System.* Stanford, CA: Stanford University Press.

Ferlie, E. 1992. The creation and evolution of quasi markets in the public sector: A problem for strategic management. *Strategic Management Journal* 13: 79–97.

Ferlie, E., Ashburner, L., Fitzgerald, L., & Pettigrew, A. 1996. *The New Public Management in Action.* Oxford: Oxford University Press.

Gerth, H. H., & Mills, C. W. 1968. *From Max Weber: Essays in Sociology.* New York: The Oxford University Press.

Grand, J.L., Mays, Mulligan, J (Eds). 1998. *Learning from the NHS Internal Market, A Review of Evidence*. London: King's Fund Publishing.

Greener, I. 2009. *Health Care in the UK, Understanding Continuity and Change.* Bristol & Portland: The Policy Press.

Gu, X. 2008. *Zouxian quanmian yibao: Zhongguo xinyigai de zhanlue yu zhanshu* (*Toward Comprehensive Medical Care Insurance: Strategy and Tactic in China's New Medical Care Reform*). Beijing: Zhongguo laodong chubanshe.

Ham, C. 1994. *Management and Competition in the New NHS.* Oxford & New York: Radcliffe Medical Press.

Ham, C. 2009. *Health Policy in Britain.* New York: Palgrave Macmillian.

Henderson, A. M., & Parsons, T. 1947. *The Theory of Social and Economic Organization.* New York: The Free Press. London: Coller-MaCmillan Ltd.

Henry, N. 1989. *Public Administration and Public Affairs.* Englewood, NJ: Prentice-Hall International, Inc.

Hughes, O. E. 1998. *Public Management and Administration, An Introduction.* Houndmills & New York: Palgrave.

Le Grand, J. 1991. Quasi-Markets and Social Policy. *The Economic Journal* September: 1236–67.

Le Grand, J., & Bartlett, W. (Eds.) 1993. *Quasi-Markets and Social Policy.* Houndmills & London.

Lee, P. N. 1987. *Industrial Management and Economic Reform in China.* Hong Kong, Oxford & New York: Oxford University Press.

Lee, P. N. 2019. *Re-engineering Affordable Care Policy in China, Is Marketization a Solution?* London & New York: Routledge.

Lindblom, C. E. 1977. *Politics and Markets, The World's Political-Economic Systems.* New York: Basic Books.

Lowery, D. 1998. Consumer Sovereignty and Quasi-Market Failure. *Journal of Public Administration Research* and *Theory* 2: 137–72.

Massey, A. *Managing the Public Sector, A Comparative Analysis of the United Kingdom and the United States.* Aldershot, England & Vermont: Edward Elgar.

Myrdal, G. 1939. *Monetary Equilibrium.* London: W. Hodge.

Naughton, B. 1996. *Growing out of Plan, Chinese Economic Reform, 1978–1993.* Cambridge: Cambridge University Press.

Ostrom, V. and Ostrom, E. 1977. Public goods and public choices in *Alternatives for Delivering Public Services towards Improved Performance.* Indiana University: Workshop in Political Theory and Public Analysis.

Porter, M. E., & Guth, C. 2012. *Redefining German Health Care, Moving to Value-Based System.* Springer, London & New York: Springer.

Propper, C. 1993. Quasi-markets, contracts and quality in health and social care: The US experience. In Le Grand, J. & Bartett, *Quasi-Markets and Social Policy.* Houndmills & London: The Macmillan Press, Ltd. 35–67

Rowley, C. K. (Ed.) 2005. *The Rent-Seeking Society, Gordon Tullock.* Indianapolis, IN: Liberty Fund, Inc.

Savas, E. S. 1978. *Privatization, The Key to Better Government.* Catham, NJ: Chatham Publishers, Inc.

Starr, P. 2011. *Remedy and Reaction, The Particular American Struggle over Health Care Reform.* New Haven, CT & London: The Yale University Press.

Shonfield, A. 1965. *Modern Capitalism: The Changing Balance of Public and Private Power.* New York: Oxford University Press.

Sultz, H. A., & Kristina, M. Y. 2006. *Health Care USA, Understanding Its Organization and Delivery.* Boston, MA, Toronto, London & Singapore: Jones and Bartlett Publishers.

Webster, C. 1998. *The National Health Service, A Political History.* Oxford & New York: Oxford University Press.

Williamson, O. E. 1975. *Markets and Hierarchies: Analysis and Antitrust Implications.* New York & London. The Free Press.

Williamson, O. E. 1996. *The Mechanisms of Governance.* Oxford & New York: Oxford University Press.

3 Policy Legacy and Vested Interests

Accompanying with the topmost priority of pro-growth policy as well as its impressive results during economic reform, the proliferation of social security initiatives has engendered the quest not only for entirely new definitions on relevant programs regarding social security policy in China, but also a fresh round of research endeavors.[1] While authors and policy analysts tried to examine the overall developmental tendency of social security policy, they often began by focusing on the evolutionary path of each selected program. For example, some are obviously rooted in the legacy of CPE, such as retirement pension, housing, and healthcare, while some others were newly introduced amid building a mixed economy, for instance, unemployment insurance and social relief (Qian 2021). To fill the gaps of the current research, the study is concerned with health care insurance, the demand for which is time sensitive and is activated increasingly with advancement of age of the enrollee. Prior to economic reform, health care was treated as non-wage compensation, chargeable to the budget of the work unit, and marking a fresh departure of public policy, it was funded through insurance programs introduced during the mid 1990s–2000s.

Scholars have lately started to launch some pioneering research on China's social security and healthcare, and each adopted an interesting theoretical approach, producing meaningful research results on well-selected themes. For example, J. Duckett was focused on the changing role of the state in health policy (Duckett 2011); Y. Huang endeavored to capture the dynamic interaction among policy actors within the party-state hierarchy (Huang 2013); P. Lee dealt with the market-oriented reform in introducing user charges as well as the undertaking responsibility system (URS) (Lee 2019); X. Huang tried to analyze public welfare and political loyalty in the authoritative location of interests in the midst of rapid program expansion (Huang 2020); and Qian's main concern rested on a rich inventory of administrative tools in policymaking and implementation (Qian 2021). To propose an alternative theoretical angle regarding social security in China, the study is devoted to examining how marketization of health care is rooted in the centrally planned economy (CPE), as policy actors are confronted with challenges in search of fresh policy options and novel managerial approaches in public medical care insurance.

DOI: 10.4324/9781003389934-4

The study suggests that the inauguration of public medical care insurance represents an unprecedented and innovative change from the conventional public funding of healthcare, wrestling with the issue of continuity and discontinuity. While one may observe some entirely new types of services, mechanisms of operations, and style of management, some continuity is still discernable. The study argues that public medical care insurance is path dependent in the sense that both policy legacy and vested interests carry weight in making the new policy of social security in general and health care. The remaining passages will first lend a general profile of conventional public funding of medical care. Then the study proceeds to make a review of three approaches to analyze conventional funding models of social security as follows: The work-unit centered approach, the corporatist approach, and the remuneration approach.

Crises and Diagnoses

Social security (including health care) policy encountered crises amid the launching of economic reform. To monitor the sequence of social security reform in various programs, a general pattern of policy initiation emerged from the crises themselves as well as responses from policy actors at various levels of the party-state hierarchy. It is pertinent for the study first investigate into the crises and then make diagnoses to be followed by an analysis regarding how policy actors at the provincial/local level and central level responded to very severe situations.

As an illustration among conventional funding programs in social security, it appears that the reform arrived first in the policy territory of public financed medical care (PFMC) that performed a role for financing healthcare for civil servants and other personnel of public organizations during the CPE era, to be followed by labor insurance medical care (LIMC) that shouldered the financial burden of curative care for staff and workers in public enterprises. The rural cooperative medical care (RCMC) that was financed and managed by agricultural collectives in rural China, remained the next.

The impetus of health care reform was first generated in a context where health care funding was adversely impacted by radical politics under Maoism. In a series of price cuts to medical care for about two decades from 1958 to 1979, for example, the party-state moved toward absorbing more and more of the costs for healthcare, but it did not seem that the government's growing budget could catch up with the increasing spending demands among users. During economic reform, the provincial/local jurisdictions began to find remedy to the financial burden of healthcare through introducing the spending control measures, as no pending control measure had been installed prior to economic reform. It was soon found, moreover, no independent and institutionalized funding system had been established to honor the medical care entitlements of the enrollees in the programs of LIMC and PFMC.

Instead, the work unit had to handle the medical care expenses by relying on its budgetary and accounting procedures commonly adopted for handling items of expenditures in the regular categories of expenses. While the funding for LIMC relied heavily on revenue generated at the public enterprise level, subject to the performance fluctuations of each enterprise and varying economic situations throughout the country, PFMC suffered less from the instability of funding sources because it relied upon public revenue appropriated to various echelons of the government. Overall, health care funding was considered as a form of non-wage compensation and derived from "supplementary wage" that was again subject to tight budgetary control of the government. Under austerity as well as the low wage policy for decades, the quest for the improvement of remuneration through the expansion of non-wage compensation represented a safer avenue that could minimize ideological controversy. Thus, this exacerbated the financial pressure on various echelons of the government.

Moreover, not all enrollees in PFMC were immune from the crisis of funding health care, despite applying spending control measures. In PFMC, two classes of personnel were entertained. Under the "full-quota appropriation" (*quane bokuan*) system, a small pocket of civil servants (and party cadres) who worked at the ministerial level and provincial level enjoyed full reimbursement of expenditure financed by the government. It is often called "government insurance." Under the "partial-quota appropriation (*chae bokuan*)" system, however, an overwhelming majority of public personnel who worked for the service units such as in research units, colleges and schools, warfare and health establishment only enjoyed partial reimbursement of medical bills. This is taken as so-called "work unit insurance" (Zheng 2011: 109). Overall, PFMC could not overcome a shortage of funding either amid of a stagnating national economy during the period of radical politics.

During the early years of the post-Mao era, it was a pressing task for sovereign planners to address some serious financial issues within LIMC and PFMC in view of the soaring, uncontrollable expenditure and unbearable financial burden on both enterprise and government units alike (Peng, Cai & Zhou 1992; Lee 2019). In addition, the funding for medical care in public enterprises, namely, state-owned enterprises (SOEs) and collective-owned enterprises (COEs), developed into a serious problem during economic reform for several reasons, major part of which were the inadequacy of program specificity, for example, lacking spending control measures and some others attributable to contextual variables such as the disintegration of LIMC in many financially troubled SOEs, the changing profile of illness, the felt impacts of an aging population, and the arrival of the first cohorts of retirees beginning in the 1980s (Peng, Cai & Zhou 1992; Lee 2019).

Despite common standards and the types of medical care entitlements to enrollees nationwide in the public sector, conventional public funding programs were characteristically "work-unit centered" in the sense that each was managed and even financed by the respective work unit largely in a fragmented fashion. For instance, risk-pooling centered on the enterprise, government unit, and production brigade levels, beyond which no apparatus was made responsible for coordinating the essential functions of a medical care program in terms of financing, management, and organization. In addition, the scale of risk-pooling was simply too small to be effective in coping with HESI cases. For example, LIMC was taken as an "enterprise insurance" or enterprise-managed insurance (Zheng 2009). Formally, enrollees in LIMC were not required to make a premium contribution, and their medical care was charged to a medical care account (included as part of a welfare fund). It was considered as part of non-wage compensation, and ultimately derived from the wage fund (chargeable to retained revenue and/or production costs). In addition, PFMC was handled by various echelons of government where budgetary accountability rested. In the case of PFMC, enrollees did not have to contribute insurance premiums either; instead, public revenue through the state budget was its sole funding source. PFMI and LIMC were considered types of "proto-insurance" in stark contrast to a full-fledged insurance program such as BMCI formally introduced later as of 2001.

Similarly in the case of RCMC, funding and budgeting were organized by the work unit of another sort, that is, mainly the production brigade where medical care benefits were charged to relevant accounts at the production brigade level. That is to say, the work unit itself performed the risk-pooling function, and neither a system of premium contribution nor a payment scheme was in place in accordance with a standard insurance design rigorously implemented through the IRF system.

Taken together, LIMC and PFMC were made available only to a privileged few who were employed in the public sector during CPE, resulting in considerable distortion in the distribution of healthcare resources, namely, approximately 10 percent of the population of China enjoying 40 percent of the health care resources in the country (Peng, Cai & Zhou 1992: 5).

RAMC offered members of agricultural collectives a limited package of public health services as well as clinical care often tied to referral services as being claimed. While Duckett makes RAMC as a case of "state retreat", the statistics about it is fragmented, suggesting that the strength of RAMC fluctuated (Duckett 2011). Starting in 1958, brigade-managed RAMC programs, number-wise, reached a zenith in the mid-1980s when 90 percent of production brigades had established such programs, but the number fell drastically to about 5 percent of brigades retaining RAMC in the late1980s in tandem with the disintegration of the collective economy in the countryside (Gu, Gao & Yao 2006: 141–3).

Above all, the study suggests that the conventional funding of health care is characterized as alienation of entitlements from funding in terms of program design. In other words, although health care funding packages that had been made available to people in China prior to 1979, all these packages such as LIMC, PFMC, and RCMC were fundamentally deficient on the funding side. Medical care entitlements were enacted in accordance with laws and regulations nationwide, but they were not supported by an independent financing system beyond the work unit level. Payments for medical care bills were treated as one of common items on the budget of the work unit, and covered by finance of the respective work unit. In practice, moreover, the work unit was often too small to sustain risk pooling effectively to honor entitlements so offered as just mentioned. Besides, neither an accountability system nor the required program specificity pertaining to spending (e.g., spending control, co-payment and payment-ceiling, catalog and listing of services, drugs and devices, etc.) was in place. How did the policy dimension of social security interface with politics? This study will examine that question next.

For the last several decades there have been three approaches in China studies that address how politics related to public policy in general and medical care within the CPE framework in the PRC. It is germane here to analyze all three approaches to shed light on the extent to which politics had a bearing in public policy (including medical care) during economic reform. In effect, public policy is inseparable from the exercise of power while accommodating interests, and it is not neutral in terms of making choices by a supposedly impartial policymaker through a pure evaluation of apolitical pros and cons. In one way or another, these approaches try to characterize how social security packages (including healthcare) are designed, how they are implemented, and how they are dictated by politics.

By and large, the work unit approach and corporatist approaches are concerned with the relational, political, and cultural dimensions of social security packages (including medical care). Besides, neither are they policy oriented nor time-sensitive. Nonetheless, they are complementary to the remuneration approach which highlights the public policy perspective.

The Work-Unit Centered Approach

The work-unit-centered approach represents one of the earliest attempts to shed light on social security at the work unit, an essential component of the Leninist party-state. This approach is an intellectual and theoretical endeavor to explain how much "work-unit collectivism," a set of cultural and behavioral attributes, is weighted in political life at the work unit level in China. By and large, the researche covers such subject-matters as life chances in the workplace, compensation and industrial relations, and political life in industrial settings among others.[2]

There have also been authors endeavoring to examine the phenomenon of "work-unit collectivism" by gauging the impact of contextual and/or institutional variables. From a comparative perspective, for instance, Chan addresses how the government can shape remuneration packages at the enterprise level. And she draws attention to the interesting parallels between large-sized Japanese firms and Chinese SOEs regarding their "organization-oriented" rather "market-oriented" character in matters of wages, job security, permanent employment, and corporate loyalty (Chan 1997). Also, specialists on the former USSR suggest, from a comparative perspective, that the work-unit-centered provision of services and benefits is closely related to the developmental pattern of industrialization preceding urbanization, as service provisions, amenities, facilities and infrastructure were being organized in the midst of building industry in the former USSR during the CPE period (Sil 1997; Straus 1997).

Building on the existing research on the work unit, it is argued here that one needs to go beyond the work unit at the micro level to identify and examine features of the whole system of social security at the macro level. Since the work unit constitutes a component of the party-state hierarchy, all work-unit-centered functions in remuneration, welfare, and subsidies are attributable to the policy and directives, laws and regulations, and programs that the party-state entity establishes at the macro level. Moreover, not only were all these key features of work-unit collectivism reinforced by financial incentives inherent in CPE, but also all policy changes of wage and non-wage compensation were explicitly defined, regulated, and mandated by the government above the work unit during the process of economic reform.

A narrow focus on the work unit is not enough. As this study argues, even if all parts were added up, they still do not make up the whole. The so-called "work-unit collectivism" is likely the result of policy imposed from above. In many cases, the informal relational network, behavioral patterns, and cultural elements at the work unit level are often derivatives of the formal dimensions of the party-state organization rather than the other way around. Given the complexity of parallel hierarchies between the party committee and administration/management at the work unit level and in each echelon above, it is likely that the powerholders at respective levels within the totalitarian party-state system, for instance, branch party secretaries, are able to build up political loyalty to particular individuals and the party by making use of government resources informally (Whyte 1974; Walder 1986a). In the structure of parallel hierarchies, however, the government apparatus in all echelons can still maintain a considerable degree of independence in the institutional and managerial realm, given the possible overlapping between the government and party organization as well as the changing weight of each overtime.

It is evident that formal and institutional arrangements rather than merely cultural and behavioral variables also play significant parts in managing and providing social security benefits. According to Max Weber, the state operates with impersonality in coordination of its organizational activities with a scale beyond the face-to-face level, making written communication, rules and regulations, command and hierarchy, incentive, and contractual recruitment requisites to the so-called "legal-bureaucratic ideal type" (Parsons 1947: 329–40; Bendix 1962: 385–457; Hughes 1998: 26–32). Taking the public enterprise as an example, three main institutional actors play significant parts in the implementation of remuneration packages (including subsidies, welfare, and insurance, etc.) at the work unit level: Enterprise management (i.e., director with his/her staff), the Congress of Representatives of Staff and Workers (hereafter, CRSW), and the Labor Union (Yuan 1985: 169–91; Lee 1987; Chan 2000). All three operate at the formal and institutional setting where impersonality is the name of the game.

In institutional terms, the work unit is at the receiving end of a vast and long chain of command building above it. The work unit operates under the dual command of both the party committee and the government apparatus within the parallel hierarchies of the party-state organization. The work unit is merely an enforcing unit whose head is appointed by the supervisor at the next higher level. On the government side mainly dealing with policy issues, the work unit is directly responsible to the bureau in charge in the respective functional area, but it is also made accountable to several other relevant bureaus on some other policy issues that are pertinent to its day-to-day management (Yang 1989: 38). In other words, the work unit is managed by multiple bureaus, one from each functional area.

Moreover, one may identify the taxonomy of three types of work unit within the party-state hierarchy: Administrative work unit, service work unit, and production work unit. And each type carries out its respective functions assigned from above by the party-state (Lu 1996: 455, 1997; Lu & Perry 1997: 5; Yang 1999: 38–70).

In managerial terms, as a rule, an organizational sub-unit is *not* taken as a work unit within the party-state hierarchy unless it has acquired full-fledged accounting unit status as well as the power to appoint and manage public personnel whereas the work unit enjoys relative independence in financial management acting as an accounting unit, coupled with the status of legal person assuming obligations arising from transactions and financial responsibility to all parties concerned within the CPE framework. Moreover, oversees allocation (including meeting employment quotas) and appointment of staff and recruitment of workers that are not shared by sub-units below the work unit. Also, in analytical terms, the work unit differs from the workplace (i.e., the work site) in a public enterprise (Bian 1994: 1–21). The latter is normally placed one level lower than the former, being merely assigned technical and production tasks, coupled with a marginal and often auxiliary role in the management of personnel, wages, bonuses, and welfare in CPE.[3]

Overall, the locus of authority over public policy, including medical care, is normally situated at the bureau level and/or above within the CPE framework. As such the work unit level is given responsibility over policy implementation and day-to-day management, but is given no policymaking, legislative, or regulatory power over the same subject-matter (Yuan 1985: 169–91; Lee 1987: 138–40; 169–91; 1991). When it comes to medical care, moreover, each work unit plays the role of employer who must shoulder major funding responsibility, for example, partial reimbursement of medical bills and/or payment of insurance premium depending on the concrete situation.

So far, Dittmer and Lu have made their first conceptual and theoretical attempts to address the issue of the changing role of the work unit during economic reform (Dittmer & Lu 2000). To what extent has the role of the work unit been redefined and re-structured during the reform era? And how has it changed managerially and institutionally? What are key factors leading to these changes? Based on some rather solid empirical research, Naughton points to the paradoxically simultaneous tendencies of both expansion and shrinkage of the role of the work unit with special reference to social security entitlements during the reform era (Naughton 1997). Focusing on the divergent directions of the change at the work unit level, this study offers some preliminary discussion as follows. First, it is noteworthy that major impetus for restructuring the work unit, institutionally and managerially, stemmed from the bureau, provincial, and ministerial levels. Examples include the changing balance between the party committee and one-man management, several restructuring efforts of the revenue retention scheme, and policy changes affecting wage and non-wage compensation, among others.

Second, there has been an obvious expansion of "collective welfare," for instance, amenities and facilities, housing and dormitory, nurseries and kindergartens, primary and middle schools, and other amenities and facilities at the work unit level as noted by Naughton, coupled with the increase of enterprise-managed hospitals and clinics as mentioned previously (Lee 2019). This current study argues that most of the expansion is derived from the remuneration policy change at the macro level, allowing the enterprise unit to take advantage of retained revenue to increase funding of non-wage compensation, while adhering to strict wage control during rapid economic growth. In other words, this kind of work-unit collectivism mainly resulted from economic reform. For instance, large-sized public enterprises expanded enterprise-managed hospitals and medical care facilities relying upon retained revenue (and/or account of production costs) as just noted. In addition, the work unit continued to play a significant role in the expansion and improvement of housing and other amenities and facilities (Bian et al. 1997: 223–50; Naughton 1997).

Third, there has been a noted shift in relative weight from the work unit to outside public organizations in coordinating and organizing the provision of new categories of social security benefits and entitlements, coupled with the adoption of entirely new managerial mechanisms and institutional innovation. Upon the arrival of the first cohorts of retirees in the 1980s, for example, local governments had to intervene, as the enterprise level was not able to provide funding for retirement due to the limited scale of the financial pool for retirement programs at the work-unit level (Lee 2001). It is evident that neither local government nor work unit was able to cope with increased demand for funding to cover social security entitlements in a fragmentary and piecemeal fashion in the absence of an independent and institutional funding apparatus. Through a series of remedial measures, attempts were made to improve program specificity of the then existing PFMC and LIMC, for instance, in the listing and categorization of services, drugs, and devices, and in the introduction of spending control measures such as deductibles, co-payments, and payment-ceilings—still this did not address the fundamental issue of the alienation of entitlements from funding, which problem was not to be tackled until the introduction of BMCI in the public sector during the early 1990s–2000s.

The Corporatist Approach

The second approach, namely, the corporatist approach, highlights the allocation of resources in the arena of social security through the exercise of the mandatory power of the state. These resources are defined, mandated, and allocated through the legal form of rights, claims, benefits, and entitlements (e.g., social security), as they are bestowed on various individuals, groups, sectors, and strata in the public sector. From the corporatist perspective, the relationship between the party-state entity and society is conceptually characterized in two alternative formulations: Either through interest representation at the societal level or the unilateral exercise of mandatory power by the state.[4] In analyzing the Chinese CPE, it is appropriate to adopt the latter by treating the benefits and entitlements for various individuals and groups as categories of mandated interests from the corporatist perspective rather than to treat them as represented interests from a pluralistic-liberal point of view. In Walder's early study, it is suggested that the Chinese proletarian class, whose status is defined in terms of a bundle of rights and entitlements, created politically, legally, economically by the party-state entity amid of building CPE.[5] Conceptually speaking, corporatism cannot be reduced to liberal-pluralism. Interest representation is neither a necessary condition, nor a sufficient condition for the allocation of state-mandated interests in the context of corporatist politics in China where workers' rights, such as an eight-hour work-day, retirement pensions, housing, medical care, and industrial democracy in the workplace, etc., were granted unilaterally by the party-state under the CPE framework.[6]

How is the relationship of the party-state entity to society in the context of CPE characterized from the perspective of corporatism? This study highlights two principal roles of the state: Forging ideological narratives, and exercising mandatory power. In Stepan's formulation, first, the logic of command economy and the logic of corporatism share a common ideological root in terms of the formulation of "whole and parts" (Stepan 1978: 3–45). In ideological terms, the party-state entity acts on behalf of the interests of all the people, while sectors, groups, work units, and individuals represent and assert the interests of constituent parts.[7] Second, the party-state played a principal role in defining and forging its relationship with its constituent units and also the members within the constituent parts. As CPE rapidly industrialized China, for example, work units emerged as constituent units in a corporatist structure and as vehicles of mandated interests (Lee 1991). Consequently, in making social security policies, not only has the division of labor between government and work unit been explicitly stipulated in laws and regulations, it has also been reinforced by culture and convention evolving from the process of economic growth and forced modernization (Dangdai Zhongguo Bianjibu 1987: 191–388).

Thus, through the process of historical evolution, a community of shared interests took shape in two interlocking realms: The work unit and the party-state entity. Right after the promulgation of the "1951 Regulations" (as amended in 1953), Liu Shaoqi was among the first top leaders who promoted a brand of "work-unit collectivism" that was anchored in labor insurance programs. In Liu's view, the state was too abstract and remote to common members of the working class, and, as a component of the socialist state, the work unit was closer to and more tangible to workers and staff. Thus, the work unit was a better, more appropriate entity to embody the interests of the working class with regards to the benefits provided and services rendered. In a series of speaking engagements to public enterprises in the Beijing area in the late 1950s, Liu advocated that the enterprise unit ought to build a community of shared interests at the work-unit level where staff and workers were able to enjoy together dormitories, housing, canteens, and other public facilities in the name of "collective welfare" (Lee 1987: 55–6).

At the behavioral and perceptual level, one can identify the respective roles of the work unit and the party-state. According to Lu, the work unit is taken as the "minor public" and the party-state as the "greater public" in the Chinese context (Lu 1997: 29–32). Accordingly, in so far as claims, benefits, and entitlements are concerned, the party-state entity should be held responsible to employees in CPE, such as civil servants, staff and workers, and personnel of other public organizations. In the public sector, however, the work unit also acts on behalf of the party-state entity in policy implementation, management, and funding for the programs of benefits and entitlements at the micro level. While the government normally shoulders financial responsibility for these programs for civil servants and public personnel in other public organizations, which are funded by tax revenue, public enterprises manage and finance similar programs for staff and workers by charging the costs to the accounts concerned (i.e., as items of production costs and/or retained revenue depending on the time period).

During the reform era, there existed a salient trend that the role of social security moved from work units to public organizations. For example, the local government undertook greater responsibility coping with the disintegration of the programs for benefits, welfare, and social security in the industrial sector during financial shortages at the work-unit level. Prior to the reform of public funding of health care from the late 1970s onward, as another example, local governments experimented with the building of risk-pooling mechanisms in order to absorb financial risks through "social unified funding" (*shehui tongchou*) in response to a weakened financial capacity at the enterprise level due to a variety of factors (Lee 2001; Guo 2003; Duckett 2004).

Focusing on perceptual data, as early as 1993, Lee and Wong conducted two comparable sets of surveys with approximately one thousand respondents each in Guangzhou and Shanghai respectively on the eve of launching the BMCI reform. Their findings appear in full congruence with Lu's conceptualization of "minor public" and "greater public" as just noted. They tried to find out how urban residents felt about where the responsibility for social security should rest—for example, the individual resident, work unit, or party-state—as issues surrounding benefits, welfare, and social insurance were emerging as serious concerns during the era of social security reform. In the said two surveys, respondents expressed overwhelmingly that the work unit ought to subsidize the payment for their medical bills, that is, 74.4 percent in Guangzhou and 81.9 percent in Shanghai (including "agree" and "strongly agree"). By the same token, a large majority of urban residents felt that, in addition to one's own obligation, the party-state entity should be held responsible for medical expenses for each person, that is, 70.1 percent in Guangzhou and 74.2 percent in Shanghai. A similar attitude about the responsibility of the party-state and work unit was held with reference to financing other social security programs such as pension retirement and housing (Lee & Wong 2001).

As far as the relationship of "work-unit collectivism" to corporatism is concerned, Lee observes that the work unit is a constituent unit of the party-state, so the former is institutionally embedded in the latter from a corporatist perspective (Lee 1991). By the same token, Bian's study observes that the work unit does *not* operate independently to make its own policies about employment, wages, benefits, and welfare; rather, the work unit always acts as an integral part of the party-state, if not subordinate unit, and the party-state is a very powerful element in shaping life chances for each worker (Bian 1994).

To examine social security policy in China, so-called "work-unit collectivism" was only part of the story. The study argues that social security can better be characterized as duality in institutional and managerial sense. On the one hand, the state intervened in establishing entitlements and benefits, determined the budgetary and accounting procedures, and controlled the percentage of revenue for it at the work unit level. On the other hand, the work unit oversaw day-to-day management of social security. In its early origin under the CPE prior to economic reform, the state and work unit jointly shouldered policy and managerial responsibility for each category of social security and welfare, for example, pensions, health care, "collective welfare," etc.

As the work unit is theoretically taken as a component of the party-state hierarchy, it is appropriate to treat its relationship to other departments/echelons of the government as the relationship between the two parts within a larger institutional whole, for instance, regarding the issue of restructuring at the institutional level and at the functional/ managerial level. From a broad analytical perspective, the study is concerned with the transfer of managerial and financial responsibility from the work unit to the local government. To put it in another way, the introduction of public medical care insurance involved the transformation from a public funding mode of social security (including medical care) affiliated with the work unit in the context of a centrally planned economy (CPE) to an entirely new funding system operating at the level of local jurisdiction in a mixed economy for a time span about three decades from the late 1980s to the present (Huang 2020; Lee 2019; Qian 2021).

The Remuneration Policy Approach

From political-economics analysis, the remuneration policy approach tries to examine the social security reform considering legacy and vested interests associated with the wage policy of the CPE period. And it is theoretically focused on the "monopolized production" that characterizes the high accumulation rate through franchise, low wage policy in the public sectors (including staff and workers in public enterprises and public personnel in the government and other public organizations), and disparities between the industrial and agricultural sectors produced by the "scissors effects" (Lee 1987; Naughton 1996). It mainly covers the two sectors of the CPE: The planned sector (embracing staff and workers of public enterprises, public personnel in and members of other public organizations in the case of BMCI), and the non-planned sector mainly including the unemployed in URMCI and peasants in NRCMCI.

Here the remuneration approach tries to focus on the issue of vested interests from the interpretative framework of reference among policy actors and to account for it in terms of "historical debts." It is well taken that the social security reform not only has produced disparities among different programs, but also has raised the issue of distributive justice in China. And vested interests (including various forms of privileges) are often the intended policy outcome. For example, Premier Zhu Rongji, in his talk about the forthcoming medical care security reform on October 27, 1997, took an explicit stand to explain why government officials and party cadres should be offered better terms than the staff and workers in public enterprises, albeit the two groups followed the common standards and types of services in social security. He also added that veterans and cadres of revolutionary war periods deserved even more consideration in view of "historical compensation." As Zhu added, above all, the public finance ought to cover all these privileged provisions as mentioned (Zhu 2002b: 271). By the same token, Xian Huang tried to address the issue of vested interests in terms of "stratified expansion of social welfare provision" (Huang 2020). Given the relevance of social security policy to the maintenance of political loyalty of some selected groups and even the general population, it is pertinent to address how vested interests enter the exercise of program specificity, for example, packaging and product/service specificity, funding and spending, the scale risk-pooling, among others.

The remuneration approach addresses both alienation of entitlements from funding and historically rooted obligations (so-called "historical debts") in conjunction with the social security (including health care) reforms. The two concepts remain analytically distinguishable, but they are often intertwined with each other in reality. The former pertains to the kinds of entitlements that have already been enacted by the government and stipulated explicitly in the laws and regulations of the party-state. The latter is concerned with how, in policy terms, to compensate the deserving but underpaid personnel prior to economic reform, some of whom were devoted to the revolutionary seizure of state power, and others worked under forced modernization through the CPE developmental strategy. In one way or another, however, neither institutional apparatus nor managerial and financial instruments were installed to build, maintain, and manage a reservoir of risk pooling and ensure payments for the entitlements in the arena of social security prior to economic reform.

In the interpretive frame of reference of policy actors, the notion of historically rooted obligations (often taken as "historical debts" *lishi qianzai*) has several shades of meaning and has yet to be clearly defined in operational terms. Conceptually speaking, its main portion refers to undefined categories of benefits and entitlements to the early generations of the workforce who were employed, but inadequately compensated under the low wage policy during the period of forced modernization preceding economic reform. This main portion falls into the arena of non-wage compensation, some of which needs to be paid to the senior members of the workforce of the CPE era, representing a manifestation of corporatism. The other smaller portion, pertains to the idea of reciprocal relationship regarding veterans and cadres who took part in the war efforts in seizing the state power. And some scholars take it as "neo-traditionalism," which is often crystalized legally and institutionally into privileges and entitlements granted to a special group of people who made sacrifices and extraordinary contributions to building the Leninist party-state during the revolutionary seizure of power in the case of the former Soviet Union and China (Jowitt 1983; Walder 1986a). In the Chinese context, examples include programs like "leave for recuperation" (*lixiu*) and privileged retirements for senior cadres and veterans, coupled with privileged medical care (Melanie 1993: 45–76).

With reference to the idea of historically rooted obligations involving social security, for example, Former Vice-Premier Wu Bangguo made an observation about the mutual relationship among the state, public enterprises, and staff and workers in a speech about social security and the resettlement of redundant employees at the enterprise level given in September, 1995, he pointed to the fact that, conceptually speaking, in such a mutual relationship, the state, public enterprises, staff, and workers share a common revenue pool with regard to social security. According to Wu, the government needed to address the matter of "historical debts," for example, retirement and other social security benefits such as medical care, housing, etc., about employees of public enterprises during social security reform. He underscored that credit had to be given to all enterprises, together with staff and workers, for they had made financial contributions to the growing wealth of the state under the low wage policy. Moreover, Wu stated that and at a time when funding for social security had been diverted in some cases, presumably for investments and economic growth. Additionally, the alienation of entitlement from funding took place concurrently in that payment for benefits and entitlements had been withheld, and no funding was institutionally set aside for them (Wu 2002: 183).

In attempts to diagnose the causes of alienation of entitlement from funding, often manifested in terms of a funding shortage for social security programs, on the eve of formally inaugurating the BMCI policy in the late 1990s, Li Tieying, the State Councilor and Director of the State Institutional Reform Commission, explained that the early generations of staff and workers created wealth but received low wages under the CPE framework while most of the social security funds were converted into capital for economic construction, and eventually crystallized into state assets (Li 1999: 16–7). Moreover, former Premier Zhu Rongji argued that since the enormous amount of assets that the government withheld came originally from the people, it was fair to return such assets to the people, considering the option of converting part of the state assets into social security funds through the release of shares in SOEs to the stock markets (Zhu 2002a: 451).

Policy analyst Wang reiterated the view that the large holding of state assets stemmed from the "high accumulation rate" under the CPE framework that mandated not only the low wage policy for workforce in industry, but also meager income and other sacrifices for peasants. Wang argued further that from the beginning of the People's Republic to 1978, the average annual rate of wage increase stood at 0.38 percent while the average annual rate of capital accumulation climbed from 21.4 percent in the 1950s up to 43.8 percent in later periods (Wang 2003: 336–7).

Focusing on the non-planned sector, furthermore, some authors and policy analysts argued that, because of "the compensation gaps" affecting the peasantry created under the CPE developmental strategy, peasants should not be left behind in terms of an entitlement to a fair share of benefits and social security. Such a view prompted the introduction of new rural cooperative medical care insurance (NRCMCI) programs for the peasantry starting in 2003 (Chapters 10 and 11). Wang added, moreover, that in fact peasants also made contributions and sacrifices for a large portion of the high accumulation rate of capital. It was therefore fair, as Wang argued, to compensate for the "hidden debts" (meaning historical debts) of retirement pension and other welfare expenditures to the peasantry while doing the same for staff and workers. He also suggested that not only should the party-state compensate the peasantry in equal terms, but also it should not treat peasants as second-class citizens of the People's Republic. In addition, Wang advocated for several alternatives to compensate peasants, for example, including proposals for bond measures, funding through taxation and public revenue, sale of public assets, etc. According to Wang, the worst scenario involved "a reverse subsidy," namely, an unfair fiscal policy favoring urban residents at the expense of the rural population. Also, he considered it "unreasonable" to introduce retirement insurance to the urban population without giving the peasantry the same sorts of subsidy that the urban dwellers currently enjoyed (Wang 2003: 338–9).

Nominally early cohorts of staff and workers were entitled to social security entitlements, but the social security accounts remained empty when it was time for them to make claims to such entitlements, for example, during old age and retirement and when they had to pay for their medical bills. In Li's view, it was warranted for the state entity to act on behalf of society and honor [historically rooted] obligations for social security benefits to the early generations of staff and workers, and one way to accomplish that was to build up a portion of the fund either from state assets or from public land (Li 1999: 16–7). Upon the introducing phase of the BMCI package starting 2001, Premier Zhu offered an elaborate explanation on why the state did not maintain savings for social security when it first launched the ambitious CPE developmental strategy in its early years. He admitted that the government "made use of the funds that stemmed from the measure of low wages and all of the profit-remittance from the enterprises for the expansion of capital investment in construction and, therefore, there was no saving for social security" (Zhu 2002a: 442).

Further to the same theme of "historical debts," policy analysts made elaboration on how the alienation of entitlement from funding took place. According to Zheng, for instance, so-called the "deficit in social security" (or taken alternatively as "debts in welfare") referred to a large sum of public funds that were intended for benefits, welfare, and social security, but withheld by the government and used for other purposes instead. He argued that the root of the problems surrounding benefits and social security was attributable to the exploitation of surplus value provided by staff and workers and its conversion into state assets from 1949 to the late 1980s. In Zheng's view, the "deficit of social security" was often manifested in the following ways: A shortage of funding for retirement pension, a deficit in the "welfare" of the old system (e.g., medical care, housing, amenities, facilities, and other "collective welfare"), a lack of disaster relief and subsidies to the needy, and a shortage of operational funding for the new social security system (Zheng 1998: 57–60). Echoing Zheng, Wang added that the high rate of accumulation included a portion of saved retirement funds, coupled with funds for other social security entitlements for staff and workers, and that the accumulation was turned into state assets controlled by the government (Wang 2003: 336–7). Under the circumstances, how did the government come to honor social security entitlements through the making of new programs of public medical care insurance? This study will try to answer this question in the remaining chapters.

Concluding Remarks

In the foregoing analysis, this study has examined the cultural, relational, and political dimensions of social security policy in general and healthcare policy in the wake of the economic reform. This study has reviewed the legacy of social security policies and vested interests built in echelons of government and various sectors of society during forced modernization under the CPE developmental strategy prior to economic reform era. Moreover, this study has discussed three main approaches articulated by scholars, policy analysts, and practitioners to deal with public policies, including basic medical care. Each approach represents an interpretative frame of reference, but they jointly shed light on how politics enters the designing, packaging, and implementation of health care reforms in China. It appears that policymaking is largely dictated by politics often manifested in ideological forms (e.g., controversy concerning "historical debts"). How was politics fused with policy in the actual process of policymaking? To what extent did the philosophy behind policy issues weigh in during the formation of new policies and program designs? To address the above questions, this study needs to examine how the merits and demerits of a policy enter policymaking, coupled with managerial and institutional issues of new medical care insurance packages during economic reform.

Notes

1 For the operational definition as well as the programs of social security in China during the economic reform, one may find a textbook version of discussion in the following volume (Dangdai Zhongguo caizheng bianjibu 1988: 204–37).

2 For example, some early pieces of serious research highlight the role of work units in determining the life chances of members of an organization located at the lowest reach of the party-state hierarchy in the public sector (Whyte 1974; Whyte & Parish 1984). Moreover, there are other pieces of relatively extensive survey research dealing with life chances pertaining to employment, wages, benefits, and industrial relations at the work unit level in China (Whyte & Parish 1984; Bian 1994; Tang & Parish 2000). Walder contributed a brilliant piece of work characterizing "work-unit collectivism" in terms of the "organized dependence" of organizational members of the work unit for satisfying all-round needs (Walder 1986a). Since the 1980s, a group of prominent authors have followed the work-unit-centered approach, trying to analyze various aspects of wage, welfare, subsidies, and social security (Walder 1986b, 1987, 1989; Huang 1990). Not long ago, Malcom took the lead to organize research on industrial relations, human resource management, and business management in the "work place," conceptually the equivalent of "work unit" (Warner 2000). Focusing on the origin and evolution, some analysts suggest that work-unit collectivism owes its origin to the legacy of the supply system of the Yan'an period (Lu 1997).

3 One may define "workplace" using two criteria: First, as the sphere where task performance is organized and coordinated by taking into consideration the convenience of the locality; and second, as the locale where face-to-face interpersonal relations emerge

as a key ingredient of coordination. Examples include a work section (*gongduan*) or workshop (*chejian*) in an enterprise, or wards (*bingfang*) or an emergency room (*jizhenshi*) in a hospital. To illustrate, one workshop at Beijing No. 1 Lathe Factory includes 18 work sections where its total number of staff and workers is 1,334. The number of personnel in a major work section ranges from 85 to 251, a size considered to be larger than the ideal for forming face-to-face relations because of the increasing difficulty for members to get to know one another. The smaller work sections include about 50 or fewer (Beijing diyi jichuangchang diaocha 1980: 111–24).

4   In defining "corporatism," there are two schools of thought: One tends to treat "interest representation" as a necessary condition for the phenomenon of corporatist politics, while the other suggests that the state-mandating act is both a necessary and sufficient condition. Schmitter has been one of the pioneering authors who advocates the former (Schmitter 1974). In China studies too, some authors are inclined to the former position, characterizing the key relationship between the state and society in terms of interest representation (Chan 1993; Unger 1995). The former often encounters an unsolved operational issue in drawing a demarcation between "interest representation" of the liberal-pluralistic tradition on the one hand and the state-mandating process of interests, as well as the creation of an organization for mandated interests, on the other hand. The latter position tries to build the linkage of the state to its constituent units not only through ideological ties, but also through the exercise of mandatory power in granting legal rights, benefits and entitlements as well as by being the official channel of communication and relationship (Stepan 1978; Chalmers 1991; Wiarda 1997). Lee makes one of the earliest theoretical attempts to apply the latter to highlight the relationship between the government and enterprise units in China (Lee 1991).

5   In Walder's view, all aspects of working-class existence, including employment and wage, job security and social security, as well as other benefits and perhaps industrial democracy, are creations of the power of the Chinese Communist party-state (Walder 1984).

6   There are institutions of representation (e.g., ACFTU, CRSW) in China similar to their counterparts in Western democratic countries, but they do not play the same roles of representation (e.g., participation in electoral politics and legislative politics). Empirical studies of China confirm that the state can fulfill its corporatist purposes, for example, by assuming rights to settle labor disputes, to redress grievances, etc. unilaterally by the state, without taking advantage of institutions of representation such as ACFTU and CRSW (Chen 2004: 27–45).

7   For instance, Lenin applies the metaphor of "the whole country as a factory and the work unit as a workshop" to characterize the relationship between the state and an enterprise unit in a CPE framework. By the same token, the sovereign planners used to apply the metaphor of "the whole country as a chessboard" to the Chinese case from an economic-managerial perspective as much as an ideological-political point of view (Lee 1991).

References

Beijing diyi jichuangchang diaocha 1980. *Beijing diyi jichuangchang diaocha (The Investigation on Beijing No. 1 Lathe Factory)*. Beijing: Zhongguo shehui kexue chubanshe.

Bendix, R. 1962. *Max Weber, An Intellectual Portrait*. New York: Anchor Books.

Bian, Y., Logan, J. R., Lu, H., Pan, Y. & Guan, Y. 1997. Work units and housing reform in two Chinese cities. In Lu, X. & Perry E. J. (Eds.), *Danwei, the Changing Chinese Workplace in Historical and Comparative Perspective*. New York: M. E. Shape. 223–50.

Bian, Y. J. 1994. *Work and Inequality in Urban China*. Albany: State University of New York.

Chalmers, D. 1991. Corporatism and comparative politics. In Wiarda, H. J. (Ed.), *New Directions in Comparative Politics*. Boulder, CO: Westview. 56–81.

Chan, A. 1993. Revolution or corporatism? Workers and trade unions in post-Mao China. *The Australian Journal of Chinese Affairs* 29: 31–61.

Chan, A. 1997. Chinese danwei reforms: convergence with the Japanese model. In Lu, X. & Perry, E. J. (Eds.), *Danwei, the Changing Chinese Workplace in Historical and Comparative Perspective.* New York: M. E. Shape. 91–140.

Chan, A. 2000. Chinese trade unions and workplace relations in the state-owned and joint venture enterprises. In Waner, M. (Ed.), *Changing Workplace Relations in the Chinese Economy.* Houndmills & London: MaCmillan Press Ltd; New York: St. Martin's Press, LLC. 34–56.

Chen, F. 2004. Legal mobilization by trade unions: the cases of Shanghai. *China Quarterly* 52: 27–45.

Cheng, X. Problem of urbanization under China's traditional economic system. In Kwok, R. N. (Ed.), *What Urban Reform, What Model Now?* Amonk & London: M. E. Sharpe. 3–15.

Dangdai Zhongguo caizheng bianjibu 1988. *Dangdai Zhongguo caizheng, Xia (Financial Policy in Contemporary China, Vol. 2).* Beijing: Zhongguo shehui kexue chubanshe.

Dangdai Zhongguo congshu bianjibu 1986. *Dangdai Zhongguo de weisheng shiye, xia (The Health Care Enterprises in Contemporary China, Volume ll).* Beijing: Zhongguo shehui kexue chubanshe.

Dangdai Zhongguo congshu bianjibu 1997. *Dangdai zhongguo gongren jieji he gonghui yundong, xia (The Working Class and Labor Union Movements in Contemporary China Vol. II).* Beijing: Dangdai Zhongguo Chubanshe.

Dittmer, L. & Lu, X. 2000. Organizational involution and socialpolitical reform in China: an analysis of the work unit. In Dittmer, L., Fukui, H. & Lee, P. N. (Eds.), *Informal Politics in East Asia.* Cambridge: Cambridge University Press 185–214.

Duckett, J. 2004. State, collectivism, and worker privilege: a study of urban health insurance in China. *China Quarterly* 177: 155–73.

Duckett, J. 2011. *The Chinese State's Retreat from Health, Policy and the Politics of Retrenchment.* London & New York: Routledge.

Guo, B. 2003. Transforming China's urban health-care system. *Asian Survey* 43.2: 385–403.

Gu, X., Gao, M., & Yao, Y. 2006. *Zhengduan yu chufang, zhimian Zhongguo yiliao tizhi gaige (Diagnosis and Prescription, Confronting China's Medical Care Reform).* Beijing: Shehui kexue wenxian chubanshe.

Huang, X. 2020. *Social Protection under Authoritarianism.* New York: Oxford University Press.

Huang, Y. 1990. Web of interests and pattern of behaviour of Chinese local bureaucracies and enterprises during reforms. *China Quarterly* 123: 431–58.

Huang, Y. 2013. *Governing Health in Contemporary China.* London & New York: Routledge.

Hughes, O. E. 1998. *Public Management & Administration (2nd ed.).* Houndmills: Palgrave.

Jowitt, K. 1983. Soviet neotraditionalism: the political corruption of a Leninist regime. *Soviet Studies* XXXV. 3.

Kallgren, J. K. 1969. Social welfare and China's industrial workers. In Doak, B. A. (Eds.), *Chinese Communist Politics in Action.* Seattle, WA and London: The University of Washington Press. 540–73.

Lee, P. N. 1987. *Industrial Management and Economic Reform in China. 1949–1984.* Hong Kong, Oxford and New York: Oxford University Press.

Lee, P. N. 1991. The Chinese industrial state in historical perspective: from totalitarianism to corporatism. In Womack, B. (Eds.), *Contemporary Chinese Politics in Historical Perspective.* fixedNew York: Cambridge University Press. 153–79.

Lee, P. N. 2001. The provision of occupational benefits in the Chinese industrial sector: the case of Guangzhou. In Lee, P. N. & Lo, C. W. (Eds.), *Remaking China's Public Management.* Westport, CT & London: Quorum Books. 115–32.

Lee, P. N. 2020. *Re-engineering Affordable Care Policy in China, Is Marketization a Solution?* London & New York: Routledge.

Lee, P. N. & Wong, C. 2001. The tale of two cities: rolling back the boundary of the welfare state during the reform era. In Lee, P. N. & Lo, C. W. (Eds.), *Remaking China's Public Management.* Westport, CT & London: Quorum Books. 67–95.

Li, T. 1999. Jianli juyou zhongguo tese de shehui baozhang zhidu (To establish the social security system with the Chinese characteristics). In Xu, D., Yin, Z. & Zheng, Y. (Eds.), *Zhongguo shehui baozhang tizhi gaige (The Reform of Social Security System in China).* Beijing: Jingji kexue chubanshe.

Lu, F. 1996. Zhonguo danwei tizhi de qiyuan yu xingcheng (The origin and formation of work unit system in China) (originally published on *China's Social Science Quarterly* Zhongguo shehui kexue jikan). In Li, D. (Ed.), *Zhongguo xiandai qiye zhidu zhilu* (The road to modern enterprise system in China). Beijing: Guoji Wenhua Chubanshe Gongsi. 439–57.

Lu, X. & Perry, E. (Eds.) 1997, *Danwei, The Changing Chinese Workplace in Historical and Comparative Perspective.* Armonk, NY: M. E. Sharpe

Lu, X. 1997. Minor public economy: the revolutionary origins of the danwei. In Lu, X. & Perry, E. (Eds.), *Danwei, The Changing Chinese Workplace in Historical and Comparative Perspective.* Armonk, NY: M. E. Sharpe. 21–41.

Melanie, M. 1993. *Retirement of Revolutionaries in China: Public Policies, Social Norms, Private Interests.* Princeton, NJ: Princeton University Press.

Naughton, B. 1996. *Growing out of Plan.* Cambridge: Cambridge University Press.

Naughton, B. 1997. Danwei: the economic foundations of a unique institution. In Lu, X. & Perry, E. (Eds.), *Danwei, The Changing Chinese Workplace in Historical and Comparative Perspective.* Armonk, NY: M.E. Sharpe. 169–94

Parsons, T. 1947. *Max Weber: The Theory of Social and Economic Organization.* New York: The Free Press; London: Collier-Macmillan Ltd.

Peng, R., Cai, R. & Zhou, C. (Eds.) 1992. *Zhongguo gaige congshu* (The Encyclopedia of China's Reform). Dalian: Dalian chubanshe.

Qian, J. 2021. *The Political Economy of Making and Implementing Policy in China.* Singapore: Palgrave Macmillan.

Schmitter, P. C. 1974. Still the century of corporatism? *The Review of Politics* 36: 85–131.

Sil, R. 1997. The Russian "village in the city" and the Stalinist system of enterprise management: the origins of worker alienation in Soviet state socialism. In Lu, X. & Perry E. J (Eds.), *Danwei, the Changing Chinese Workplace in Historical and Comparative Perspective.* New York: M. E. Shape. 114–41

Stepan, A. 1978. *The State and Society, Peru in Comparative Perspective.* Princeton, NJ: The Princeton University Press.

Straus, K. M. 1997. The Soviet factory as community organizer. In Lu, X. & Perry E. J (Eds.), *Danwei, the Changing Chinese Workplace in Historical and Comparative Perspective.* New York: M. E. Shape. 142–68.

Takahara, A. 1992. *The Politics of Wage Policy in Post-Revolutionary China.* Houndmills & London: Macmillan Press Ltd.

Tang, W. F. & Parish, W. 2000. *Chinese Urban Life under Reform, The Change of Social Contract.* Cambridge, New York & Melbourne: Cambridge University Press.

Unger, J. 1995. China, corporatism, and the east Asian model. *The Australian Journal of Chinese Affairs* 33: 29–53.

Walder, A. G. 1984. The remaking of the Chinese working class, 1949–1981. *Modern China* 10.1. 3–42.

Walder, A. G. 1986a. *Communist Neo-traditionalism: Work and Authority in a Chinese Factory.* Berkeley: The University of California Press.

Walder, A. G. 1986b. The informal dimension of enterprise financial reform. In the Joint Economic Committee, *China's Economy Looks Toward the Year 2000, Vol. II. The Four Modernizations.* Washington, DC: The US Government Printing Office. 630–45.

Walder, A. G. 1987. Wage reform and the web of factory interests. *China Quarterly* 109: 22–41.

Walder, A. G. 1989. Factory and manager in an era of reform. *China Quarterly* 118: 242–64.

Wang, X. 2003. *Fenpei Zhengyi yu shehui baozhang (Distributive Justice and Social Security).* Shanghai: Shanghai Caijing Daxue Chubanshe.

Warner, M. 2000. *Changing Workplace Relations in the Chinese Economy.* Houndmills & London: MaCmillan Press Ltd; New York: St. Martin's Press, LLC.

Wiarda, H. J.(Ed.) 1997. *New Directions in Comparative Politics,* Boulder: Westview.

Whyte, M. K. 1974. *Small Groups and Political Rituals in China.* Berkeley: University of California Press.

Whyte, M. K. & Parish, W. L. 1984. *Unban Life in Contemporary China.* Chicago, IL: University of Chicago Press.

Wu, B. 2002. Zai kunnan qiye zhigong shengho baozhang he fenliu anze gongzuo zuotanhui shang de jianghua (Speech at the work conference of assurance of livelihood of staff and workers and streams of job reassignments in difficult enterprises). In Laodong he shehui baozhangbu (Eds.), Xinshiqi laodong shehui baozhang zhongyao wenxian xuanbian (*The Collection of Important Selected Documents on Social Security during the New Era*). Zhongguo laodong baozhang chubanshe & zhongyan wenxian chubanshe. 178–90.

Yang, M. M. 1989. Between state and society: the construction of corporateness in a Chinese socialist factory. *Australian Journal of Chinese Affairs* 22: 31–60.

Yang, X. 1999. *Zhongguo danwei zhi du (The Danwei System in China).* Beijing: Zhongguo jingji chubanshe.

Yuan, B. 1985. Zai quanguo changzhang fuzezhi shidian gongzuo zuotanhui shang de jianghua (Talk at the meeting on pilot program on the national factory directory responsibility system). Guoying gongye qiyefa diaochazu (ed.) *Changzhang fuzezhi cankao ziliao (Reference Material for the Factory Directory Responsibility System).* Zhenjiang: Zhongguo jingji chubanshe. 112–31.

Zheng, G. 1998. Zhongguo shehui baozhang gaige de hongguan sikao (A macro consideration on the social security reform in China). In Yu, G. & Song, X. (Eds.), *Wei shichang jingji de lieche pugui (To build Rail for the Train of Market Economy).* Beijing: Xueyuan Chubanshe. 85–92.

Zheng, G. 2009. *Cong qiye baoxian dao shehui baoxian: Zhongguo shehui baoxian zhidu bianqian yu fazhan (The Change and Development of the Social Security System in China).* Beijing: Zhongguo laodong shehui baoxian chubanshe.

Zheng, G. 2011. *Zhongguo shehui baozhang gaige yu fazhan zhanlue, yiliao baozhang pian (The Reform and Developmental Strategy of Social Security, the Volume on Medical Care Security).* Beijing: Renmin chubanshe.

Zhu, R. 2002a. Jiakuai wanshan shehui baozhang tixi, queshi quojia changzhi jiuan (Accelerate the building of a perfect social security system, ensure stability and peace in the nation). In Laodong he shehui baozhangbu (Eds.), *Xinshiqi laodong shehui baozhang zhongyao wenxian xuanbian (The Collection of Important Selected Documents on Social Security during the New Era).* Zhongguo laodong baozhang chubanshe & Zhongyan wenxian chubanshe. 438–54

Zhu, R. 2002b. Guanyu zhigong yiliao baozhang zhidu gaige wenti (The issue regarding the reform of medical care security system of staff and workers). In Laodong he shehui baozhangbu (Eds.), *Xinshiqi laodong shehui baozhang zhongyao wenxian xuanbian* (*The Collection of Important Selected Documents on Social Security during the New Era*). Zhongguo Laodong baozhang chubanshe & zhongyan wenxian chubanshe.

Zhuang, Q. 1984. *Laodong gongzi shouce* (*Manual of Labor and Wages*). Tianjin: Tianjin remin chubanshe.

4 Early Origins and Policy Precedents

In building the centrally planned economy (CPE) during the 1950s, two public funding programs of medical care were first made available to all personnel employed in the planned sector of the economy, namely, Labor Insurance Medical Care (LIMC) and Public Financed Medical Care (PFMC) (Dangdai Zhongguo congshu bianjibu 1988: 232–7). In one of the most ambitious and innovative efforts in public policy, sovereign planners made use of the basic medical care insurance (BMCI) to replace the said two conventional funding programs as an integral part of health care reform that began as early as the late 1980s (Song & Gao 2001: 2–40; Zheng 2011: 102–3).

The restructuring of the said two programs of medical care was intended to be part of a large health care reform and to be further consolidated under a comprehensive social security system, broadly including retirement benefits, medical care benefits, unemployment pensions, and social relief (He 2005: 3–26; Qian 2021). In what is taken as path dependency, the study will examine PFMC and LIMC to address two issues. First, to what extent the designs of the two conventional public funding programs have bearing on that of the basic medical care insurance (BMCI) programs introduced during the 1990s and 2000s? Second, how did the entrenched interests that were invested in the said two programs affect the shaping and implementation of the BMCI?

In this chapter, the study will first discuss the early origins and subsequent evolution of the said two conventional programs of medical care from the 1950s to the late 1970s, providing highlights on the main features of each program (Yang 2004: 105–33). Then the discussion will then dwell on the policy outcomes and key issues of two programs as well as remedial responses that paved the way later to designing, packaging, and implementing BMCI.

Inaugurating the PFMC Program

The PFMC program evolved incrementally and built upon preceding social security policies and programs that had been adopted in the base areas where medical care and preventive care services were provided to public personnel working in government and service units prior to the establishment of the PRC (Yang 2004: 105–33). It is fair to suggest, overall, that the Yenan Way, albeit with root in a

DOI: 10.4324/9781003389934-5

revolutionary war, cast a long shadow on the development of the PFMC packages (Dangdai Zhongguo congshu bianjibu 1987: 301–4; Zheng 2002: 120–3). Beyond the "supply system", social security packages incorporated certain "privileges," that is, compensation for extraordinary contributions under extraordinary circumstances, including a privileged retirement system called "leave for recuperation" (taken as *liuxiu* in Chinese) during the early years of the PRC (Dangdai Zhongguo congshu bianjibu 1987: 324–7).

The scope of the PFMC program then covered essential (or basic) medical care services, adopting a simple reimbursement procedure to cover expenditures for various medical care services, including both hospital care for inpatients and clinical visits for outpatients, coupled with diagnosis, examinations, prescription drugs, treatments, and operations. It also covered work injuries, work disability, and planned childbirth, in addition to food services for inpatients and transportation costs for cases of referral, clinical visits, and hospital care. As the earliest precedent of user charges, patients had to pay for such items as registration fees, as well as non-essential items, such as health supplements, cosmetic and corrective surgery (Dangdai Zhongguo Congshu Bianjibu 1987: 301–4).

To enrol in PFMC, individual membership was adopted, while family membership was not entertained in the program design. As a result, the government needed to work out the issue of the entitlement of spouses, children and dependents in the case of PFMC because they were excluded for lack of employment status in the government and other public organizations. Accordingly in September 1952 the Ministry of Finance, Ministry of Health, and Personnel Bureau jointly announced the ruling to authorize funding to cover the medical care entitlements of spouses and children of public personnel. Furthermore, in another policy paper promulgated in September 1955, children and dependents of public personnel who enjoyed the PFMC were given two options: Either in a "unified funding" scheme (a form of risk pooling limited to the work unit) or a co-payment option coupled with financial assistance through the welfare fund of the work unit (Dangdai Zhongguo congshu bianjibu 1987: 311–2).

As a long-term trend starting from 1953, there came about decentralization from the Ministry of Finance (MOF) to the provincial and local governments about financial appropriation for medical and preventive care to public personnel affiliated with respective central government units and provincial and local jurisdictions (Zheng 2002: 120–1). In a financial term, all categories of medical and healthcare entitlements and benefits for public personnel in PFMC were funded by public revenue appropriated through state budgetary procedures, and government units and other fully budgeted units at various levels provided funding for medical and preventive care services to public personnel. While public personnel of the government and party at the ministerial level and provincial level enjoyed the privileges of full reimbursement, the other personnel of service work units such as education and research institutes, welfare and medical care only enjoyed partial reimbursement of medical bills as previously noted (Zheng 2011). It is noteworthy in view of limited and insufficient exercise of program specificity that neither funding was independently established, nor budgetary systems were separately built for the handling of such entitlements in case of PFMC.

Characteristic of the ORF system within the hierarchy mode of governance, the budgetary and accounting connectivity between funding and spending was relatively weak as being inherent in the financial management pertaining to PFMC (Chapter 2). And the spending control measures were often lacking. Moreover, spending pressure aggravated in PFMC amid an expanding scope of coverage, an increase in membership, the improvement of living standards, wage reforms, and a changing economic environment over years.

By the early 1960s, it became evident that the expenditure of the PFMC program always exceeded budgetary limits by large margins.[1] To cope with the uncontrollable increase of expenditure, accordingly, a measure for co-payments was first introduced in 1965, on the eve of the Cultural Revolution (Zheng 2002: 121–2). The phenomenon of growing expenditure in medical care services persisted in the post-Mao era.[2] During the early phase of economic reform, it was found that no policy and measure of effective spending control was in place, resulting in considerable irregularities and abuses, together with inadequate supervision, lax financial discipline, and an unauthorized expansion of the scope of benefits and entitlements and of the perimeters of reimbursement (Dangdai Zhongguo congshu bianjibu 1988: 232–5; Zheng 2002: 121–9). And this paved the way for first attempts of reform during economic reform.

The Beginning of the LIMC Program

Parallel to the PFMC program, the LIMC program was an integral part of the social security platform advocated by the Chinese Communist Party (CCP), reflecting the labor movements as well as ideological commitment associated with the early phase of the Chinese Communist movement back in the 1920s and 1930s (Dangdai Zhongguo congshu bianjibu 1988: 288–301). It was first introduced into the Northeast provinces and, subsequently, North China as the CCP further consolidated its territorial gains during the Civil War period, 1945 to 1949 (Kallgren 1969: 540–73; Lee 1987: 32–8). It was then extended throughout China from the early 1950s to the late 1950s.

Focusing on its historical origin, one may consider the "labor insurance" (or social security to be precise) package as a product of "societal corporatism" in the sense that it was created partly by impetus from below, while the PFMC can be taken as an example of "state corporatism" to the extent that it was built mainly through the initiatives of the party-state. Operating with egalitarianism and coordinated through the central command under the party-state, the LIMC and PFMC programs were comparable in terms of benefits and entitlements that were made available to the enrollees who were employed in the public sector prior to the reform (Dangdai Zhongguo congshu bianjibu 1987: 302–10).

As sovereign planners inaugurated the social security packages for staff and workers in the early 1950s, relatively comprehensive coverage of entitlements and benefits to staff and workers (including childbirth and maternal benefits, medical care, sick leave, work injury benefits, benefits for the disabled and invalids, death benefits, retirement payments, etc.) were incorporated into the Regulations of Labor Insurance (hereafter, the 1951 Regulations; amended in 1953) as promulgated on February 26, 1951 (Dangdai Zhongguo congshu bianjibu 1987: 302–7). The title of "social insurance" is ill-defined, referring to social security in general, while only a part of it (e.g., retirement pension) relies upon risk pooling mechanisms at the inter-enterprise level coordinated by the All-China's Federation of Labor Unions. The 1951 Regulations laid the foundation for the social security system in China for many decades to come and even continued into the reform era, as illustrated by Professor Bian Yanjie in his field study in Tianjin (Bian 1994: 177–208).

The LIMC was generous. Not only did it cover the main part of medical care benefits (e.g., the expenses of diagnosis and treatments, basic prescription drugs, and hospitalization), but also collateral benefits (e.g., sick leave). However, inpatients still had to pay for their own transportation in the case of referrals, food services in the case of hospitalization, and expensive drugs beyond the ceilings of the basic categories. Taken as "half insurance" just like PFMC, LIMC covered one half of the expenses of the spouses and dependents of staff and workers when making use of the services provided by public hospitals, but they enjoyed full coverage of all expenses of diagnosis and treatments when seeking cure in enterprise-managed hospitals and facilities as well as in contracted medical care clinics (Dangdai Zhongguo congshu bianjibu 1987: 316–7; Dangdai Zhongguo congshu bianjibu 1988: 235–7).

In accordance with the 1951 Regulations, the design of the "labor insurance" system embraced three clusters of benefits and entitlements at the enterprise level. The first cluster included the labor insurance fund mainly for retirement benefits (3 percent of total wages) and labor union dues (2 percent of total wages); the second cluster had to do with a medical and healthcare subsidy amounting to 5–7 percent depending on the industry (with adjustments later on); the third cluster pertains to "welfare fund" (including "collective welfare" mainly for amenities and facilities) consisting of 2.5 percent. While the union organization administered the first cluster of benefits and entitlements, the enterprise management acted on behalf of the Congress of Representatives of Staff and Workers (CRSW) and managed the second and third clusters, often in collaboration with the union (Dangdai Zhongguo conghshu bianjibu 1988: 312–4).

It is within the power of sovereign planners at the macro level to entrust responsibility to the work unit at the micro level for managing social security in general and the medical care benefits. For instance, the public enterprise, either SOE or COE, was taken not only as a legal entity, but also as an accounting unit in the CPE framework, bearing legal and financial responsibility over the entire package of social security policy.

In a close examination of LIMC, one finds that the enterprise unit provided the funding for the essential medical care demands in accordance with the 1951 Regulations (as amended in 1953). In accounting terms, it was charged to the account of "medical care and healthcare subsidy" in the second cluster as just noted above, but it did not rely on risk-pooling mechanisms sustained by premium contributions as pension retirement does.[3] It is evident that no risk pooling mechanisms of any scale were established for medical care entitlements beyond the work unit level.

In the process of institutional evolution, the provision of medical and healthcare benefits became, formally and nominally, the responsibility of enterprise management, which acted on behalf of, and also was made accountable to the CRSW starting in the 1950s. The CRSW was supposed to be the highest decision-making body responsible for the matters of welfare, insurance and benefits within the jurisdiction of the work unit, but the enterprise management and Labor Union each had considerable say and often were given specific managerial roles. On top of industrial democracy and workers' participation, the CRSW was, by design, given the role of check-and-balance to the powerful enterprise director, to say the least (Lee 1987).

As the medical care system began to take shape, the enterprise management often had two options concerning the delivery of health and medical care services: First, it could sign service agreements with public hospitals in the respective jurisdiction to provide medical and healthcare services to staff and workers and, accordingly, cover medical care expenses through reimbursement; and second, it often built its own medical care providing facilities to cater to medical care demands of staff and workers, coupled with dependents, within the work unit (Dangdai Zhongguo Congshu 1988: 235). Continuing even up to economic reform, the latter, namely enterprise-managed hospital, was indicative of a broad tendency moving toward the direction of "work-unit collectivism" during the reform period, that is, an endeavor to make use of available financial resources to build its own clinics or hospitals for staff and workers.[4]

It is noteworthy that "work-unit collectivism" originated prior to the Cultural Revolution, but it flourished in the case of medical care at the enterprise level after Mao's era. At the onset of medical care reforms after 1979, for instance, there registered the visible growth of enterprise-managed hospitals at the work unit level, targeting primary care and clinical services. As public enterprises faced the pressure of wage control, they tended to seek better terms of remuneration through expansion of "supplementary wage," meaning more spending in social security, subsidy and welfare and "collective welfare" in terms of housing, amenities and facilities in addition to substantial portion of which consisted of enterprise-managed hospitals. As of 1983, the number of enterprise-managed hospitals at the county level or above was counted as one half of the national total (i.e., 5,061 in the national total of 10,466), and the number of hospital beds is counted as less than one sixth of the national total (i.e., 433,721 in the national total of 2,341,609).[5]

Sovereign planners were able to introduce the policy and programs of social security in general and basic medical care to the SOEs and COEs incrementally from 1951 to 1956 (Dangdai Zhongguo congshu bianjibu 1987: 307: Zheng 2002: 123). For policy implementation, the policymakers drew a boundary between SOEs and COEs (depending on ownership), allowing the latter more autonomy and flexibility. Indicative of a corporatist tendency, economic reform ushered in a new phase of public policy by formally bringing the benefits and entitlements of social security for COEs into the state arena from 1977 onward. By 1984, 17 million staff and workers of COEs—or 62.9 percent of the total—had been included in social security schemes comparable to those of SOEs (Dangdai Zhongguo congshu bianjibu 1987: 329–32).

Macro-Managing the Social Security (Including Medical Care)

Conceptually speaking, social security was treated as non-wage compensation in the context of CPE. Taking a close look at the managerial and financial issues of social security packages in general and the LIMC package in particular during the pre-reform era, one can gauge how broad and how deep the party-state intervened in management at the work unit level. In the CPE in the Chinese context, the social security packages, including medical care, were closely related to the remuneration policy in the public sector as previously mentioned (Chapter 3). In accordance with the 1951 Regulations, the social security benefits and entitlements are conceptually understood as "workfare," an integral part of non-wage compensation for staff and workers employed by SOEs.[6] As part of non-wage compensation, however, the programs of benefits, welfare, and insurance represented a group-oriented incentive scheme. Once an individual was included in a workfare program, he/she was, in principle, given benefits, etc. equal to any other personnel within the same category or rank. During radical politics such as the Cultural Revolution, group-oriented incentive was politically safer than performance-oriented incentive, because the former stressed some kind of collectivism generally immune from political assault, while the latter was subject to criticisms of "individualism and materialism."

There were four periods of change about the financing of social security benefits (including basic medical care) at the work unit level from the 1950s to the 1980s. The first period lasted from 1951 to 1968, while a coherent and well-integrated design of the social security system was adopted and implemented in the industrial sector. This design was managed by the three-way collaboration of the party committee, enterprise management, and labor union at the enterprise level. Not only did the union organization acquire a significant leadership role in organizing the CRSW and overseeing the agenda as well as issues relating to wages, subsidy and welfare, and industrial relations, but also it took charge of union dues and the labor insurance fund (relating to retirement pension), positioning itself to perform a well-defined set of functions (Dangdai Zhongguo congshu bianjibu 1987: 307–10; Lee 1987).

Like other social security benefits, funding for the LIMC program was proportionally tied to the total wage and the supplementary wage of a given enterprise. It is noteworthy that the account of "medical and healthcare subsidy" constituted a substantial portion of the supplementary wage to cover benefits and entitlements of medical care services for staff and workers as just noted (Dangdai Zhongguo congshu bianjibu 1988: 213). In addition, an enterprise unit could draw from various funds and subsidies to cover not only the regular kinds of medical care services but also all collateral expenses, such as sick leave and medical care expenses for retirees, coupled with some adjustments of social security funding among various industrial sectors (Dangdai Zhongguo congshu bianjibu 1988: 204–37).

In the second period from 1969 to 1977, the government dismantled the All-China Federation of Labor Unions (hereafter, ACFLU), resulting in the abolishment of some social security programs pertaining to the 1951 Regulations (Zheng 2002: 126–7). Under Maoist assault during the Cultural Revolution, the Ministry of Finance (MOF) made its retreat by proposing to terminate, for example, the labor insurance fund that had been managed by the union organization at the enterprise level till 1969. Instead, retirement payments, paid sick leave (long term beyond six months), and other "labor insurance subsidies" were to be absorbed by the "extra business expenditure" to be calculated according to the actual amount spent. As a result, financial management such as planning, budgeting, accounting, and auditing of social security were weakened considerably. Nonetheless, the MOF issued some policy guidelines to require enterprise units to appropriate the welfare fund of staff and workers under the budgetary item of supplementary wage, the proportion of which remained at 11 percent of total wages. For more than one decade from 1966 to the late 1970s, the so-called "work-unit collectivism" prevailed, as enterprises were allowed discretion in finding other ways to meet the needs of medical care services and other welfare benefits (Dangdai Zhongguo congshu bianjibu 1988: 214–6).

Despite all merits of "work-unit collectivism" just noted, social security entitlements in general and medical care entitlements in particular were conceptually treated as a form of non-wage compensation, and much less than a component of an established program of public insurance. Nor an independent funding source was built institutionally and managerially to ensure the payments for such entitlements.

The third period witnessed a shift from radical politics to reform-oriented policy by placing emphasis on productivity, revenue, and incentive in handling issues of wages, bonus, and benefits. Beginning in 1979, the State Council decided to finance security benefits solely through "retained revenue" at the work unit level. In July 1979, the State Council promulgated a set of regulations known as the 1979 Regulations, which divided retained revenue into three portions: A production development fund, a welfare fund for staff and workers, and a reward fund for staff and workers.[7] This means, overall, that staff and workers were pressured to generate enough retained revenue to pay for their own social security expenses (including medical care benefits) which were normally charged, in budgetary terms, to the accounts of health and medical care subsidy (of welfare fund) in accordance with the 1979 Regulations as noted.

In the fourth period starting in 1983, a new balance was struck between retained revenue and "welfare" demands, making sure that those enterprises running at budgetary deficit would be provided with a protective cushion and not drown financially. Above all, not all SOEs were able to attain their revenue goals for reasons beyond their control, e. g. technical depreciation, change of product market, aging of workforce, etc. It was, therefore, not feasible to continue the provision of benefits and entitlements if retained revenue remained the sole source of the social security funding according to budgetary and accounting rules. Accordingly, sovereign planners worked out a compromise by taking care of the basic needs of welfare, subsidies and "labor insurance," even if some public enterprises could not fulfill revenue targets, meanwhile ensuring incentives to those SOEs which were able to fulfill revenue targets. In the absence of property rights concept in a market economy, it was a matter of fairness regarding the rightful share of retained revenue that was generated by public enterprises. It was well argued that lack of funding for social security at the work unit level might have to be attributed to the accumulation of enormous public funds and assets held at the local government level in view of excessively large profit remittance from the enterprise level (Chapter 3).

Taken as a whole, the SOEs were given considerably more room to spend in the social security packages than ever before from 1983 onwards, resulting in visible expansion in non-wage compensation, such as amenities, facilities, housing, "collective welfare," and health care etc. The MOF promulgated a policy paper in April 1983, allowing all SOEs to set aside social security funding from two sources: For the first portion, namely supplementary wage (e.g., normally 11 percent of total wage), could be charged as production costs, and if this was not sufficient, for the second portion, the remaining could be charged to the account of retained revenue. Moreover, SOEs would be allowed to use part of the "enterprise reserve fund" for welfare expenditure for staff and workers if they experienced inadequate retained revenue when failing to fulfill revenue targets.[8]

It is evident that throughout approximately three decades from the early 1950s to the 1970s, a comprehensive and elaborated system of entitlement and benefits of social security was legislated by the party-state entity but managed at the work unit level. And they were funded by conventional public finance channels of the CPE, for example, either retained revenue and production costs for public enterprises, or taxation revenue for the government units and service work units. Neither had any independent funding system ever been built, nor program, mechanisms and managerial and financial tools had been in place to ensure that social security entitlements including medical care were to be met. In terms of the program specificity, entitlements of social security were institutionally alienated from funding vehicles.

Remedial Policies and Measures

In the aftermath of Mao, the entire medical care system faced a host of complex issues, among which financial management was most pronounced and urgent, for instance, the pressure of uncontrollable spending in both the PFMC and LIMC (Zheng 2002: 131). And it was estimated that the expenditure for medical care increased by 20 percent or even reaching 30 percent in some cases, on average annually from the early 1980s to the late 1990s (Peng, Cai & Zhou 1992: 16–7). To cope with the financial difficulties of the PFMC and LIMC, the government units began to make remedial responses to the overspending and shortage of financing sources in the PFMC and LIMC programs across jurisdictions. Despite relatively comprehensive coverage of entitlements, above all, the full range of financial issues of medical care were rooted in two dimensions of program specificity: Spending and funding.

They were inseparable from each other in maintaining budgetary balance as well as continuous operation of the funding of basic medical care (Song 2001: 89–90; Zheng 2002: 131–9; Yang 2004: 106; Zheng, Gao & Yu 2010: 17–20).

Overall, a new variety of the spending measures regarding PFMC and LIMC were recommended and introduced in conjunction with staging for the reform of public funding of healthcare from the 1980s to 1990s. To begin with, various jurisdictions were focused on spending control through the repackaging of services, deductibles and co-payment schemes, payment-ceiling, and accountability systems as well as the establishment of offices/bureaus in charge. Centering on product/service specificity, for example, the various governments endeavored to curtail spending through repackaging medical care services by including those essential and cost-effective types of medical care services while excluding those less essential and less efficient ones (Dangdai Zhongguo congshu bianjibu 1988: 233–5; Zheng 2002: 127–8; Zheng, Gao & Yu 2010: 17–8). The focus was often placed on "negative listing" by identifying non-essential categories of medical care services that were to be excluded, that is, those secondary and tertiary categories of medical care services as well as those non-listed items such as nutrients, cosmetics, obesity, etc. (Cheng & Dong 1999: 397).

To instill cost-awareness and make each enrollee accountable to the choice of medical care, the government introduced a co-payment scheme of medical care in the transactions between the enrollee and providing units aiming at containing the runaway increase of expenditure by both the PFMC and LIMC programs (Dangdai Zhongguo congshu bianjibu 1987: 316–7; Cheng & Dong 1999: 397–8; Zheng 2002: 120–1). For example, the 1984 Circular recommended provincial and municipal jurisdictions to begin their pilot experiment of co-payment in the PFMC program by requiring both inpatients and outpatients to shoulder a given "self-paid portion" (*zifu bilie*), equivalent to the commonly used concept of "co-payment" in the West (Zheng 2002: 133). As the 1985 Circular was being implemented, three options about co-payments were tried out (Song 2001: 89). These accountability policies were extended throughout the country from 1989 onward, and by 1993 the co-payment measures were introduced to all units covered by the PFMC programs (Song 2001: 89).

Also, the same set of co-payment measures was subsequently extended to the LIMC programs in various jurisdictions. For example, some enrollees affiliated with public enterprises with better productivity would have to pay 10–20 percent of their medical care bills, while those users in difficult enterprises might have to shoulder up to 50 percent on average. It is estimated that 80 percent of enterprises adopted co-payment schemes under the LIMC program by 1993, when the BMCI reform reached its staging period (Song 2001: 89).

Furthermore, various jurisdictions experimented with several versions of the accountability system, namely, the so-called "undertaking" (*baogan*) systems in common Chinese expression, to strengthen accountability pertaining to the PFMC. These systems include : (1) the so-called "fixed-quota current expenditure undertaking" (*jingfei dinge baogan*; abbreviated as FCEU) version, whereby the work unit was made accountable for a fixed amount of appropriation, and thus it was allowed to retain any surplus but to absorb any deficit; (2) the hospital-managed version, whereby a service agreement was signed with a chosen hospital, and making it accountable for expenditure within the given financial targets coupled with built-in financial incentives; and (3) the joint management version whereby there was a joint management among several units (e.g., the work unit, the providing unit and the funding unit) based upon a service agreement to delineate responsibility, rights, and obligations, in addition to financial schemes for sharing savings but shouldering deficit (Song 2001: 90; Zheng 2002: 134–5).

In addition, the government at various levels endeavored to devise new organizational tools and managerial mechanisms to strengthen spending control and cope with the overly rapid increase of expenditure by the PFMC program (Peng, Cai & Zhou 1992: 17–8; Zheng 2002: 134). In accordance with the 1989 Circular, for instance, various jurisdictions were required to establish a PFMC managing committee, and/or set up a PFMC program office within the jurisdiction's healthcare bureau. In some jurisdictions, however, surveys suggest that the PFMC office was established in and affiliated with the finance bureau. Accordingly, the new PFMC offices were given an active role in managing and controlling the spending of medical care services in various jurisdictions throughout the country (Zheng 2002: 134). How are the above-mentioned measures implemented in a jurisdiction? It is appropriate to examine a concrete case next.

The Prelude to the Reform

During economic reform, various jurisdictions started to address the policy issues of healthcare by making remedial responses, and some ingredients of the reform were entertained already in these remedial responses. Taking advantage of the author's many field investigations, it is here to dwell on the case of Guangzhou to illustrate what took place empirically with regards to spending control measures in healthcare, amidst the lack of funding in healthcare at the local level. Before Guangzhou was in a position to consider financial sources for healthcare, uncontrollable spending was posed as the first challenge for the municipal government. Guangzhou is one of most representative cases of spending control during rapid growth of expenditure in the PFMC, for example, an increase of spending in healthcare normally higher than 20 percent of annual growth rate on average, and in some years higher than 30 percent (Interview, Morning December 28, 1922). As early as the mid-1980s, the municipal government made the first move to introduce spending control measures systematically for PFMC programs in Guangzhou (Chen 1995). Guangzhou also adopted managerial measures recommended by provincial authorities for strengthening the financial accountability of the work unit, hospital, and individual subsequently in 1987 (Guangdongsheng yiliao baozhang zhidu gaige yanjiu xianmu bangongshi 1999: 191).

According to policy analyst Cai, the municipal government continued to reform the management of the PFMC program in 1994. The government started with a systematic review of entitlements within each category of cadres and officials, together with the types, standards, and quotas for medical care services in light of available financial resources. Accordingly, the municipal government took its own initiatives to introduce a few spending control measures. In accordance with one measure adopted, for example, the work unit had to shoulder a certain portion of the deficit when it had exceeded fixed quotas and standards of spending in health-care, meaning that the finance bureau was not to absorb excess spending automati-cally as it had used to be (Cai 1996; Dong 1999).

Meanwhile, the provincial government put forth yet another policy paper, the 1994 Plan, in order to break excessive spending for the PFMC program in June 1994.[9] To implement the 1994 Plan, the municipal government accordingly intro-duced a joint-management version of "undertaking system" among several units involved (such as the financial unit, work unit, and hospital), allowing these three units jointly to share 50 percent of the surplus from the preceding year and, con-versely, shoulder the deficit from the preceding year in the following proportions, say, 5, 4, 1. In addition, the 1994 Plan proposed a co-payment scheme requiring employed personnel to shoulder co-payment of 20 percent of expenses for clinical visits and 5 percent for hospital care services, and retirees 10 percent for clinical visits and 5 percent for hospital care. Also, the government introduced the scheme for a deductible (also known as the "payment-starting criterion," *qifu biaozhun*; hereafter, PSC) for employees and retirees. The work unit would also consider advancing reimbursement after the patient fulfilled PSC (for employees, up to 500 RMB, and for retirees, 400 RMB). As a manifestation of "neo-traditionalism" mentioned previously (Jowitt 1983; Chapter 2), however, all senior cadres, per-sonnel with privileged retirement (or called "*liuxiu*"), and disabled veterans were exempted from both co-payment and the PSC requirement (Cai 1996; Dong 1999: 192–3).

Indicative of the phenomenon of alienation of entitlements from funding, some public enterprise units were brought to court by staff and workers for failing to honor full reimbursement for medical care in accordance with the 1951 Labor Regulations in spite of remedy measures introduced as noted above (Interview December 29, 1992). And the controversies and litigations were not subsequently put to rest until 1998 when the State Council acted upon the situation, formally announcing the 1998 Decision, the landmark document signaling the inauguration of the BMCI, and ensuring that all entitlements and benefits to staff and workers to be funded and honored properly (Guowuyuan 1998).[10]

While trying to cope with the financial crisis of the LIMC program in Guang-zhou as early as 1984, the Labor Bureau issued a series of rulings to authorize various enterprise units to work out reimbursement quotas for medical expenses of employees when the units were no longer able to meet requests for reimbursement of medical payments in full. Also, in 1985 the Labor Bureau promulgated catalogs for drugs covered by PFMC and LIMC. In 1987 the Labor Bureau issued a policy permitting enterprise units to propose reimbursement schemes according to age and seniority, and endorsed proposals as submitted, except for simple and indis-criminate reimbursement quotas (Interview May 11, 2000).

Regarding public enterprises, a survey of SOEs in Guangzhou attests that the lack of control measures over excessive and uncontrolled expenditure for medical care resulted in the widespread disintegration of the LIMC programs throughout the municipality during 1990 and 1991. The survey indicates that, of the SOEs assessed, only 7 out of 29 SOEs were able to finance LIMC programs in accordance with the 1951 Labor Insurance Regulations, that 15 (more than one half) simply paid staff and workers a fixed sum for medical care under the "fixed norm undertaking system," that 6 worked with reimbursement schemes according to age brackets, and that 2 covered a portion of clinical care coupled with a reimbursement scheme for hospital care according to seniority (Interview December 29, 1992). Although the sample of the survey is small, it provides an illustration of the general lack of spending control measures throughout Guangdong Province (Dong 1999).

It did not appear optimistic among policy analysts regarding the ability of SOEs to cope with the financial crisis, as they had to shoulder big medical bills for staff and workers in Guangzhou during the 1980s and 1990s. According to policy analyst Chen, neither was there any set of spending control mechanisms in place to check excessive and uncontrollable demands for medical care services from users, nor were effective spending control measures adopted to counter the over-provision of drug prescriptions and overuse of medical devices at the public hospital level. According to Chen's estimate, LIMC medical bills normally, on average, consisted of 13 percent of total wages in public enterprises in Guangzhou, but often reached 17 percent when including reimbursements for part of the expenses for hospital care (say, ranging from 50 to 90 percent). Taken together, Chen suggested that the "financial liability" for all kinds of benefits and insurance (including the LIMC program) could easily reach 45 percent of the total wages, meaning public enterprises alone were confronted with an excessively heavy financial burden under the conventional public funding system (Chen 1995). As the inadequacy of spending control measures posed a serious problem for the delivery of basic medical care prior to the BMCI reform, the absence of funding mechanisms to sustain the provision of entitlement was another crucial issue to be dealt with.

Local Experiments of Risk Pooling Mechanisms

As one of the most significant landmarks of policy innovation in public funding in China, various echelons of government took the initiatives to experiment with the new packages of risk-pooling mechanisms across various jurisdictions to tackle the financing issue of medical and healthcare with regard to so-called high expenditure and serious illness (HESI), including catastrophic medical care events, during the late 1980s and early 1990s (Zheng, Gao & Yu 2010: 18–9). In tracing the roots of risking pooling mechanisms, a core component of the BMCI program today, one finds that the often-cited case of the Vegetable Company of the East City District in Beijing represents an embryonic design of risk-pooling mechanisms in the late 1980s, addressing the issue of HESI for the first time (Lee 2019). Prior to 1989 there had been reform initiatives to build up the so-called "social unified funding" (*shehui tongchou*; hereafter, SUF) of basic medical care expenditure for retired personnel (including the category for those on "*lixiu*," leave for recuperation, i.e., privileged retirement scheme,) in such places as Mushi in Shandong Province and Jingxi in Liaoning Province (Zheng 2002: 135–6). It appears that all ingredients of a public medical care insurance are found present in the design of the package for the first time. This package required participant enterprises to pay for an annual contribution in full to the SUF account for the enrollees to cover expenses of retired ("*lixiu*") personnel for clinical visits, hospitalization, physical checkups, and transportation costs for referrals. The package also incorporated the feature of co-payment that followed the principle of a three-way sharing of medical care expenses (government, work unit, and patient) with or without a spending cap (exceeding the "payment-ceiling" criterion) (Zheng 2002: 135–6).[11]

The policy initiatives of SUF for retirees were formally endorsed for the first time on November 28, 1990, when the Ministry of Labor (MOL) held a work conference about labor insurance medical care reform with the participation of various provinces and municipalities. The work conference marked the beginning of pilot programs and policy experiments on a large scale, formally promoting SUF designs across the country. Some statistical surveys suggest that SUF was then shown to be feasible despite limitations and shortcomings. Subsequently, in 1992, the MOL started not only to solicit opinions on public (or social) medical care insurance at the enterprise level, but also to authorize the experiments of one of the earliest risk pooling designs called "social unified funding" (*shehui tongchou*; hereafter, SUF) for HESI. The SUF pilot programs for HESI were adopted in Dandong, Shiping, Huangshi, Zhuzhou, and other cities. By the end of 1994, the same measure was extended to an additional twenty jurisdictions, covering 3,746,000 staff and workers, coupled with the potential to grow further (Lee 2019; Zheng 2002: 131–6).

In 1994 SUF programs were implemented in 14,000 enterprises in fourteen jurisdictions, and 357,000 retirees subscribed to SUF in one form or another, representing a 26.1 percent increase over the one-year period from 1993. In the same year, the total sum of collection amounted to 60 million RMB with outgoing payments of 70 million (meaning a shortfall of 10 million). However, the accumulated savings reached 6.72 million, with a decrease of 12.31 million from 1993. Besides, relevant social (or public) insurance institutes experimented with building clinics and hospitals for retirees, which proved effective in containing cost increases as well (Zheng 2002: 135–6).

In his field investigations to Guangzhou and Shanghai, the author was able to have a close look at the HESI cases (including catastrophic medical events) in the two cities during the staging phase of the BMCI reform. In Guangzhou, an interviewee detailed the circumstances where Guangzhou's public enterprises took the first step to experiment with risk-pooling mechanisms to build a funding source for HESI among the staff and workers of public enterprises. In the view of the Guangzhou government, the major illness insurance (*dabing baoxian*, hereafter, MII, major illness insurance), mainly covering hospital care in Zone II and HESI (or equivalent to those cases above payment-ceiling) in Zone III, was found most appropriate and feasible among the various options. It was repeatedly reported that many public enterprises faced financial ruin when having to shoulder the enormous costs for HESI cases of staff and workers. The interviewee made mention of the policy paper (No. 17, 1992) of the MOF, reissued by the MOL, suggesting that there was a way to finance HESI by injecting additional funds into the welfare fund for staff and workers (Chen 1995). To lessen the financial burden of the enrollees, however, policy actors appeared to prefer to drop clinical care from the then-existing LIMC program.

As a prelude to the adoption of a centrally sponsored BMCI in 2001, Shanghai experimented with its own versions of risk-pooling mechanisms beginning in 1996. Shanghai's experimental insurance scheme mainly dealt with the cases of retirees in addition to HESI cases. Also in 1998, a version of risk-pooling mechanism for special clinical services for retired staff and workers was first established, to be financed jointly by the hospital care insurance fund, the retirement fund, and the wage fund (calculated according to the average wage of currently employed staff and workers). This program allowed the work units and patients to shoulder 50 percent of the expenditure for special clinical services at chosen hospitals in the second and third tier, with the remainder to be absorbed by the medical care insurance bureau (Zuo 2000).

To introduce risk-pooling mechanisms such as SUF pilot programs for major illness, policymakers had to come to terms with the issues of conceptualization and operational definition, constituting integral part of the exercise of product/service specificity (Lee 2019). During the early phase of health care reform in the early 1990s, there existed some ambiguity about the operational definitions of "major illness," that concerns two shades of meaning. From the medical-scientific perspective, the term, "major illness" (*dabing*) refers to serious illness. And from financial vantage point, it often refers to "expenditure of medical care for major illness" (*dabing yiliao feiyong*) or more precisely, "medical care of large sum expenditure" (*dae feiyong yiliao*), underscoring the priority of cost containment (Liu & Liu 1999: 62–4, 87). As proposed by PN. Lee, one may conceptually divide expenditures for medical care services into three zones as follows:

> Zone I: clinical care that involves a relatively small expenditure;
> Zone II: hospital care that requires a relatively large expenditure; and
> Zone III: HESI cases (including a catastrophic medical event; normally exceeding the payment-ceiling limit) pertaining to a large and potentially uncontrollable expenditure (Lee 2019).

In various jurisdictions, policymakers appeared able to differentiate Zone I from Zone II and III, but they did not normally draw a distinction between Zone II and III, which became an issue for product/service specificity later, from the mid-1990s onward. It appears that the SUF programs were intended to cover Zone II and III mainly for alleviating the financial burden of public enterprises and of ensuring essential medical care services to staff, workers, and retirees when the LIMC programs were in disintegration during the post-Mao era.

Considering the "interpretative scheme" of policy participants and analysts, the scope of SUF programs and the principles of payments are as follows: First, the scope of expenditure of the SUF programs shall be determined both by considerations of medical science and the actual amount of expenditure; secondly, the deductible (so-called payment starting criterion, or PSC) and classes of payment are to be governed by the consideration of financial capacity of the established fund; thirdly, various jurisdictions have discretion to include dependents into the SUF programs; and finally, the reimbursement of expenditure for organ transplants shall follow the regulations and schemes of cost sharing established by each jurisdiction (Liu & Liu 1999: 87).

Among those jurisdictions that established the SUF program for major illness, enterprise units with different affiliations (e.g., central, provincial, prefectural/ municipal unit, and county) were, in principle, required to follow the residential principle to enroll in the SUF program on behalf of staff and workers. The SUF program normally covered a county at the beginning, but it was expected to expand to the prefectural/municipal jurisdiction whenever feasible. Accordingly, the local authorities concerned created non-departmental public entities (NDPEs) for medical care insurance that were separate from government and public enterprises. These public entities served as holders of the SUF account for insurance for major illness among staff and workers and participant enterprises. They also took charge of collection, management, and payment pertaining to the SUF for serious illness. They represented one of the earliest attempts of "one-arm's length" style of public management in China in the sense that they were legally independent of the government and not subject to interference from any government unit (Zheng 2002: 131–2).

Emerging from SUF pilot programs in medical care services were several novel methods and managerial approaches adopted by various jurisdictions. For example, transaction-centered management was adopted in many cases: Participant enterprises and providing units jointly signed a service agreement for basic medical care services to prescribe the standards for charges, scope, items, expenses and norms of services, and measures of saving and incentives, under the auspices of the social labor insurance bureau/institute in a given jurisdiction. Additionally, the relevant bureaus developed administrative instruments to control the delivery of medical care services at the basic level through the enforcement of well-defined scope and standards and rules of reimbursement. The relevant authorities also worked together to devise a mechanism for regulatory control over entry into the medical care insurance market. For instance, the bureau of labor, bureau of health, and trade union jointly established standards, procedures, and mechanisms to evaluate the qualifications and eligibility of various kinds of clinics and hospitals about their application for the licensing and listing in the SUF catalog of medical care services (Zheng et al. 2002: 136–7).

It is noteworthy that both the SUF program for major illnesses among staff and workers and the program for medical care expenditure for retired personnel grew in their enrollments from 1993 to 1996. For example, the former enjoyed a rapid expansion from 2,679,094 in 1993 to 7,911,835 in 1996; and the latter from 225,182 in 1993 to 664,715 in 1996 (Zheng et al. 2002: 137–8). As one of its first steps during the early 1990s, the MOL drafted the "Opinion regarding the Trial Implementation of Unified Social Funding for the Expenditure for Major Illness" on March 19, 1992 (Zheng et al. 2002), indicative of the emergence of a medical care insurance to integrate entitlement with funding, a proto type of BMCI, before the commencement of the BMCI reform.

Concluding Remarks

The foregoing analysis has tried to examine early origins of public funding of medical care and first policy precedents regarding basic medical care in conjunction with the introduction of PFMC and LIMC, coupled with discussions on the other types of benefits and entitlements, designs of funding mechanisms, issues of management and institution as well as implementation at the beginning of CPE. Furthermore, the study is devoted to an analysis of various remedial responses to the spending issues as well as the new proposals to deal with financing problems across jurisdictions that prepared the ground for launching of the basic medical care insurance. Through remedial responses in terms of spending control measures and policy experiments of funding through risking pooling designs, And, these represent the embryonic concepts and programs for BMCI took shape for the first time prior to the BMCI reform from 1994 onwards, the topic to be discussed in next four chapters.

Notes

1 For instance, there was an actual expenditure of 24.6 RMB on average for each individual public employee over the budgeted sum of 18 RMB in 1960 and 34.4 RMB over the budgeted sum of 26 RMB in 1965 (Zheng 2002: 120–1).

2 For example, it was reported that in 1982 the expenditure of PFMC exceeded the budgetary limit by 3,700 million RMB (Zheng 2002: 128).

3 In accordance with the 1951 Labor Insurance Regulation (as amended in 1953), by design, the branch of the Labor Union at the work unit level was expected not only to assume responsibility for managing retirement pension at the work unit level but also to join the larger financial pool at the next higher level to diversify financial risks. The early design of the retirement pension system features an arrangement of financial pooling involving a cluster of enterprise units under the All-China Federation of Labor Unions, but it was not put into practice fully because of the dismantlement of labor unions during the Cultural Revolution. Consequently, local governments had to shoulder the financial burden of retirement of staff and workers when they retired after the economic reform era until the introduction of an entirely new retirement scheme (Dangdai Zhongguo Chongshu bianjibu 1987: 302–14).

4 In China, "collective welfare" (or known as "collective welfare facilities/enterprises") refers to a well-defined category of benefits in terms of amenities and facilities made available to members of a work unit, for example, canteens, nursery school (or even primary school), sports facilities and theaters, dormitories and housing units, etc. (Dangdai Zhongguo congshu bianjibu 1987: 210–40; Bian 1994: 183–208).

5 These enterprise-managed hospitals cover only a portion of the ordinary cases (e.g., emergency cases and cases of simple, common, and frequent illness) with the remaining cases normally being treated in public hospitals at the municipality and county levels (Dangdai Zhongguo congshu bianjibu 1986: 17–28).

6 "Workfare" differs from "welfare" in that the former is tied to work performance and the latter is mostly tied to needs. Both can be taken as a form of social security.

7 The full title of the 1979 Regulations is the Regulations of the Implementation of Retained Revenue of the State-Owned Enterprises (Dangdai Zhongguo congshu bianjibu 1988: 216).

8 The title of the policy paper is the Provisional Regulations Concerning the Issue of Financial Solution of Tax for Revenue in State Owned Enterprises in Industry and Transportation (Dangdai Zhongguo congshu bianjibu 1988: 216–7).

9 The full title of the policy paper is the "Plan for the Reform of Public Financed Medical Care for Directly Administered Units and the Municipality of Guangzhou" (abbreviated as 1994 Plan) (Cai 1996; Dong 1999: 192–3).

10 The 1998 Decision is known among the policy circle as Document Guofa No. 44, the full title of which is as follows: The "Decision Concerning the Establishment of a Basic Medical Care Insurance System for Staff and Workers in Cities and Towns," promulgated by the State Council in 1998 (Guowuyuan 1998).

11 In some cases, "*lixiu*" personnel were given leeway in claiming reimbursement according to actual expenses, meaning no capping limit (Zheng 2002: 135–6).

References

Bian, Y. J. 1994. *Work and Inequality in Urban China.* Albany: State University of New York.

Cai, G. 1996. Cong gongfei laobao yiliao dao shehui yiliao baoxian (From public financed medical care to social insurance medical care). *Gaige daobao (Journal of Reform).*

Chen, T. 1995. Qiantan Guangzhou yiliao baoxian zhidu gaige qibu de shiyong moshi (A preliminary discussion on the applicable initiating model of the reform of medical care system). *Guangdong laodong bao (Guangdong Laodong Journal).* May 28.

Cheng, L. & Dong, S. 1999. Guanyu yiliao baoxain feiyong kongzhi wenti yanjiu (A research on the expenditure and control of medical care insurance). In Zheng, D., Liu, D. & Zhang, B. (Eds.), *Shehui baozhang zhidu gaige zhinan (Guidelines for the Reform of Social Security System).* Beijing: Gaige chubanshe. 391–401

Dangdai Zhongguo congshu bianjibu 1986. *Dangdai Zhongguo de weisheng shiye, xia (The Health Care Enterprises in Contemporary China, Volume ll).* Beijing: Zhongguo shehui kexue chubanshe.

Dangdai Zhongguo congshu bianjibu 1987. *Dangdai zhongguo de gongzhi fuli he shehui baoxian (The Wage, Welfare and Social insurance of Staff and Workers in Contemporary China).* Beijing: Zhongguo shehui kexue chubanshe.

Dangdai Zhongguo congshu bianjibu 1988. *Dangdai Zhongguo Caizheng, Xia (Finance in Contemporary China).* Beijing: Zhongguo shehui kexue chubanshe.

Dong, B. 1999. Guangdongsheng chengzhen yiliao baozhang gaige yanjiu (Research on medical care security reform in cities and towns in Guangdong Province). In Guangdongsheng yiliao baozhang zhidu gaige yanjiu xianmu bangongshi (Eds.), *Guangdongsheng yiliao baozhang zhidu gaige (Reform of Medical Care Security System in Guangdong Province).* Shenzhun: Guangdong renmin chubanshe.

Guangdongsheng yiliao baozhang zhidu gaige yanjiu xianmu banggongshi 1999. *Guangdongsheng yiliao baozhang zhidu gaige yangjiu zong baogao (The General Report of the Research on the Reform of Medical Care Security System in Guangdong Province).* Shenzhun: Guangdong remin chubanshe.

Guowuyuan 1998. Guowuyuan guanyu jianli chengzhen jiben yiliao baoxian zhidu de jueding (The decision of the State Council concerning the establishment of basic medical care insurance in cities and towns). *Guowuyuan gongbao (Bulletin of State Council)* 33: 1250–4.

He, P. 2005. Wanshan chenzhen shehui baoxian tizi yanjiu (To perfect the social insurance system. in cities and towns). *Shehui Baoxian Yanjiu (Social Insurance Research)* 7: 3–26.

Hu, S. 2001. *Yiliao baoxian he fuwu zhidu (Medical Care Insurance and System of Services)*. Chengtu: Sichuan remin chubanshe.

Interview (one interviewee, Guangzhou) December 29, 1992.

Interview (two interviewees, Guangzhou), morning May 11, 2000.

Jin, W. 1996. Laodong jiaohuan yu guoyou qiye zhigong de laodong jijixing (The labor exchange and labor incentive of staff and workers in the state-owned enterprises) (originally published in Zhongguo Shehui Kexue. 1993. 6). Li, D. (Eds.) *Zhongguo de xiandai qiye zhidu zilu (Road to Modern Enterprise System in China)*. Beijing: Guojia wenhua chubanshe gongsi. 78–85.

Jowitt, K. 1983. Soviet neotraditionalism: the political corruption of a Leninist regime. *Soviet Studies* XXXV.3: 275–97.

Kallgren, J. K. 1969. Social welfare and China's industrial workers. In Doak, B. A. (Eds.), *Chinese Communist Politics in Action.* Seattle and London: The University of Washington Press. 540–73.

Lee, P. N. 1987. *Industrial Management and Economic Reform in China. 1949–1984.* Hong Kong, Oxford and New York: Oxford University Press.

Lee, P. N. 1991. The Chinese industrial state in historical perspective: from totalitarianism to corporatism. In Womack, B. (Eds.), *Contemporary Chinese Politics in Historical Perspective.* New York: Cambridge University Press. 153–79.

Lee, P. N. & Wong, C. 2001. The tale of two cities: rolling back the boundary of the welfare state during the reform era. In Lee, P. N. & Lo, C. W. (Eds.), *Remaking China's Public Management.* Westport, CT & London: Quorum Books. 67–95.

Liu, G. & Liu, X. 1999. *Zuixin shiyang yiliao baoxian zhengce huida (The Most Recent and Practical Q & A of Medical Care Insurance Policy)*. Beijing: Jingi kexue chubanshe Zhongguo shehui kexue jikan). In Li, D. (Ed.), *Zhongguo xiandai qiye zhidu zhilu* (The Road to Modern Enterprise System in China). Beijing: Guoji wenhua chubanshe gongsi. 439–57.

Melanie, M. 1993. *Retirement of Revolutionaries in China: Public Policies, Social Norms, Private Interests.* Princeton, NJ: Princeton University Press.

Peng, R., Cai, R. & Zhou, C. (Eds.) 1992. *Zhongguo gaige congshu (The Encyclopedia of China's Reform)*. Dalian: Dalian chubanshe.

Qian, J. 2021. *The Political Economy of Making and Implementing Social Policy in China.* Singapore: Palgrave Macmillan.

Song, X. 2001. Yiliao boxian zhidu gaige jipeitao cuoshi (The reform and complementary measures of medical care insurance system). In Song, X. (Ed.), *Zhongguo shehui baozhang tizhi gaige yu fazhan baogao (The Report on the Reform and Development of the Social Security System in China)*. Beijing: Zhongguo remin daxue chubanshe. 84–105.

Song, X. & Gao, S. 2001. Zhongguo shehui baozhang tizhi gaige: zhuyao jinzhan, yanjun xinshi yu zhengce jianyi (The reform of social security system in China: major progress, serious situation and policy proposals). In Song, X. (Ed.), *Zhongguo shehui baozhang tizhi gaige yu fazhan baogao (The Report on the Reform and Development of the Social Security System in China)*. Beijing: Zhongguo remin daxue chubanshe. 2–40.

Walder, A. G. 1986. *Communist Neo-traditionalism: Work and Authority in a Chinese Factory.* Berkeley: The University of California Press.

Wang, X. 2003. *Fenpei Zhengyi yu shehui baozhang (Distributive Justice and Social Security)*. Shanghai: Shanghai caijing daxue chubanshe. 112–34.

Wang, Y. 2008. Jianli quanmin yiliao baozhang zhidu—Shanghaishi de tansuo (To establish medical care security system—the exploration of Shanghai municipality). In Wang, Y. (Ed.), *Zhongguo weisheng gaige yu fazhan de shizheng yanjiu (Empirical Research on China's Health Care Reform and Development)*. Beijing: Zhongguo laodong baozhang chubanshe.

Yang, T. 2004. Wanshan yiliao baozhang zhidu de silu he duice (The thought and proposal on how to perfect medical care system). In Chen, J. & Wang, Y. (Eds.), *Zhongguo Shehui Baozhang Fazhan Baogao (Report on the Development of Social Security in China)*. Beijing: Shehui kexue wenxian chubanshe. 105–33.

Zheng, B., Gao, Q., & Yu, H. 2010. Xinzhongguo shehui baozhang zhidu de bianqian yu fazhan (The change and development of social security in China). In Zou, D. (Eds.), *Zhongguo shehui baozhang fazhan baogao, No. 4 (The Report of Development of Social Security in China, No. 4)*. Beijing: Shehui kexue wenxian chubanshe. 26–8.

Zheng, G. et al. (Eds.). 2002. *Zhongguo zigong yiliao baozhang zidu bianqian yu pingu (The Change as well as Assessment of Medical Care Insurance System of Staff and Workers in China)*. Beijing: Remin daxue chubanshe.

Zheng, G. 2002. Zhongguo zhigong yiliao baozhang zidu bianqian yu pingu (The change as well as assessment of medical care insurance system of staff and workers in China). In Zheng, G. et al. (Eds.), *Zhongguo zigong yiliao baozhang zidu bianqian yu pingu (The Change as well as Assessment of Medical Care Insurance System of Staff and Workers in China)*. Beijing: Remin daxue chubanshe. 3–28.

Zheng, G. 2011. *Zhongguo shehui baozhang gaige yu fazhan zhanlu (The Reform and Developmental Strategy of Social Security in China)*. Beijing: Remin chubanshe.

Zou, H. 2000. Zai 1999 nian Shanghaishi weisheng gongzuo huiyi shang de jianghua, zhaiyao (Speech at the 1999 work conference on health care task in Shanghai municipality), Liu, J. (Eds.), *Shanghai weisheng nianjian 2000 (Shanghai Yearbook of Health Care 2000)*. Shanghai: Shanghai kexue jishu wenxian chubanshe. 85–92.

Part II

Basic Medical Care Insurances in the Planned Sector

5 Inaugurating Basic Medical Care Insurance

This chapter is devoted to an analysis of the policy initiation as well as new program designs pertaining to social security in general and healthcare during economic reform in China. In this chapter, the focus will be the BMCI reform, representing an entirely new departure for public funding of healthcare in the urban sector (Zheng 2002; Deng & Li 2008: 113–48; Zheng 2011: 37–44; Lee 2019). Introducing BMCI in a financial and managerial term, the main thrust of the BMCI reform was concerned with a movement toward marketization in the realm of public policy, and an endeavor of building the risk pooling mechanisms that works in providing protection to the residents at the community level against medical care events, especially expensive ones. As just noted in the last chapter, all policy precedents and experimentation of spending control and risk-pooling measures served as a prelude to the current BMCI system (Zheng, Gao & Yu 2010: 26–8).

In addition, this chapter is concerned with how the central policy actors politically reconciled with their provincial/local counterparts with reference to the divergent views on optional designs regarding social security (including healthcare) as well as the vested interests of different cohorts of the workforce in the transformation during economic reform. The BMCI design was intended to cover the enrollees of all age cohorts of the workforce in urban China, including both senior personnel and retirees who had been previously covered by conventional funding packages such as PFMC and LIMC, and fresh recruits to the emerging mixed economy (Wang 2008). A political dimension entered the packaging of BMCI, as the main emphasis was placed on funding entitlements to the enrollees who had previously subscribed to PFMC and LIMC, namely, those employees in the public sector who had worked through forced modernization under the CPE.

The study will first lend an account on the general characteristics about the policymaking process about public policy in China, and then proceed to highlight the dynamic interaction between the central government and provincial/local jurisdiction in the realm of social security (including healthcare) during economic reform. To be followed, the study will examine how politics was intertwined with public policy issues in the case of public medical care insurance. To account for the general pattern as well as its variations, finally, the study will further examine selected

DOI: 10.4324/9781003389934-7

cases, such as Guangzhou, Shanghai, and Shenzhen, to assess the variations of broad policy trends at the provincial/local level.

The Policymaking Process

As healthcare reform moved on during the 1990s and 2000s, the policymaking process regarding healthcare became exceedingly complex involving numerous policy actors, resulting in nearly 3000 insurance plans at the county, prefectural/municipal, and metropolitan level (Zheng 2011: 102–78; Lee 2019). In drafting and packaging public medical care insurance, overall, the loci of power rested at both the central and provincial/local level, and they each played their respective roles in the policymaking process. It is noteworthy, however, that provincial/local jurisdictions carried weight in case of funding of social security owing to their financial "undertaking" (*chengbao*) to some explicit delegation of responsibility and assignment of task (Ge & Gong 2007; 46–70; Gu 2008: 109–29; Lee 2019; Huang 2020; Qian 2021).

In China studies, some pioneering works have endeavored to tackle the issues on the defining features of the public organization with reference to institutional, policymaking, and managerial arenas (Schurmann 1968; Lieberthal & Oksenberg 1988; Lieberthal & Lampton 1992). Two analytical dimensions are found theoretically relevant in the existing literature on organization and management in China: The first cluster of salient characteristics of the Leninist Party-state hierarchy, for instance, the parallel hierarchies between the party committee and administration, monitoring system, political mobilization, etc., and the second cluster regarding the public organizations that operate with the monopoly and franchise and are armed with administrative/managerial tools in the context of CPE. While the first cluster is concerned with the regime's endeavor to maintain its political stability and survival, the second cluster tries to account for how public policy is made and implemented. It is well argued that the crisis of the welfare system poses as the crisis of the regime's stability and survival (Huang 2020). However, it is necessary for analysts to go beyond the concern about the exchange between social security benefits and political loyalty, and to address the concrete issues of public policy and management.

To account for the policymaking process in China, one needs to focus on the relevant ministries and provincial status jurisdictions that played pivotal roles in designing, packaging and implementing policies and programs of social security (including healthcare) (Lee 2019; Huang 2020; Qian 2021). In a formal and institutional sense, provincial governors are placed under the command of the Premier who is assisted by the staff and ministers of the State Council. Conceptually speaking, both are taken as an integral part of the formal organization, albeit they each operate independently and differently in public policy. And provincial governors are of equal rank with ministers. In the case of conflicts, each can appeal for the Premier to arbitrate among ministerial units and also in the relationship between ministries and provincial jurisdictions (Schurmann 1968; Lieberthal & Oksenberg 1988; Lieberthal & Lampton 1992).

Taken generally as the legal-bureaucratic ideal type, the public organization, including the government, differs from the economic organization in goal orientation, institutional structure, resource management, and the use of other managerial tools.[1] By and large, the policymaking process takes place in what Downs calls it as "flat hierarchy" (Downs 1967), meaning in China's case that central policy units interact with a relatively large number of subordinate units at the provincial level. The party-state hierarchy formally consists of four echelons: The central government, the provincial jurisdictions (or those with the equivalent status), the prefectural/municipal jurisdictions, and the county/urban district jurisdictions. The central government oversee 34 provincial status jurisdictions, embracing 23 provinces, four directly administered metropolitan cities, five autonomous regions, and two special administrative districts. Under the governance of the provincial jurisdictions, coupled with four directly administered mega-cities, there are 333 prefectural/municipal jurisdictions and 2,852 counties/urban districts, including 967 urban districts, 1,323 counties, 391 county status municipalities, and nearly 400 other units of autonomous counties as well as those of the same status, etc. (Zh.m.wikipedia.org, 3:32 pm, 7 October 2020; Huang 2020).

On the vertical dimension, each organizational unit in charge exercises command over its subordinate units within the framework of the party-state hierarchy. As the wording of "bargain" normally refers to the relationship between equals in both market and non-market context, it does not seem likely that the superordinate and subordinate are often in position to "bargain" with each other on an equal footing in a hierarchical relationship. To exercise command in the policymaking and implementation, theoretically speaking, the superordinate employs an inventory of administrative and managerial instruments in the case of social security policy, as noted by various authors (Lee 2019; Huang 2020; Qian 2021). However, it is likely that at the operational level, the policymaker would apply a mix of administrative and managerial instruments in different policy arenas (Qian 2021). And therefore, it is warranted to address the operational issues of policymaking and implementation in chosen empirical cases to account for particularity as well as variations in various policy arenas.

On the horizontal level, the organizational units of equal status interact with one another to attain common policy goals and carry out assigned tasks through an exchange of information, consultation, and coordination. As a rule, however, the relations between the government units of equal status rely upon neither market transactions nor the exercise of property rights. Bargaining takes place as a quid pro quo exchange of equal values often in the because the central authorities had but it is very limited in the administrative context both in China and elsewhere (Lee 2019). Nonetheless, the government unit and other public organizations often rely upon transactions (often including the element of bargaining) when they interact with non-governmental units in the marketplace in certain economic functions, such as procurement, purchasing, and contracting. Also, the government unit and other public organizations may impose user charges on some categories of services rendered to citizens in a relationship characterized as quasi-transactions. In the party-state hierarchy as just examined, the relationship between the central government and provincial/local jurisdiction constituted the core of the policymaking process in the case of public medical care insurance to be tackled in the next section.

The Central Government versus Provincial/Local Jurisdictions

When building an entirely new system of public medical care insurance, questions arise as to the roles the central government and provincial/local government each assume respectively. To begin with, the central government had the final say over the BMCI in a formal sense, while the provincial/local jurisdictions still had a share of policy responsibility, commanded financial resources, and enjoyed relatively large room of autonomy in the process of policymaking and implementation. In the matter of drafting, packaging and policy implementation, the central government tended to resort to a combination of persuasion, coordination, and, to some extent, the exercise of command in relation to provincial/local governments. It is well taken, that as a final resort, the central authorities were able to extract compliance from their provincial subordinates, because the central authorities had a say over appointment, promotion, and dismissal of the top-ranking officials and cadres at the provincial/local level, in addition to evaluation and supervision (Lee 2019; Huang 2020; Qian 2021).

In principle, provincial/local governments were given considerable financial resources commensurate with the policy responsibilities in the arena of social security, including medical care. In practice, however, the provincial/local government had to assume the policy responsibility often without sufficient financial resources for implementation throughout the healthcare reforms. Often taken as "load shedding," it was often observed in some cases of irregularity within the hierarchy of a provincial/local jurisdiction. For example, as policy responsibility was delegated downward to the lower echelons of the government, financial resources did not follow (Lee 2019). Like other cases of social security policy, moreover, the progress of the BMCI reform was dictated by the availability of financial resources.

The financial reforms had profound impacts on the social security reforms in general and health care reform during economic reform on two accounts. First, the central government assigned most of the responsibility of social security policy, together with the tasks of implementation, to the provincial/local jurisdictions, albeit the central government assumed a general leadership role in policymaking and implementation. Examples included policy initiation and policy direction, authorization of experimentation and pilot programs before each a given episode of policymaking, as well as evaluation and supervision after implementation and enforcement in what is taken as "ex ante and ex post interventions" (Qian 2021).

Second, the central government was able to establish considerable dominance over provincial/local jurisdictions through the financial reforms from 1980s to 1990s during economic reform, but it did not have any obligation to provide funding for social security reform, including the case of BMCI, URMCI and NRCMCI. The financial reforms were marked by two major policy episodes in a long-term trend starting from 1980: The "financial undertaking system" (FUS) of 1980 and the "revenue sharing system" (RSS) of 1994 (Ge & Gong 2007; 46–70; Gu 2008:109–29; Lee 2019). Starting in 1980, FUS allowed provincial/local governments a relatively large share of financial resources, thereby risking the excessive expansion of financial power at the provincial/local level from 1980 onward. The balance of financial power between the central and provincial/local level was not restored until the introduction of RSS in 1994. Consequently, there was registered a dramatic increase of revenue remittance to the central government, approximately in the range of 20 percent higher from 1994 onward, amid a corresponding shrinkage of revenue at the provincial/local level. It is estimated overall that after 1994, the provincial level was able to retain a range from 40 percent to 50 percent of total revenue, depending on the provincial unit (Gu 2008: 109–29; Duckett 2013; Lee 2019: 75–89; Huang 2020; Qian 2021). RSS of 1994 appeared to strengthen the central government's overall policymaking role but undermine the financial capacity of provincial/local jurisdictions to meet funding crisis of social security in a long run.

In such a restructuring of public financial management, the provincial/local jurisdictions found themselves heavily loaded in financing health care amid of overemphasis on economic growth at the expense of social security concerns (Ge & Gong 2007: 46–70; Lee 2019). This led to a relative shrinkage of public funding and a drastic increase in out-of-pocket payments (OPP) by patients in the health care sector, the climax being reached during the late 1990s and early 2000s (Ge & Gong 2007: 46–98; Duckett 2011; 35–58; Huang 2013: 53–81; Lee 2019: 75–97). The central government could not lend much help to funding of BMCI at the provincial/local level during economic reform. In the cases of URMCI and NRCMCI, however, the central government assumed a significant role to provide enrollees subsidy to premium contribution for the first time. Meanwhile, it played an entirely new role in maintaining some measure of equality among jurisdictions, mainly, to assist the less developed and more disadvantageous regions and provincial jurisdictions as well as marginalized sectors of the population (Lee 2019; Huang 2020; Chapters 9–11).

As a review of the concrete situation, it was apparent that provincial/local jurisdictions were caught in the dilemma between the conventional funding programs of social security and lack of financial resources for any move in the direction of social security reforms, including healthcare reform. First, in many existing PFMC and LIMC programs, neither a set of managerial and financial mechanisms, nor an institutional entity was established to ensure an independent funding source for the provision of basic medical care benefits as just noted (Chapter 4). Second, it was not likely to make public financial resources available because the pro-growth policy enjoyed higher priority than social security. Also, it was not readily possible either to convert public assets to meet the funding needs for social security reform (Chapter 3; Lee 2019). Third, the financial stringency for social security policy was further aggravated by the increasing number of employees moved to the senior age bracket of the workforce as the matter of the natural age cycle (Peng, Cai & Zhou 1992: 3–25; Lee 2001: 115–31; Zheng 2011: 102–8; Chapter 4).

Besides, was no easy task in the transformation from the conventional funding mode of health care to the newly introduced BMCI. Policymakers had to ensure that the entitlements and benefits of the BMCI are made comparable with those of what the conventional funding had previously offered, if not in better terms, to honor the existing remuneration policy as well as historically rooted obligations that it entailed. Taken as "rigidity of welfare," accordingly, policymakers had to navigate through a narrow path of policy change by making the BMCI reform acceptable to enrollees of conventional funding programs, taking into full consideration of their vested interests, and thus minimizing social costs of large-scale restructuring. Moreover, in qualitative terms, BMCI represented a higher hurdle for policymakers to cross for it was an upgrade in all design, financing, and managements, for instance, the new component of HESI to be included for the new funding plans and to be managed with new form of risk pooling mechanisms (Chapters 8 and 12). At all levels of the party-state hierarchy, policy actors had to address HESI through SCMI (Chapter 8). With great financial difficulties and complicity of policy and management, provincial/local policy actors thus entered a new political arena where the BMCI was introduced.

The Political Dimension of Policymaking

Like other social security policy issues, the BMCI reform was concerned with a political maneuvering between the central government and provincial/local jurisdictions. Under the circumstances, the provincial/local jurisdictions were held financially responsible for making up funding gaps for the provision of medical care entitlements for all employees who had been originally hired under the CPE. The situation turned worse during the increasing proportion of senior members and retirees as well as financial difficulties of enterprise units under economic fluctuations during economic reform. Confronted with the policy crisis of social security, both the central government and the provincial/local jurisdictions were expected to find solutions to deal with the issues at hand. To deal with "historical debts" of the party-state entity, it appeared that the central policymakers tried hard to convince and cajole their provincial/local counterparts to set aside funding out of the available funds and fixed assets they held in order to finance social security entitlements, including basic medical care, in the transformation from the conventional funding mode to BMCI (Chapter 3).

Regarding the basic characteristic of the relationship between the central government and provincial/local jurisdictions, some evidence allows preliminary analysis on the theoretical alternatives as follows. First, can the relationship be taken as some sort of "bargaining" in the transaction in the marketplace, or rather a pure exercise of command within the party-state hierarchy? The study argues that so-called bargaining in public policy arena differs from that in the market situation. Here the central-local/provincial relationship was concerned largely with the game of how to allocate the shares of responsibility among echelons of the government, together with financial burden. The case of social security policy is not the same as the case of investment projects as noted several of authors on the subject-matter (Lieberthal

& Oksenberg 1988; Lieberthal & Lampton 1992). The former targeted the allocation of financial burden (responsibility) in making social security policy, not in
terms of "gain" in common usage, while the latter involved fighting for share of revenue derived from investments. Above all, the object of bargaining was not like the
commodity that carries material values as in case of market transactions. Second,
characteristic of "fragmented authoritarianism," multiple ministerial units and pro-
vincial/local governments were involved in the policymaking process, coupled
with overlaps in jurisdiction and responsibility in each policy arena (Lieberthal &
Lampton 1992: 1–30). However, In the case of health care reforms, there witnessed
considerable coordination in the policy initiation phase and beyond, just opposite
to disintegration and paralysis as entailed by "fragmented authoritarianism." And
often a top level leader was in charge of policymaking while a designated ministerial unit was responsible for overall coordination among other ministerial units and
provincial jurisdictions (Qian 2021).Third, it is likely that there existed some asymmetric information in the central-local/provincial relationship in the sense that the
latter had upper hands in terms of better access to information of the local situation
of each local/provincial jurisdictions (Huang 2020; Qian 2021). To a certain extent,
however, the gaps of asymmetric information could be bridged through the open
access of information and the dynamic of interactions within the group of policy
actors, for instance, participation in pilot programs and policy experimentation as
well as a series of meetings and conferences at the vertical and horizontal levels.

Working within the institutional framework and financial structure as just portrayed, policymakers at the central and local level had to act upon the policy issues of
public medical care insurance at hand through some form of coordination emerging
from economic reform. To begin with, there were four phases of policy evolution
from the early 1990s to 2010s, demonstrating how the central government tried to
take the initiative and coordinate the work of drafting as well as control the policy
agenda for the BMCI reform. And adjustments were made from one phase to another in view of the information gaps to be bridged (Zheng 2002: 119–59; Deng &
Liu 2008: 106–10; Zheng 2010: 18–20; Chen & Yi 2011: 1–56).

The first phase extended from 1993 to 1996 when the core ideas of the BMCI
reform were first articulated and tested through selected pilot programs conducted
by central policymakers based on research reports filed by the State Institutional
Reform Commission with input from other ministerial units. The said reform formally commenced in 1994, focusing on staff and workers in public enterprises.[2]
Meanwhile, provincial/local governments were given considerable room to par-
ticipate in policymaking. In the same year, accordingly, pilot programs were introduced in Jiujiang Municipality in Jiangxi Province and in Zhenjiang Municipality
in Jiangxu Province (Wang 2008). In substance, then, the main issue revolved
around the respective roles as well as the relationship of two accounts of the proposed basic medical care insurance (BMCI), namely, the Personal Account (PA)
and the Unified Social Funding Account (USFA), considering the types of services
and sources of payment for basic medical care.

The second phase lasted from 1996 to 1998, as the State Council authorized
further extension of pilot programs to more provincial and municipal jurisdictions,

in addition to making needed adjustments and refinement of policy stands and taking clues from feedback regarding previous policy experiments. During the second phase, policymakers at the central and provincial/local level appeared to reach a consensus to propose policy alternatives to fill two funding gaps: One had to do with the gap between the level of conventional funding modes (i.e., LIMC and PFMC) and the level of BMCI, and the other was concerned with the gap of above payment-ceiling, including HESI cases. These funding gaps were left uncovered by the PA USFA scheme in the first phase. It was evident in the second phase that the policy actors were confronted with the dilemma between the thrifty version and enriched version of BMCI. While policy actors (especially provincial/local jurisdictions) found the former preferable in terms of less financial burden, they could not easily forfeit the claim for non-wage compensation by the workforce in the public sector (to be elaborated in Chapter 8).

The third phase began in 1998 when the central policy leadership worked out a full-fledged program for basic medical care insurance (BMCI), signaling that its final draft was ready for a trial implementation throughout China (Zheng 2002: 139–48, 2010: 18–20). Ambitious as it was, the fourth phase starting in 2001, endeavored to integrate health care insurance with a broad social security system (Zheng 2002: 119–59; Deng 2008: 106–10; Chen & Yi 2011: 1–56). Finally, the fourth phase was coincided by debates on the controversy of "marketization" beginning in 2005, and in fact engendered much uncertainty about the central policymakers' intention in the minds of policymakers at the provincial/local level, leading to further amendments to their policy. But a clear picture emerged after the announcement of a "new medical care reform" in 2009.[3]

It appears that through four phases of policymaking exercises, there were several salient issues of policy deliberation involving policy actors at both the central and provincial/local levels, for instance, the linkage of PA to USFA, the supplementary medical care insurance (SMCI), and the dilemma between the a comparable version of conventional funding and a scaled-down design only to cover the portion of funding beyond the above payment-ceiling. However, these issues represent varying degrees of politicization with regard to the weighting of vested interests entailed in each type of choice, and it is worthwhile to dwell on it in the analysis of the following three empirical cases in the remaining passages.

Shanghai and Guangzhou Compared

As this study argues that the provincial/local governments were largely responsible for drafting, packaging, and implementation of their own versions of BMCI, it is pertinent to examine selected empirical cases, namely, Shanghai, Guangzhou and Shenzhen, to shed light on how the provincial/local governments took part in the policymaking process to formulate BMCI.

Among the three cases chosen for discussion, Shanghai enjoyed considerable autonomy of discretion because of its national reputation considering widely reported policy experiments of "total volume control and structural adjustment" as well as the "three synchronized reforms" of insurance, delivery, and drug management in

2000 (Hu 2001). Overall, the Shanghai municipal policymaking team treated the BMCI reform as an integral part of an overall restructuring of the healthcare system. Not only did the team have its own concerns about the healthcare system, but also, team members adopted their own distinctive approaches toward medical care insurance reform. First, they lent priority to spending control rather than merely to funding during the introduction of BMCI. For Shanghai's policymakers, in other words, the cutting of waste was no less important than the fundraising. Second, they sought to curtail medical expenditure by channeling patients to low-tier hospitals and community clinics at the urban district level, and by addressing the distorted allocation of health care resources featuring a "reverse pyramid" at the municipal level. They tried to overcome the excessive concentration of the cases of common and frequent illnesses at the higher-tier public hospitals that were better funded and equipped with better trained doctors for medically difficult cases, while under-utilizing lower-tier hospitals that were poorly funded and equipped with less trained personnel for common and frequent illnesses (Lee 2019). And third, they endeavored to control spending by strengthening managerial reform of public hospitals as well as tightening regulatory control over the pricing of pharmaceutical products. The Shanghai municipal policymaking team pertinently tackled the issue of abuse of drug franchises at the hospital level, for example, tendency in earning an excessively large portion of revenue from sale of drugs and imposing unfair burden on the patients during economic reform (Wu, Li & Li 2008: 70–1).

In Shanghai, the main thrust of the BMCI reform, featuring the urban insurance program (UIP), focused on the workforce conventionally employed within the perimeter of the CPE, including civil servants in the government, the personnel of service units, as well as the staff and workers in public enterprises in October 2000.[4] After some preparatory work, BMCI was put fully into practice beginning in 2003. It appears that the financial burden was heavy for building a solid foundation with an appropriately large scale to anticipate the funding requirement for a sizable cohort of senior personnel and retirees in an industrial base beginning early in the country. And its implementation was slower than expected, and lasted for more than 15 years, as the Shanghai municipal policymaking team built a solid deposit of funding to sustain the risk-pooling mechanisms of BMCI programs (Wu, Li & Li 2008: 70–1).

In Shanghai, the municipal policymaking team had to be confronted with the choice of either a higher or lower hurdle of funding. The higher hurdle meant an expensive option to comprehensively cover all types of services such as HESI cases, hospital care and clinical care (in Zone III, II & I). And the lower hurdle was a less expensive one, for instance, hospital care insurance (Zone II) and hospital insurance for retirees (Zone II and III; equivalent to HESI) short of clinical care in Zone 1. The higher hurdle appeared to be closer to the funding level of the conventional funding mode of PFMC and LIMC (Zone I, II & III). Under financial strains and pro-growth policy, the policymakers in Shanghai originally leaned toward a lower hurdle of funding for BMCI in choosing a design focusing on the HESI.

In fact, Guangzhou echoed Shanghai regarding the preference of a smaller budget for BMCI. And this was reflected in public opinion at the grassroots level during the staging period for BMCI. According to two surveys conducted in Guangzhou and Shanghai respectively in 1996, residents of both municipalities were generally receptive to an early thrifty version of BMCI centering on the major illness insurance (MII,) program only (namely hospital care in Zone II only, not above ceiling payment). In the two surveys on Shanghai and Guangzhou each in the eve of inaugurating BMCI, residents were asked how much they agreed with the following statement: One ought to be responsible for one's own expenses for minor illness, while for major illness one should take part in a "unified social funding" (*shehui tongchou* or USF) arrangement (i.e., a form of risk pooling at the municipal level). Those who registered either "agree" or "strongly agree" in Guangzhou totaled 69.8 percent compared to 14.6 percent who responded with "disagree" or "strongly disagree." By the same token, the responses of residents in Shanghai indicated that 69.6 percent were in favor ("agree" or "strongly agree") while 21.9 percent were not in favor ("disagree" or "strongly disagree") (Lee & Wang 2001). Despite this general attitude toward a smaller budget, they could still go along with the PA-USFA design, provided that the government and work unit were willing to shoulder the financial burden.

Guangzhou, subordinate to Guangdong province, serves as a good illustration of the decision-making role of a sub-provincial jurisdiction. According to the author's field investigations, the Guangzhou municipal leadership made two rounds of attempts to take part in the BMCI reform (Interview April 28, 2000; Lu 1999: 2–6). In the first round, Guangzhou had not seriously knocked on the door to join the club of BMCI reformers until May 1996 when it filed an application to take part in expanded pilot programs under the auspices of the Guangdong Provincial Government.[5] Meanwhile the Guangzhou municipal government drafted and submitted three separate sets of proposals with related policy papers to address medical care insurance reform in November 1997, early 1998, and January 1999, respectively; but for one reason or another, none of these draft proposals was taken seriously and translated into any formal policy (Interview April 28, 2000; Lu 1999: 2–6).

In the second round, the Guangzhou government acted upon a formal State Council request for the BMCI reform to be transmitted through the provincial authorities to the Guangzhou municipal level in the late 1990s (Interview April 28, 2000; Interview Mornings May 11, 2000; Interview Afternoon May 11, 2000). Accordingly, on April 2, 1999, the Guangdong provincial government put forth a formal request to the municipal government on the basis of the 1999 Proposal to governments at the municipal and county levels to draft and submit their plans for the BMCI reform.[6] Subsequently, the Guangzhou municipality government was able to introduce the BMCI reform covering employees of the planned sector by toeing the line of the State Council in 2001.[7] It took more than one decade, steadily from 2001 to the mid 2010s and beyond, for Guangzhou Municipality to incorporate public employees group by group into the BMCI program.[8] It appears that the funding foundation for BMCI was built upon premium contributions by enrollees (including senior employees and retirees) over a lengthy period of time, formally 15 years, although senior employees and retirees were helped by the municipal government and work units, a development to be addressed later in Chapters 6 and 7.

Based on the author's assessment in the field, it appears that Guangzhou municipal government inaugurated its own version of BMCI but not without facing the choice between the high hurdle and low hurdle type of funding just noted. On the one hand, the municipal policymaking team favored a cost-effective proposal by addressing the narrower but essential medical demands of the employees, namely, major illness insurance (or taken as MII, hospital care) in Zone II only, an option involving any amount less than the payment-ceiling. This means that the municipal policymaking team was reluctant to opt for the higher hurdle of financing (including both Zone I & II) in line with the previous policy commitments to conventional funding programs (e.g., PFMC and LIMC). While the work unit and provincial/ local government were held responsible for the financing of LIMC and PFMC, no financial reservoir had been built institutionally in the work unit or any other echelon of the party-state hierarchy to meet the entitlements of basic medical care under PFMC and LIMC prior to the BMCI reform. When the enrollees of conventional funding programs had to shift into the BMCI programs, question arose on how to pay for their enrolment in BMCI given that the work unit and local government had transferred revenue accumulated through saving—brought about by paying low wages to enrollees—for investments and economic growth over a long stretch of forced modernization. On the other hand, the municipal policymaking team had to consider the State Council's position regarding the AP-USFA design that combined the personal account (AP) with the unified social funding account (USFA), and it was finally incorporated into the version of BMCI falling into the types of medical care demands pertaining to both Zone I and Zone II. However, the State Council's position in favor of a PA-USFA design for BMCI was closest to the level of funding of, if not equivalent to, the conventional funding programs of PFMC and LIMC. By sheer force of command from higher echelons, the municipal government finally yielded to the position of the State Council, and, as a result, had to shoulder a heavier financial burden by accepting basic medical care falling in both Zones I and II in the name of "historical debts" (Chapter 2).

The Guangzhou case reflects an interesting twist in the evolution of BMCI from an early thrifty version of lower funding level to an enriched version of higher funding level. As the study suggests, the BMCI design started with the lower hurdle of funding and moved to a higher hurdle subsequently. Zhu Rongji made a statement on October 27, 1997, by advocating that basic medical care insurance ought to be low funding level and broad in coverage (*di shuiping guangfugai*), but he did not close the door to an enriched package embracing SMCI (Zhu 2002: 266–74; Huang 2020: 88; See Chapter 8).

According to Lu, a former ranking official of Guangzhou Bureau of Labor and Social Security, when the BMCI reform was discussed by the Standing Committee of the State Council at the end of 1998, Premier Zhu made clear his position for defending the vested interest of employees working within the planned sector. As Lu quoted, Premier Zhu stated, "Neither scaling down [of the service] nor reducing the funding level [of BMCI]," meaning to maintain both the level of medical care entitlements for staff and workers and, the level of the work unit's expenditure for medical care benefits unchanged (Lu 1999: 4). This clearly explains why the Guangzhou policy team turned away from their preceding policy preference for MII and instead adopted the PA-USFA design finally to better accommodate the vested interests of public employees in the CPE regime. Arguably, in other words, it is not warranted to forfeit the unfulfilled claims for social security (e.g., of LIMC or PFMC) for public personnel in the planned sector even though new social security funding programs, including BMCI, were introduced. Besides, in what is taken as the integration of entitlements with funding, the BMCI is managed by a non-departmental public entity and sustained by a full-ledged funding program consisting of risk pooling mechanisms.

Two Generations of BMCI in Shenzhen

Shenzhen represents one of the earliest examples of policy experimentation with regards to social security policy that began in the municipality in 1992, and the focus subsequently shifted to basic medical care in response to the central government's BMCI reform initiatives in the widely published pilot programs in Jiujiang and Zhenjiang implemented in 1994. Overall, Shenzhen worked with two generations of BMCI reform, the first generation lasting from 1996 to 2013 while the second generation starting from 2014 onward. Shenzhen's BMCI reform endeavored to cover both employees in the planned sector and those hired in the non-planned sector, such as flexibly employed personnel (including temporary workers, contractual workers, and "outside personnel") and agricultural laborers. The latter consisted of two-thirds of the labor force in Shenzhen. In terms of financial resources, however, the principal concern was still focused on BMCI, including a thrifty version introduced earlier, and an enriched version (with insurance for HESI events added subsequently). In common with Shanghai and Guangzhou, Shenzhen has the core features of the BMCI design, indicative of the emerging pattern of reform efforts across various jurisdictions.

For the first generation of the BMCI design, Shenzhen joined Jiujiang and Zhenjian to launch a policy experiment in 1996, and was able to reach the maturity of its policy development resulting in a full-fledged program of health care insurance (Hong 1995a, 1995b; Shenzhenshi shehui baoxiaozhi bianzhuan weiyuanhui 2004: 87–108; Qiu 2010: 272–4). In funding and managerial terms, Shenzhen's thrifty version of BMCI began by establishing a basic medical care insurance foundation (hereafter BMCIF, or the foundation) that played a pivotal role in financially managing the embryonic BMCI system (Shengzhenshi renmin zhengfu 2004: 246). On the one hand, the said foundation oversaw collecting premium contributions from enrollees as well as work units (e.g., government units, political parties, service units, and public enterprises) that had previously been covered by the PFMC and LIMC programs. On the other hand, the foundation was responsible for payment, together with co-payments from enrollees, to providing units for curative care and dispensary services rendered to enrollees, according to well-defined payment schemes.[9]

The first generation of BMCI offered three programs as follows: The hospital care insurance (hereafter, HCI), the comprehensive care insurance (hereafter, CCI), and the special care insurance (hereafter, SCI) (Shenzhenshi renmin zhengfu 2004). CCI catered to the basic medical care of those who had originally subscribed to PFMC and LIMC. In what is taken as "neo-traditionalism," SCI was reserved for veteran cadres who had taken part in the revolutionary undertaking prior to 1949 (as previously noted in Chapter 3). Both CCI and SCI were generous by providing not only insurance benefits for clinical care but also hospital care, and SCI had even better terms. By contrast, HCI served those enrollees who were only entitled to hospital care (i.e., Zone II), while they made their own out-of-pocket payment (OPP) for each clinical visit (i.e., Zone I), as in the case of temporary workers (or flexibly employed personnel, mostly manual laborers) and hired agricultural laborers. Hospital care normally commanded higher costs in cases of major illness. As a rule, the work unit made premium contributions on behalf of the enrollee. HCI operated with a set of risk-sharing mechanisms suitable to temporary workers and agricultural laborers who were, by and large, younger, and less likely to fall ill than enrollees of CCI normally at a higher age bracket, but still needed protection for more expensive medical events requiring hospital care. No less important was that enterprise units needed a basic medical care insurance operating with risk pooling mechanisms to cushion the impact of a financial burden unexpectedly caused by hospitalization of temporary workers and agricultural laborers (Shengzhenshi renmin zhengfu 2004).

Like other jurisdictions, Shenzhen faced the choice between the two hurdles of funding, namely, either higher hurdle or lower hurdle. For example, closest to the conventional funding mode, CCI, which was considered a "higher hurdle," was offered to all employees and retirees who had a household registration in Shenzhen. CCI embraced both clinical care and hospital care (in Zone I and II), two major areas equivalent to the funding level of the pre-reform programs of medical care (i.e., PFMC and LIMC). At the point of having to decide during the BMCI reform, the Shenzhen policymaking team also paid deference to the central government by accepting CCI, taking into consideration of the vested interests of existing employees within the planned sector (Shengzhenshi renmin zhengfu 2004).

Amid of public debates over health care reform after 2005 as well as the proposed "new medical care reform" in 2009, the Shenzhen government made several attempts to draft new versions of BMCI from 2008 to 2012, paving the way for the second generation. The second generation of BMCI was based upon the policy paper, the 2013 Measures, promulgated by the Shenzhen municipal government in September 2013, taking effect on January 1, 2014.[10]

The second generation consisted of three packages, named here as Scheme I, Scheme II, and Scheme III.[11] Scheme I superseded the early CCI scheme (in Zones I and II as noted), while still catering to the demands of employed personnel who had previously subscribed to the PFMC and LIMC in the planned sector within CPE. Scheme I covered both clinical visits and hospital care (i.e., Zones I and II) intended for personnel permanently employed in work units of the planned sector (i.e., government, quasi-government units, and public enterprises). They were normally residents and, therefore, holders of permanent household registration (called "blue ink" household registration) in Shenzhen (Shenzhenshi renmin zhengfu 2013). With corporatist coloring, it also embraced retirees from the public sector who were used to enjoying the benefits of the PFMC and LIMC with slightly better terms than younger and freshly employed personnel.[12]

The second generation of health care insurance was intended to tackle the public funding of medical care for the workforce in the non-planned sector too. Scheme II covers flexibly employed personnel, while Scheme III serves agricultural laborers (*nonmingong*).[13] Shenzhen, a fast-growing metropolitan city with exceedingly high labor mobility, relies heavily on this flexibility employed personnel and agricultural laborers for all kinds of services, construction and industries in the jurisdiction. The two schemes, which overlap in hospital care insurance (HCI) for the first generation prior to 2013, are mainly designed, though not exclusively, to meet the demands of personnel who came to work in the jurisdiction and had yet to establish permanent household registration in Shenzhen. Schemes II and III were concerned with employees in the non-planned sector to be saved for further analysis in Chapter 9.

Concluding Remarks

The foregoing analysis endeavored to examine the policymaking process regarding the healthcare reform. The study argues that the provincial/local governments tended to assume both policy responsibility and heavy financial burden. While facing uncertainty, overall, policymakers worked with a sequential decision-making model whereby policymaking was guided by feedback culled from trial implementations, pilot programs and policy experiments. Based on the case study across jurisdictions, it was found that some common features of BMCI were shaped and put into practice nationwide, coupled with some variations among different jurisdictions.

In the policymaking process pertaining to BMCI, top policymakers at the central and provincial/local level were not purely policy-oriented. They had to face political decisions regarding vested interests of various sectors as well. In the foregoing analysis, the study tackled the issue of alienation of entitlements from funding, namely, unfunded, and under-funded programs for basic medical care that were a legacy of the past, for example, PFMC and LIMC, and reviewed how the issue was resolved as the BMCI was introduced. It became an exercise for the central government to persuade provincial/local governments to find the ways and means to take care of vested interests of the former enrollees of PFMC and LIMC in the designing and packaging of BMCI. Accordingly, this study undertakes to examine the issue of "historical debts" in the designs and implementation of BMCI in some detail in Chapters 6–8.

Notes

1 The public organization (including the government) differs from the economic organization in many ways, but the former entertains multiple policy goals while the latter normally works with narrowly chosen economic goals, for example, profit/revenue pursuits (Downs 1967; Rainey 1991; Gortner, Mahler & Nicholson 1997; Hughes 1998). In addition, both need to depend on resource management to attend to the goals. By and large, resources carry greater weight in the economic organization than the public organization. Theoretically speaking, when the public organization needs to learn from

the economic organization, it tends to be more relevant and successful to focus on the issues of resource management. As a rule, the economic organization does not address the issue of externality—a policy concern of the public organization. Health care is a case on the point (Lee 2019).

2 The first phase began with the policy paper "Opinion Concerning the Reform of the Health Care System of Staff and Workers" (hereafter, the 1994 Opinion) issued jointly by the State Institutional Reform Commission, the Ministry of Finance, the Ministry of Labor, and the Ministry of Health Care on April 14, 1994 (Chen & Yi 2011: 1–56).

3 The new medical care reform is based on the policy paper titled "Opinion on Further Reform of the Medical and Health Care System" (hereafter, 2009 Opinion) issued on March 17, 2009 (Chen & Yi 2011: 8–22).

4 The full title of the 2000 Measures reads as follows: The Measures regarding Basic Medical Care Insurance for Staff and Workers in the Cities and Towns of Shanghai Municipality (hereafter, 2000 Measures), promulgated on October 20, 2000 (Shanghai remin zhengfu 2001).

5 Accordingly, at the municipal level, a medical care reform leadership team was formed, and the Office of Medical Care Reform that included participating units (such as the Health Care Bureau, Finance Bureau, Social Insurance Bureau, Pricing Bureau, Personnel Bureau, Planning Commission, Institutional Reform Commission, Federation of Labor Unions, and the Academy of Social Science) was established in November 1996 (Interview April 28, 2000).

6 As issued and circulated, the draft is called the "Proposal for Planning Reform of the Basic Medical Care Insurance System for Staff and Workers in Towns and Cities in Guangdong Province" (hereafter, 1999 Proposal) on April 2, 1999 (Guangdongsheng remin zhengfu 1999). To follow the 1999 Proposal, the Guangzhou government had to work within the framework as outlined by two main policy papers, one from the State Council in 1998 (Guofa [1998] No. 44) and the other from the provincial government in April 1999 (Yefu [1999] No. 31) (Interview April 28, 2000).

7 In official terms, the Guangzhou municipal government approved the introduction of the basic medical care insurance system in June 2001, and it was put in operation in September 2001. The basic medical care insurance program works on the basis of the policy paper called the "Measures for the Trial Implementation of Basic Medical Care Insurance in the Cities and Towns of Guangzhou Municipality" (taken as the 2001 Measures), which was first issued by the Office of the People's Government of Guangzhou Municipality on November 1, 2001 (Guangzhou nianjian bianchuan weiyuanhui 2002).

8 Figures in the Guangzhou Yearbook show that in the basic medical care insurance program, enrollment began with 1,086,445 in 2002, then grew steadily, reaching 7,248,482 in 2011 (Guangzhou nianjian bianzhuan weiyuanhui 2002–2012)

9 The schemes of payment feature the following: (1) a quota for co-payment structured according to age, (2) a quota for insurance payment coupled with a co-payment at 10 percent of the entire medical bill, and (3) a deductible normally exceeding 8 percent of the average annual wage (Shengzhenshi remin zhengfu 2004).

10 The full title reads as "Measures for Social Medical Care Insurance for Shenzhen Municipality," issued by the Shenzhen Government on September 29, 2013, abbreviated here as the 2013 Measures (Shengshenshi renmin zhengfu 2013).

11 In fact, the drafters of policy papers on social medical insurance have changed their minds several times with respect to the appropriate names for packages of social medical care insurance. In the original text of the 2013 Measures, *dangci* is used, and its closest literal translation is "bracket," "class," or "grade," with a connotation of categories of higher and lower quality. Here "Scheme I, II, and III" are used in order to take away the stigma associated with the names of different packages of medical insurance (Shengzhenshi renmin zhengfu 2013).

12　For the status of retirees, their entitlements and privileges are defined in accordance with the 2013 Measures (Shenzhenshi renmin zhengfu 2013). However, the "2013 Measures" did not address "special medical care insurance" *(teshu yiliao baoxian;* abbreviated as SMCI hereafter), that is, the privileged insurance program for cadres on "leave for recuperation" *(lixiu)* (Shengzhenshi renmin zhengfu 2004).

13　While the work unit has to subscribe to Scheme I on behalf of its employees with household registration, it may choose either Scheme I, Scheme II, or Scheme III on behalf of employees without household registration (Shengzhenshi renmin zhengfu 2013).

References

Chen, W., & Yi, L. 2011. *2011 nian zhongguo yiyao weisheng gaige tizhi baogao* (*The Year 2011 Report of Medical and Dispensary Care in China*). Beijing: Xiehe yike daxue.

Cheng, L., & Dong, S. 1999. Guanyu yiliao baoxian feiyong kongzhi wenti de yanjiu (Research on the control issue of expenditure for medical care). In Zhang, D., Liu, D., & Zhang, B. (Eds.), *Shehui baozhang zhidu gaige zinan* (*The Guide for the Reform of the Social Security System*). Beijing: Gaige chubanshe. 391–401.

Deng, D., & Liu, C. 2008. Chengxiang yiliao baozhang tixi xianzhuang ji pingjia (The current state as well as appraisal of the medical care system in cities and countryside). In Deng, D., Liu, C. et al. (Eds.), *2006–2007 nian Zhongguo shehui baozhang yu fazhan baogao* (*The 2006–2007 Report on and Development of the Social Security System in Cities and Countryside*). Beijing: Remin chubanshe. 113–48.

Downs, A. 1967. *Inside Bureaucracy.* Boston, MA: Little, Brown and Company.

Duckett, J. 2011. *The Chinese State's Retreat from Health.* London & New York: Routledge.

Ge, Y., & Gong, S. 2007. *Zhongguo yiliao gaige: wenti, genyuan yu chulu* (*China's Medical Care Reform: The Issues, Roots and Solution*). Beijing: Zhongguo fazhan chubanshe.

Gortner, H. F., Mahler, J., & Nicholson, J. B. 1997. *Organization Theory, A Public Perspective.* Fort Worth, TX, Philadelphia, PA & San Diego, CA: Harcourt Brace College Publishers.

Gu, X. 2008. *Zuoxian quanmin yigai, zhongguo xinyigai de zhanlue yu zhanshu* (*Towards Universal Coverage of Healthcare Insurance, the Strategical Choices and Institutional Frameworks of the New Health Care Reform*). Beijing: Zhongguo laodong shehui baozhang chubanshe.

Guangzhou nianjian bianzhuan weiyuanhui 2002–12. *Guangzhou nianjian 2002–12* (*Yearbook of Guangzhou 2002–12*).

Hong, W. 1995a. Jianli geren yiliao zhanghui yu shehui tongchou xiangjiehe moshi de xingchangshi (New adventure in establishing the model for combining personal accounts with unified social funding). *Zhongguo weisheng shiye guanli* (*The Management of China's Health Care Enterprises*): 8.

Hong, W. 1995b. Shenzhensi yiliao baoxian gaige de nandian yu chulu (The difficulties and solution in the medical care insurance reform in Shenzhen municipality). *Zhongguo weisheng shiye guanli* (*The Management of China's Health Care Enterprises*): 1.

Hu, S. 2001. *Yiliao baoxian he fuwu zhidu* (*The System of Medical Care Insurance and Services*). Chengdu: Sichuan renmin chubanshe.

Huang, Y. 2013. *Governing Health in Contemporary China.* London & New York: Routledge.

Huang, X. 2020. *Social Protection under Authoritarianism, Health Politics and Policy in China.* New York: Oxford University Press.

Hughes, O. E. 1998. *Public Management & Administration, An Introduction.* Houndmills & New York: Palgrave.

Interview (one interviewee) April 28, 2000.

Interview (one interviewee) May 12, 2000.

Interview (two interviewees) May 11, 2000.

Interview (two interviewees) morning May 11, 2000.

Lee, P. 2001. The provision of occupational benefits in the Chinese industrial sector: the case study of Guangzhou. In Lee, P, & Lo, C. W. (Eds.), *Remaking China's Public Management*. Westport, CT & London: Quorum Books. 113–32.

Lee, P. 2013. China's health care reform in perspective. In Cheung, F., Woo, J. & Law, C. (Eds.), *Health Systems: Challenges, Visions, and Reforms from a Comparative-Global Perspective*. Hong Kong: HKIAPS, Chinese University of Hong Kong. 331–58.

Lee, P. 2019. *Re-engineering Affordable Care Policy in China, Is Marketization a Solution?* London & New York: Routledge.

Lee, P. & Wang, C. 2001. The tale of two cities: rolling back the boundary of the welfare state during the reform era. In Lee, P., & Lo, C. W. (Eds.), *Remaking China's Public Management*. Westport, CT & London: Quorum Books. 67–95.

Lieberthal, K., & Lampton, D. (Eds.) 1992. *Bureaucracy, Politics and Decision Making in Post-Mao China*. Berkley & Los Angeles & London: University of California Press.

Lieberthal, K., & Oksenberg, M., 1988. *Policy Making in China: Leaders, Structures, and Processes*. Princeton, NJ: Princeton University Press.

Liu, S. 2004. *Zhongguo yiliao gaige de zhidu fenxi (Systems Analysis of China's Medical Care Insurance)*. Taipei: National Cheng Chi University.

Lu, G. 1999. Zhongguo yigai de jinchen he Guangzhou yigai ijzhan (The progress of China's care reform and development of Guangzhou's medical care reform). *Shishi Guangdong Shuzihua de kexingxin yanjiu (The Feasibility Research on the Implementation of Digitalized Medical Care in Guangdong)*. File://D:\document\content.him April/28: 2–6.

Peng, R., Cai, R. & Zhou, C. (Eds.) 1992. *Zhongguo gaige congshu (The Encyclopedia of China's Reform)*. Dalian: Dalian chubanshe.

Qian, J. 2021. *The Political Economy of Making and Implementing Social Policy in China*. Singapore: Palgrave Macmillian

Qiu, X. 2010. Shenzhen shehui baoxian shiye fazhan lichen yu zhanwang (The progress and prospect in the development of social insurance enterprises in Shenzhen). In Le, Z., & Zu, Y. (Eds.), *Shenzhen shehui fazhan baogao (The Report of Social Development in Shenzhen)*. Beijing: Shehui kexue wenxian chubanshe.

Rainey, H. G. 1991. *Understanding and Managing Public Organizations*. San Francisco, CA: Jossey-Bass Inc.

Schurmann, F. 1968. *Ideology and Organization in Communist China*. 2nd ed. Berkeley & Los Angeles: University of California Press.

Shanghai renmin zhengfu 2001. Shanghai chengzhen zhigong jibaen yiliao baoxian banfa (The measures of basic medical care insurance for staff and workers in cities and towns of Shanghai). In Liu, J. *Shanghai wensheng nianbao 2001 (Yearbook of Health Care 2001)*. Shanghai: Shanghai kexue jishu wenxian chubanshe. 205–10.

Shanghaishi caizhengbu 2001. Guanyu zai benshi yiliao jigou zhankai yaopin jizhong zhaobiao caigou shidian gongzuo de rougan yijian (Several opinions concerning the task of pilot programs in the procurement of pharmaceutical products through unified collective bidding in the municipality). In Liu, J. (Ed.), *Shanghai weisheng nianjian 2001 (Shanghai Yearbook of Health Care 2001)*. Shanghai: Shanghai kexue jishu wenxian chubanshe.

Shanghaishi remin zhengfu 2010. Shanghaishi chengzhen zhigong jiben yiliao baoxian banfa (The measures for basic medical care insurance for staff and workers in cities and towns of Shanghai municipality). www.shanghai.gov.cn/shanghai/node2314/node3125/node3127/suerobject6a1259.himl.

Shenzhenshi renmin zhengfu 2013. Shenzhenshi shehui baoxian banfa (The measures for social medical care insurance in Shenzhen municipality).

Shenzhenshi shehui baoxianzhi bianzhuan weiyuanhui 2004. Yiliao baoxianzhi (medical care insurance system). In Shenzhenshi shehui baoxianzhi bianzhuan weiyuanhui (Ed.) *Shenzhenshi shehui baoxianzhi* (*The Journal of Social Insurance in Zhenzhen Municipality*). Shenzhen: Haitian chubanshe.

Wang, D. 2008. *Zhongguo yiliao baozhang zhidu gaige* (*The Reform of the Medical Care Security System in China*). Beijing: Zhongguo shehui kexue chubanshe.

Wu, Z., Li, Y., & Li, X. 2008. Shanghai yiliao baozhang zhidu gaige yu fazhan baogao, 2008. (The report on Shanghai medical care reform and development, 2008). In Wong, H. (Ed.), *Shanghai shehui baozhang gaige yu fazhan baogao 2008* (*The Report on Social Security Reform and Development in Shanghai 2008)*. Beijing: Shehui kexue wenxian chubanshe.

Zheng, G. 2002. Zhongguo zhigong yiliao baozhang zhidu bianqian yu pingu (The change within and the evaluation of medical care security for workers and staff in China). In Zheng, G. et al. (Eds.), *Zhongguo shehui baozhang zhidu bianqian yu pinggu* (*The Change within and Evaluation of the Social Security System in China*). Beijing: Renmin daxue chubanshe. 119–59.

Zheng, G. 2010. Gongli yiyuan chengben hesuan yu qiye chengben hesuan de bijiao fenxi (An analysis of costs accounting comparing public hospitals and enterprises). *Zhongguo weisheng jingji* (*China's Health Care Economics*) (29): 11.

Zheng, G. 2011. Zhonguo yiliao baozhang gaige yu fazhan zhanlue (The development strategy for medical care security in China). *Shehui baozhang zhidu* (*Social Security System*) 2: 37–44.

Zheng, B., Gao, Q., & Yu, H. 2010. Xinzhongguo shehui baozhang zhidu de bianqian yu fazhan (The change and development of social security in China). In Zou, D. (Eds.), *Zhongguo shehui baozhang fazhan baogao, No. 4* (*The Report of Development of Social Security in China, No. 4*). Beijing: Shehui kexue wenxian chubanshe. 26–8.

Zhu R. 2002. Guanyu zhigong yiliao baozhang zhidu gaige wenti (Issues regarding the reform medical care security system of staff and workers). In Laodong he shehui baozhangbu & zhonggong zhongyang wenxian yanjiushi (Eds.), *Xinshiqi laodong he shehui baozhang zhongyao wenxian xuanbian* (*Selected Important Documents of Labor and Social Security during the New Era*). Beijing: Zhongguo shehui baozhang chubanshe & zhong yang wenxian chubanshe. 266–74.

6 Types and Provision of Basic Medical Care

The BMCI reform represents the rise of the hybrid mode of governance in the realm of public policy. And it is concerned with the introduction of the markets into public policy, accompanying the growth of hierarchies. It is often policy-oriented, operating in the political arena, and it is not reducible to profit/revenue pursuits in the marketplace. To illustrate how the hybrid mode of governance took shape, the chapter will deal with the exercise of program specificity, examining how BMCI financially makes medical care services available and accessible to enrollees, and covering such issues as payment schemes, spending control measures, transaction-centered management, and the size of a jurisdiction among others. Meanwhile the study will try to make comparisons among public organizations within a nation by demonstrating how the hybrid mode of governance was built in some selected jurisdictions at the provincial/local level. such as Guangzhou, Shanghai, and Shenzhen

The chapter is focused on the exercise of program specificity (including product/service product) pertaining to BMCI, addressing the types and provision of basic medical care services. Moreover, the study endeavors to discuss two issues arising from the process of designing and introducing BMCI in China. First, what kinds of services ought to be included? This study will discuss issues of product/service specificity in the BMCI reform, for example, the operational definition of basic medical care, and the use of listings and catalogs to ensure that enrollees have access to the right kinds of services. And second, how is the insurance funding to be provided? The kind of insurance funding not only dictates the available sum of spending but also the choices of services. Also, in theoretical terms, the main concern here rests on the balance between the financing side of BMCI and the spending side amidst the process of marketization.

Analytical Dimensions of Program Specificity

While inaugurating BMCI, the central policymakers made the first attempt to address the issue of program specificity in 1994 in connection with pilot programs in Jiujiang municipality at Jiangshu province and Zhenjiang municipality at Jiangxi province. As summarized in the "1994 Opinion," the central policymakers put forth guiding principles covering four analytical dimensions as follows: (1) the

DOI: 10.4324/9781003389934-8

"low level" of medical care services, (2) the broad coverage of membership, (3) co-insurance with premium contributions by both the employer and employee in a given work unit, and (4) the proposed two-account scheme of PA-USFA combining the Personal Account (PA) with the Unified Social Funding Account (USFA).[1] Each of four dimensions just noted highlights some distinct characteristics of market transactions associated with BMCI, albeit some issues of operational definition as well as theoretical concerns remain to be tackled.

It is germane to dwell briefly on the four analytical dimensions regarding the program specificity of BMCI and then proceed to examine policy implications on each. Here "low level" refers to both the funding level and types of curative care service (including drugs and devices), namely, essential (or "basic" so to speak) curative care services rendered at the least funding level. "Broad coverage" is concerned with membership, that is, the eligibility of enrollment of all employees (both public and non-public sectors) in each jurisdiction, normally coupled with the broadest fundraising base. Co-insurance means that both employer and employee must contribute a share of the insurance premium. The combination of "two accounts" pertains to the PA-USFA scheme that combines the personal account (PA) for outpatient services (i.e., clinical care) with the "unified social funding" account (USFA) for inpatient services (i.e., hospital care). Theoretically speaking, the two accounts are interlocking, and an operational linkage between the two accounts was subsequently worked out in the process of implementation (Guojia Tigaiwei et al. 1999a: 100–3; Wu & Chen 1999: 364; Song & Liu 2001: 116–7).

Centering on "low level" medical care, extensive discussions among members of the policy circle were devoted to the issue of product/service specificity although it is conceptually intertwined with program specificity—the means and ways (e.g., skills and knowledge, managerial and marketing designs, financial schemes, production technology, etc.) pertaining to the production of products and delivery of services. Often product/service specificity goes beyond the adoption of an operational definition, and it could amount to the choices of policy alternatives (Du & Ding 2008; Du et al. 2008: 13–8).

To begin with, one finds several shades of meaning for "basic" medical care services relevant to the operational definition of the "low level," and these shades of meaning often overlap. First, the so-called "low level" is defined as a bare minimum but adequate level of services in medical, professional, and technical terms. Second, "low level" is taken as identical with the government's policy choice of affordable care at a given funding level as mandated, for example, the funding levels, types, and standards of curative care services mandated by the state and often funded by public finance, including revenue remittance and tax revenue. By the same token, it may refer to a "reasonable" funding level of medical care provision in accordance with the scope and standards as stipulated by the state, as the state's policy is an unspecified category. Third, from a specific social security vantage, low-level medical care is treated as a form of social welfare, of which the funding level is normally lower than that of insurance, therefore equivalent to social relief. Fourth, "low level" is culturally defined in terms of criteria and norms of social acceptability among the residents of a community (Peng 1996; Cheng & Dong 1999; Guojia Tigaiwei et al. 1999a, 1999b; Guowuyuan 1998; Lee 2013).

It appears that "low level" created dissonance among competing interpretations in the process of marketization as the concept jeopardized maintaining common ground among various policy actors who stand on different organizational positions and represent divergent vested interests. As a result, the exercise of mandatory power over the selection of types of basic medical care often substituted for market choice as far as the transaction is concerned in BMCI markets. Here, in the case of BMCI, for example, low-level medical care was operationally treated as equivalent to the "basic medical care" that policymakers chose to endorse and finance. With pure financial concerns, would the operational definition of basic medical care mean to exclude high expenditure and serious illness (HESI) from the BMCI packages? Would it be appropriate to treat HESI as part of basic medical care? It does not seem that policymakers and analysts provided an answer during the early phase of the BMCI reform, albeit they soon made amendments (Chapter 12).

The exercise of program specificity in BMCI was marked by a transition from a thrifty version to an enriched version. With reference to the packaging exercise in the early 1990s, actors within the policy circle were inclined to choosing a thrifty version of basic medical care focusing on common and frequent cases of illness, reflecting the level of consumers' culture during the time, but a salient and strong expectation for the higher funding level and for more difficult and serious cases surfaced during later phases in drafting BMCI. Subsequently, policymakers and the public appeared to prefer an enriched version aiming to embrace HESI. At the end of the day, policymakers did not appear able to hold the funding level of BMCI at a lower level, making it to stay comparable to that of conventional funding mode of medical care.

Attesting the said transition in packaging BMCI, Premier Zhu Rongji made a statement regarding the funding level and coverage on October 27, 1997 in response to the briefing about the policy experimentation and pilot program nationwide. Zhu underscored the policy theme of low funding level and broad coverage. Concerning the low funding level, he argued on the grounds of financial burden and risk of deficit as well as China's status as a developing country. By broad coverage, he stressed that all territories, all enterprises, and all residents had to be included, with an eye on the basic living standards of the workforce, the unemployed personnel as well as enterprises in deficit and bankruptcy. It is noteworthy, nonetheless, that Zhu did not close the door for accommodating SMCI, the funding level of which went beyond the payment-ceiling (Zhu 2002: 266–74; Huang 2020: 88).

Reflecting the modest expectation of the funding level during the early phases of policymaking, Wu Ritu and Chen Jinfu, ranking officials of the Ministry of Labor and Social Security, argued that financial capacity had to take precedence over the demands of enrollees to answer, in operational terms, what was meant by "basic" (or essential) medical care insurance. Echoing Zhu's statements just noted, they argued that in light of the level of productivity at the current stage of economic development in China, the benefits of basic medical care insurance had to remain financially at a low level, that is, meaning a thrifty version of essential curative care insurance. About to the level of both premium contributions and expenditures for benefits, they recommend again that neither should these match the existing level of medical care consumption, nor it needed to catch up to increasing demands or even to compete with the insurance level of any advanced country (Wu & Chen 1999).

In the process of marketization, much emphasis was placed on the financial capacity of the government as well as the affordability for the enrollees concerned when dealing with the concept of "essential" (or "basic"). According to Wu and Chen, benefits and entitlements for essential curative care insurance should be set at a "low level" principally in terms of financial requirements (Wu & Chen 1999). Accordingly, the level of premium contributions should be tailored to the financial capacity of the work units: Neither too high, nor too low for most work units concerned. For instance, within a given option of a common risk-pooling scheme, policymakers had to avoid two extremes to overcome the issue of "adverse choice" in the markets, meaning that in operational and financial terms, the scheme of premium contributions ought not to be too high to require high-performing enterprises unjustifiably to overpay, nor too low to allow poor-performing units to take advantage of a "free ride."[2] And this view was echoed later in the choice of "basic figure," the range between 300 percent and 60 percent of average annual wage, in the calculation of premium as given in the remaining passages in this chapter.

Among some jurisdictions, moreover, the heated controversies of BMCI reform were fueled mainly by the anxiety about repeated overspendings and cost-containment measures characteristic of the preceding PFMC and/or LIMC programs. To maintain its sustainability, the design of BMCI was intended to ensure that, from the long-term perspective, the funding level be commensurate with the ability of the insured to pay. In the case of Hainan Province, for example, the newly proposed medical care insurance was committed to being lower than the conventional PFMC and LIMC in three areas: The level of premium contributions, the level of expenditure, and the growth rate of the revenue of the providing unit (Gao 1999: 383).

Program Specificity Amid Marketization

Furthermore, the policymaking needed to be confronted with two interconnected sets of issues of program specificity. The first set was focused on the types of product/service in BMCI. Theoretically speaking, the services of BMCI are considered private goods in the sense that they provide benefits marketable in that the benefits are attributable to the insured/ patient, and the costs of which are retrievable from the insured/patient through premium contribution (or user charges). In other words, the insured/patient needs to pay for charges/fees for each item of service that he/she receives from the provider through both insurance and OPP (e.g., deductible, co-payments etc.). While the patient benefits personally from medical care, moreover, the third party (e.g., undifferentiated multitude of members of the community) can take advantage of its externality, for instance, enhancing labor mobility, maintaining a healthy and productive labor force, controlling medical risks while competing in expanding markets, and absorbing the spill-over social costs of economic growth in China (Song & Liu 2001: 84–106).

As Chinese policy analysts Guan Zhiqiang, Cui Bin, and Don Chaohui take pain to explain: The health care reforms (including the BMCI reform) were designed to place more emphasis on providing collective goods, and quasi-collective goods dealing with "market failure" and the negative "externality" of economic activity, while maximizing the utility of public health policy (Guan, Chui & Dong 2007: 37–63). Also, it is considered partly as "worthy goods," a form of quasi-collective goods (e.g., financial protection, security, etc.) to the extent that the government plays an important role in its provision and financing (Savas 1987: 52–6).

The second set of issue of program specificity pertained to the funding modes, i.e., making the choice of public insurance, or subsidized public hospitals, or both. In the Chinese medical care system, the provision of basic medical care relies on two parallel channels of funding, one concerning public insurance, for instance, in case of BMCI, and the other regarding the low-price service rendered by the subsidized public hospital (Lee 2019). While the former' resource management is handled through a kind of the IRF system operating with the markets, through the latter, health care is treated as a public policy concern expected to be funded or subsidized through the ORF system relying on the mandatory power of the Party-state entity. And the latter is an integral part of the low-price policy in basic medical care. According to Prof Gu Xin, the low-price policy is enforced through the policy tool of public finance and regulatory control (Gu 2010: 1–36). From public policy considerations, sovereign planners intended to incorporate both funding channels into China's health care system. Public insurance was not intended to operate in isolation, but to work with subsidized public hospitals. Complementary with the low-price policy of basic medical care through subsidized public hospitals operating with the ORF system, the BMCI reform was intended to provide insurance funding to medical care services and thereby reduce OPP through the IRF system.

With the introduction of BMCI, the exercise of program spedificy entertained a fresh issue concerning HESI (including catastrophic medical events). The issue of HESI has to do with the type of service about the funding and spending above payment-ceiling in Zone III. With regards to the funding level, Zone I and Zone II combined are roughly equivalent to the package of services under the PA-USFA scheme, while Zone III is concerned with the expenditure that exceeds the payment-ceiling in the thrifty version of BMCI. In the early pilot programs in Jiujiang and Zhenjiang in 1994, the above payment-ceiling large expenditure was subject to availability of funding as well as approval of the head of the work unit in charge on an ad hoc basis (through either public finance or enterprise revenue). For the first time, the 1998 Decision put on the policy agenda the establishment of supplementary medical care insurance (SMCI) programs financially covering a main portion of Zone III, coupled with a comparable subsidy scheme for civil servants and members of some other public organizations in accordance with a policy paper subsequently circulated in 1998 and 2000 (Guowuyuan 1998).

By and large, Zone I is concerned with clinical care paid out jointly through PA and OPP of enrollees with personal savings as a key funding mechanism, while Zone II and Zone III rely heavily upon risk pooling mechanisms among a multitude of enrollees and work units to produce externality for all. BMCI benefits, especially in Zone II and Zone III, are taken as quasi-collective goods that often engender the unintended outcome of the free ride, the control of which requires the exercise of product/specificity, spending control measures and other forms of regulatory control.

Above all, the exercise of program specificity not only needed to embrace the work of product/service specificity, but also to establish and apply actuarial and financial schemes, regulatory control and managerial measures accompanying the provision of quasi-collective goods. Also, in all three zones, a variety of spending control measures was also set in place (for instance, co-payment, deductible, a ceiling for payment, catalogs/lists of services and drugs, and designated hospitals, clinics, and pharmacies), all requisites making the BMCI more complete as a full-fledged public medical care insurance program.

Hierarchies Engendered through Mandatory Power

For the provision of quasi-collective goods in the case of BMCI, the government needed to intervene by exercising mandatory power in the realms of financing, supervision and regulatory control, thereby propelling the growth of hierarchies that were embedded in markets. Zhang Zuoyi, Minister of Labor and Social Security, argued in 1998 that it was necessary for supervisory authorities to determine the scope and standards of "basic" curative care services maintain the fiscal well-being of the BMCI foundation based on the experience from the earlier reform of conventional funding programs, for example, PFMC and LIMC. In accordance with the 1996 Opinion and the 1998 Decision, it was urged that those ministries in charge should establish the scope, standards, and methods of calculation regarding curative care service, the catalogs and listed items of prescription drugs for curative care, as well as the standards and management of facilities and medical devices (Guowuyuan 1998: 110–1; Guojia Tigaiwei et al. 1999a:107).

In theoretical terms, product/service specificity is market-oriented with its main concern being the demands of the client. Nevertheless, it is often linked with other elements of program specificity, leading to the proliferation of regulatory control and managerial mechanisms with financial implications. In the process of marketization through BMCI, the exercise of product/service specificity was, operationally and managerially, connected with concrete ways and means of provision, for example, the so-called "three major catalogs" to cover prescribed medicine, curative care services, and medical devices respectively. In the case of Hainan Province, for instance, the jurisdiction promulgated a drug prescription catalog with 1,606 listed prescriptions to be included in payment, coupled with eight major categories of medicines excluded from payments. The same methods were extended to curative care and medical devices for examinations and treatments (Gao 1999: 386). These lists/catalogs of dispensary services have been strengthened through the introduction of collective-bidding procurement procedures as well. Through the exercise of product/service specificity, overall, sovereign planners lent considerable weight to the party-state hierarchies amid of introducing markets into public medical care insurance (Du 2007; Guan et al. 2007; Gu 2008; Lee 2019).

As this study has just enunciated the central government's position with reference to the various dimensions of basic medical care insurance, it is appropriate to have a look at how BMCI was marketed at the provincial/local level. In the case of Shanghai, for instance, the municipal government took five years from 1998 to 2003 to implement medical care insurance reform at full scale. To inaugurate the 2000 Measures, the municipal government worked on product/service specificity by adopting standard formats and practices that had been utilized throughout the country. Examples of the government's efforts included, as a first step, adopting the operational definition of basic medical care and introducing the scope and items of diagnoses and treatments pertaining to basic medical insurance (Shanghai yiliao baoxianju et al. 2002). Also, it lost no time in 2002 in introducing, for managerial purposes, a set of provisional measures regarding the scope and items of prescription drugs for BMCI (Shanghai yiliao baoxianju et al. 2003).

To build BMCI, furthermore, the municipal policymaking team made efforts to integrate the task of program specificity with the restructuring of medical care delivery by tackling, for instance, the issues of revenue control, financial management, pricing and drug procurement. Emphasis was also placed on the control over the excessively large portion of revenue and pricing of drugs that contributed to a rapid growth in expenditure for basic medical care throughout economic reform. The municipal government installed a set of relevant administrative measures and regulatory controls, for example, the "two-line management" of expenditure and revenue for prescription drugs in hospitals (Shanghai weishengju & Shanghai caizhengju 2001). In addition, the municipal government enforced the policy of "collective bidding" in the procurement of generic drugs (Shanghai caizhengju 2001). Accompanying the growth of hierarchies, considerable workload was involved in tasks regarding product/service specificity and other issues of program specificity while implementing BMCI. As hierarchies thrived in the marketization of BMCI, it is germane to try to identify, analyze, and characterize, in the remainder of this chapter, the kinds of organizational apparatus and managerial tools adopted.

Organizational Apparatus and Managerial Control

To treat the BMCI reform as a case of marketization, it is pertinent to examine how BMCI was organized, coordinated, and provided for; and how it dealt with such matters as the delineation of jurisdiction, nature and type of institution as well as key managerial functions in markets. To a certain extent, BMCI represented an alternative bureaucracy that was market-oriented, differing from regular government bureaucracy.

To build a "bureaucracy" to render BMCI services, the central policymakers were first confronted with the issue of the jurisdiction of BMCI in the conjunction of choosing an institutional design and managerial system during the late 1990s

(Guowuyuan 1998: 109). The size of jurisdiction was discussed considering the number of enrollees, the volume of basic medical care services, and the scale of funding for marketization. Theoretically speaking, a reasonable choice in the size of jurisdiction has to do with an ideal scale of risk-pooling mechanisms, an optimal level of management, balancing disparate stages of development among the regions, and the appropriate range of variation in the consumption level in the population served by a BMCI program (Wu & Chen 1999: 365). Considering the scale of risk pooling the larger the size of jurisdiction, the greater the number of enrollees, the bigger the volume of medical care service, and the greater the amount of revenue and expenditure to maintain and manage.

Addressing the size of jurisdiction in connection with building a new institutional apparatus for BMCI, Wu Ritu and Chen Jinpu argued on behalf of the top policymaking circle that the prefectural/municipal unit ought to be the ideal size of jurisdiction for BMCI. They added, in theoretical terms, that if the scale of risk pooling (i.e., "unified social funding") were fixed at the county (or municipal) level, for example, the scale of the financial pool would be too small to sustain the financial risks of medical care. If the scale of risk pooling were fixed at the provincial level, regional diversity and complexity would be too great to cope with. In some exceptional cases only, however, the county (or town of the same status) could be chosen as the unit to implement "unified funding" (i.e., risk pooling), given that in some prefectural/municipal jurisdictions, the levels of economic development were obviously uneven, and differences in the level of consumption by enrollees were too large to be bridged. Also, it was appropriate to introduce risk pooling mechanisms to some metropolitan areas such as Shanghai, Beijing, Tianjin, and Chongqing where the levels of economic development were relatively even and variations of consumption within each jurisdiction were small (Guowuyuan 1998: 109).

Questions arose on the feasibility of the said recommended choice of jurisdiction for BMCI pointing to the issue of whether the prefectural/municipal level assumed responsibility to manage healthcare prior to economic reform. If the recommendation had been accepted, BMCI would have had to be established in 333 prefectural/municipal jurisdictions throughout China, rather than over 2000 counties approximately. Considering Wu and Chen's policy recommendation, there was the obvious discrepancy of choice between the prefectural/municipal jurisdiction and the county jurisdiction as the organizational vehicle for BMCI.

The choice of the county was obviously deviated from that of the prefectural/municipal level as officially recommended during the inauguration of BMCI. How one can account for such a discrepancy? So far there has been no attempt to offer an explanation for it. It is likely that the county government, together with the work unit, used to be an important vehicle of financial management in China's local administration. And it was in a better position to assume financial responsibility. Since it had withheld the larger share of public funds and assets, substantial part of which was saving for social security payments.

Furthermore, the issue of jurisdiction is concerned with the membership and eligibility of an enrollee in BMCI. As Wu and Chen have argued, the eligibility to enroll in a BMCI program ought to be tied to the residential status rather than affiliation with a work unit only. Indicative of the trend of moving away from "work-unit collectivism," policymakers could find it more effective and feasible in addressing issues of funding, spending, delivery and accessibility and convenience of services to the enrollee by organizing and coordinating medical care on residential basis. Also, the work unit was simply too small to be an appropriate scale of risk pooling, albeit it represented a managerial level promising convenience and accessibility.

Placing emphasis on residence, Wu and Chen proposed adopting residential management—rather than trade-centered management—as a "unified funding" mechanism for BMCI. They urged, in addition, that all provincially and centrally affiliated units should take part in BMCI offered at the local/municipal level. Residential management meant to work at the local community level where the enrollees resided, and it was considered favorably for the sake of better use of health care resources as well as convenient and timely access of the insured to medical care services. Even in the case of railway, electricity, and oceanic shipping where staff and workers were highly mobile, it was still recommended for them to subscribe in "unified funding" programs at the local community level, whenever it was feasible (Wu & Chen 1999: 365: Lee 2019).

Further to the issue of residential management, it is theoretically warranted to examine the proposal of the new organizational apparatus to oversee BMCI. By design, often called "executive agency" (*zhixing jigou*) or "medical care insurance institute" was recommended, but it was up to the decision taken by respective jurisdictions. An executive agency mainly played a financial and managerial role in handling the collection of premium contributions and purchasing medical care services on behalf of the insured. Beyond the responsibility of budgeting and accounting, it acted as a holder of insurance funds, maintaining the financial independence and integrity, and being insulated from changing revenue conditions and policy fluctuations of the government concerned.

To have public insurance perform effectively, the top policymakers endeavored to provide the BMCI fund some institutional safeguard, not only maintaining its long-term stability and continuity, but also acting against arbitrary interference from "outside forces," for example, ironically, the party committee and government bureaucracy at the local level. To cope with the unwelcome intrusions, for example, the executive agency was given managerial and financial autonomy to run the BMCI program thereby being made institutionally insulated from changing policies and regulatory functions of the local government. Accordingly, it was proposed to develop the division of labor and delineate the responsibility between the bureaucratic units and executive agencies to curtail the former's undue interference with the latter's work. In what was taken as "the separation of policy from management" (*zhengshi fenkai*), the division of labor was introduced: Government departments were to assume the responsibility of policymaking, institution, and standards for medical care, while the executive agency would carry out the managerial tasks in charge of collection, payment, and management of medical care insurance on a day-to day-basis (Guojia Tigaiwei et al. 1999a, 1999b).

It was also imperative for policymakers to consider seriously how to establish a new form of public organization to hold and manage social security funds, and meanwhile to maintain its institutional autonomy and managerial independence and run it in an effective and efficient fashion. Ideally speaking, policymakers could adopt either non-departmental public entities (NDPEs) or a trust or foundation that is part of the legal tradition of the market economy of the West, but it did not seem feasible in China where the legal culture was relatively weak and the CPE remained dominant in economic development. There is evidence to suggest that sovereign planners seriously considered borrowing from the West and adopting the non-profit oriented public organization to run and manage social security funds.

In addition, the executive agency acted on behalf of the "foundation" (*jijin*), the kind of public fund that was institutionally nested in a bundle of laws and regulations and maintains independence from the government (Liu 2004: 169–71). From a broad perspective, neither was the executive agency part of the bureau management, nor was it command-oriented, acting as an extension of the government. By design, the executive agency was not a "service unit" either that normally performed some auxiliary functions of the government related to policy implementation in the public sector. Instead, one might treat the executive agency's charge over the medical care insurance program as market-oriented, mainly dealing with transactions with providers as well as premium contributors by the insured (i.e., employers and employees) through the IRF system.

As the study has examined salient characteristics as well as key issues pertaining to the executive agency, it is pertinent to shift our focus to the main features of the network of transactions in which the executive agency played a leading role in the remainder of this chapter.

Transaction-Centered Management

As previously noted, BMCI bears close resemblance to the German mandatory health insurance plans in that both rely on transaction mechanisms to handle not only the spending, but also the funding side of medical care insurance (Chapter 2). On the funding side, the enrollee (often the employee) needs to contribute a share of the premium to the insurer to pay for insurance benefits, in addition to another share shouldered by the employer. The said employer's share is considered as non-wage compensation to the enrollee (or employee). On the spending side, the insurer and enrollees have to pay the provider for a category of defined medical care services based on the service agreement upon which all actors agree. In the case of BMCI, the executive agency (or so-called social insurance institute, or medical care insurance institute) represented the insurer, holder of BMCI foundation, dealing with both provider and enrollee (together with the employer) respectively through a quid pro quo exchange of equal value in a market situation.

By design, a BMCI works as a network of relationship characterizing a transactional triad: First, between insurer (i.e., the executive agency) and insured (i.e., enrollee and employer); second, between insurer and provider; and third, between insured (i.e., enrollee/patient) and provider. The operation of transactional triad was subject to considerable constraints imposed by hierarchies, for example, the room of choice, actual competition, and contestability among all actors concerned.

Comparatively speaking, in the German case, the insured were given the choices of insurer and provider, allowing a greater degree of contestability among actors in question. However, it did not appear that China went as far as the German case. As a rule, the insured (employee and employer) only faced only one insurer, remaining as a question yet to be tackled in due course.

The New Public Management (NPM) marketizers would find an interesting parallel in the BMCI reform in China with reference to adopting some forms of "contractualism" like the quasi-market experiments in the UK (Pollit & Bouchaert 2004: 83–5). While the relationship of funding unit to the provider appears to be "contractual" in Chinese case, the executive agency seemingly behaves like "trust" in terms of purchasing function in the British case (Ferlie 1992; Ferlie et al. 1997: 56–87). In the British case, authors tend to treat the relationship of "trust" (or local government with commissioning role in other incidents) to the provider as "service agreement" of administrative nature rather than a pure contract in a strict legal sense. At best, the said relationship was even taken as commissioning rather than true commercial transaction. In the British case of quasi-market experiments, the purchasing side including the trust (or local government) that never developed into a full-fledged and independent actor in the marketplace, for example, the true purchaser in market transactions. Nor have the users (i.e. patients) ever acquired an institutional role of their own, enjoying autonomous financial power to pay for one's own medical bills. Instead, the third party (e.g., the trust or local government) paid on their behalf. From a comparative perspective, China's public medical care insurances (i.e., BMCI, URMCI, and NRCMCI) differed from the British NHS to the extent that the former worked through transactions in handling both funding and spending tasks but did not employ commissioning in terms of unilateral relationship of financial appropriation of the government to the provider.

In the BMCI design, the executive agency played a pivotal role to coordinate, organize, and manage funding and spending functions, relying on a transactional network of designated hospitals (*dingdian yiyuan*) and designated pharmacies (*dingdian yaofan*) on a short list, from which enrollees were given choices as to who was to be preferred, meaning that the selected providers had to compete with one another and courted the favor of their potential users in market situation.[3] In the Chinese case, it appeared that on the spending side, the executive agency worked with two types of providers, namely, designated hospitals and designated pharmacies, in a purchasing rather than commissioning relationship. The former, normally public hospitals, often operating under the undertaking responsibility system (URS), were revenue-oriented, but still under the bureau management regarding a variety of functions such as quality and quantity of products/services, pricing, and budgeting and accounting (Lee 2019). The latter, designated pharmacies, were also revenue-oriented and assumed corporate form. As a rule, insurance funding followed the enrollees (i.e., users) who received the services rendered by chosen, designated hospitals for curative care and by designated pharmacies for dispensary services respectively.

In case of BMCI, for instance, the executive agency assumed a pivotal funding role to substitute for the work unit of pre-reform vintage (i.e., public enterprise, service unit, government unit or other public organizations in PFMC and LIMC) in the delivery of basic medical care. The executive agency acted as the holder of BMCI foundation. And it was responsible for a portion of co-payment for medical care services, together with the enrollee's share, provided that both the work unit and enrollee had fulfilled their obligation for premium contributions. The effective operation of the transaction-centered management hinged on whether there existed a legal and institutional environment favorable to the working of the market; for instance, questions arose about corporate culture, the rule of law, the application of contracts to the arena of public policy, and the adjudication by the court. To consider the question of how the new "contractual" network featuring transactional triad was built amid the lingering cultural influence of CPE, it is germane to examine some empirical cases in Shenzhen and Guangzhou as given below. The two cases represented the varying mixes between the markets and the state.

To begin with, Shenzhen represents a typical case of transaction-centered management in BMCI, characterizing the heavy reliance on the market mechanisms. And the municipal policymaking team was able to make full use of transactions as the managerial tool by which basic medical care service could be delivered, as hierarchies were operationally fused markets. For example, designated providers were still subject to considerable regulatory control, having to abide by a set of managerial rules, such as keeping records for inspection for two years, providing an open listing of prices, and enforcing pricing regulations, among other things. Meanwhile providers acquired legal status to handle accounting matters involving payments from the medical care insurance institute. Within the transactional network with designated providers, the insurance institute, acting as the sole principal in the said system, was able to exercise considerable supervisory power to enforce spending control and to minimize costs. In addition, the said system sought to prevent and/or minimize irregular medical behavior, such as over-provision, which was often responsible for uncontrollable spending and the rising costs of medical care services (Shenzhensi renmin zhengfu 2013).

Comparing with Guangzhou, overall, Shenzhen's policymakers tended to rely more heavily on market tools in financial management in the case of BMCI. In accordance with the 2013 Measures, the municipal medical care insurance institute (called "executive agency" elsewhere) needed to choose and sign service agreements with designated medical care providing units (*dingdian yiliao jigou*) and designated retail drug stores (*dingdian lingshou jigou*) to provide services to the enrollees in exchange for payment for medical care services. These designated providers were selected from among a pool of qualified ones, i.e., those having fulfilled a certain set of professional and managerial criteria on a competitive basis. As a rule, all enrollees were required to receive medical care services such as diagnosis, treatment, tests, examinations, and hospital care at designated providing units and to buy prescription drugs at designated retail stores. Through service agreements, these designated units agreed to provide curative care services and dispensary services by observing a set of regulations and principles while meeting high medical and professional standards.

The next case involves Guangzhou, a major industrial city in south China, historically leaning toward light industries, and not enjoying as much autonomy comparable with Shenzhen as a municipality under the Special Economic Zone. Guangzhou had to work under the command of the provincial government of Guangdong during the BMCI reform, when it first prepared to introduce BMCI in 1999 and started treating the system of transaction-centered management of designated hospitals and pharmacies as part and parcel of spending control measures (Lu 1999; Interview May 28, 2000). As the system was put into practice on a trial basis in 2001, the Guangzhou municipal government constructed a network of designated hospitals to render curative care services and a network of designated pharmacies to provide dispensary services based on the transactional relations (Guangzhoushi renmin zhengfu 2001). In operational terms, the Bureau of Labor and Social Security (or BLSS) acted as the insurer to sign service agreements with providers (i.e., various hospitals and pharmacies). BLSS chose to sign service agreements only with participant providers that had already been licensed by the respective authorities, and to allow these designated providers to render services to the insured in accordance with service agreements meeting the fixed criteria and standards of services (Guangzhoushi renmin zhengfu 2001).

In practice, the insured (i.e., users) normally were given insurance cards for services at the designated hospitals and pharmacies. While Shenzhen tended to use the transaction-centered management to regulate markets, the Guangzhou government took advantage of its administratively dominant position to exercise considerable control directly by restricting providers and pharmacies from engaging in certain abusive and unnecessary medical care behavior leading to over-provision. It appeared that the Guangzhou government resorted to administrative rules and heavy-handed approaches to enforce control on providing units' spending (Guangzhoushi renmin zhengfu 2001).

In the two cases analyzed above, it is apparent that the provision of BMCI was mediated through transactions in the Chinese case, and both the spending and the financing side operated with market mechanisms. However, hierarchies grew with marketization due to special types of product/services (e.g., quasi-collective goods), and program requisites (e.g., monopoly and scale of economy). The study will further elaborate on the introduction of regulatory control—a defining feature of hierarchy—to transactions on the spending side in the sections to follow.

Payment Schemes and Spending Control

It is pertinent to examine, through the lens of one chosen case of Shenzhen, how payment schemes were installed and how spending control was imposed in conjunction with the delivery of medical care in BMCI. Like many other jurisdictions, the Shenzhen municipal government tried from the very beginning to install a variety of payment schemes and spending control measures in connection with the BMCI reform. For instance, the government introduced regulatory instruments and managerial measures targeted at cost control in 1996, 2003, and 2013, respectively. In some specific ways, the Shenzhen government formulated and implemented a variety of co-payment schemes not only to ensure "value for money" but also to discourage irregular and abusive spending behavior. It is noteworthy that several payment schemes were employed to enhance cost awareness and encourage prudent choices by enrollees, for example, through having co-payment tied to each medical bill systematically for curative care services, hospital care, prescription drugs, and the use of advanced devices.

In Shenzhen and other jurisdictions throughout China, co-payment was often termed "portion of self-payment" (*zhifu bili*), "subsidy" (*buzhu*), or "reimbursement" (*baoxiao*) to a certain proportion during the BMCI reform (Song & Liu 2001: 95–6; Zheng 2002: 140–2). For those who were entitled to an insurance payment for hospital care in Scheme I, II, and III, the enrollee normally could claim a reimbursement (or "portion of payment") amounting to 90 percent of the total medical bill (or alternately, a 10 percent co-payment), regardless of the tier of hospital. For a retiree, the portion of reimbursement is 95 percent (or a 5 percent co-payment), regardless of the hospital tier. In the case of specially approved medical devices, moreover, the reimbursement for each enrollee is 80 percent (or a 20 percent co-payment) for all three schemes alike (Shenzhen renmin zhengfu 2013: Article 56). Moreover, there was a form of deductible called "payment starting line" (*qifuxian*), abbreviated as PSL; or in other cases "payment starting criterion" (*qifubiaozhun*), abbreviated as PSC. Such modalities also allowed patients to make a claim for a larger payment such as for hospital care after having made the required initial payment.

The Shenzhen policymakers adopted a co-payment system for Scheme I that was associated with the PA-USFA scheme borrowed from the pilot programs of Jiujiang and Zhenjiang (Zheng 2002: 140–1). Under the Shenzhen's version of BMCI, moreover, hospital care and major illness were chargeable to the major illness fund (MIF), while the enrollee could claim insurance benefits as stipulated in the provisions of the insurance programs. For example, through Scheme I, the enrollee was required first to make a payment going beyond the deductible limit. As soon as the total amount of deductible was paid (e.g., 100 RMB for a first-tier hospital, 200 RMB for a second-tier hospital, and 300 RMB for a third-tier hospital), the insurance institute, having charged to USFA account and local supplementary medical care (LSMC) account according to fixed proportions, had to absorb a fixed portion of the expenditure for hospital care through the MIF (Shenzhen renmin zhengfu 2013: Article 55, 56). It is noteworthy in this case that the deductible payment scheme was structured to encourage better use of health resources at the lower-tier medical facilities.

In addition, there were some noticeable changes in the PA-USFA scheme in accordance with the 2013 Measures: Like the case of Guangzhou with an "enriched" version of PA, so to speak, the use of PA in Shenzhen was broadened to allow more discretion to the enrollee to share with family members and to pay for non-basic medical care services and drug prescriptions (Shenzhen renmin zhengfu 2013: Article 39).

Finally, the second generation of Shenzhen's BMCI medical care insurance incorporate cost control into the service delivery system, trying to maximize the use of health care resources by channeling patients to community clinics, relieving congestion at the high-tier hospital facilities, and thereby maintaining a low budget and lower costs for healthcare services as noted in Chapter 5. By doing so, the workload of designated hospitals in the higher tiers was expected to be lessened, and overall costs for basic medical care were to be put under control.

Concluding Remarks

The foregoing analysis has examined the four analytical dimensions concerning the exercise of program specificity pertaining to BMCI, addressing some key issues concerning the choices of the type of services and the ways of funding in BMCI. Furthermore, the study has tried to tackle the main issues in the design-ing of organizational apparatus and managerial tools regarding BMCI, coupled with the spending control measures. The study demonstrated how market mecha-nisms were incorporated into several key spending links in a public insurance program in which essential medical care was treated as a combination of both private goods and collective goods. Characteristics of the hybrid mode of gov-ernance, hierarchies (e.g., regulatory tools, vertical coordination through com-mand, etc.) grew at each key functional link where market mechanisms were installed. Examples include product/service specificity, program specificity (e.g., co-insurance, co-payment), executive agency (e.g., insurer), and transaction-cen-tered management.

Despite the institutional and managerial autonomy bestowed on the executive agency, the CPE's tradition of bureau management had not entirely loosened its grip on medical care insurance matters. For instance, the medical care insurance fund was still subject to the budgetary control of the state financial system. To min-imize uncertainty at the institutional and financial level, existing financial sources as well as financial obligations of the state and work unit have remained intact (Guowuyuan 1995: 6, 10; Guojia Tigaiwei 1999a: 101). Moreover, the conven-tional instruments of financial control and scrutiny over collection, expenditure, management, and delivery of services continued to play important roles in super-vising the medical care insurance fund, for example, regular reviews by bureaus in charge, auditing by financial bureaus, financial scrutiny by labor unions and the CRSW, and established supervisory bodies for the medical care insurance system (Guojia Tigaiwei 1999a: 102, 1999b; 107; Wu 1999: 367–8). In the BMCI reform, one may find a Chinese brand of "quangos" (quasi-autonomous non-governmental organizations), one of the most popular of the NPM designs among OECDs in the

1990s. It marks the rising trend toward the so-called one arm-length approach in performing a chosen block of functions constituting an essential component of a modern society and requiring firm and long-time financial commitments made by a country's top policymakers.

Notes

1 Literally speaking, the principle is put as: "low level, wide coverage, shared financial responsibility by two parties and the combining of personal accounts with a unified social funding account" (dishuiping; guanfugai; shuangfan fudan; tongzhang jiehe; Guowuyuan 1998; Guojia Tigaiwei et al. 1999a: 100–3).
2 It is, therefore, recommendable in the view of Wu and Chen that the premium contributions to essential curative care should be set at 6 percent of total wages in light of the actual financial capacity of enterprises and local financial units. Given as a controlling indicator, each jurisdiction could make necessary adjustments according to actual situations (Wu & Chen 1999: 366). In fact, Wu & Chen toed Premier Zhu's suggestion about the figure of 6 percent of total wages (Zhu 2002: 268).
3 The system of designated hospitals and pharmacies was introduced as an integral part of the medical care insurance reform beginning in the early and mid-1990s (Guowuyuan 1998; 110–1; Cheng & Dong 1999; Guaojia Tigaiwei et al. 1999b). During the expansion of pilot programs from 1996, designated hospitals and pharmacies were adopted as well, for example, in Xiamen (Interview January 23, 2002).

References

Cheng, L. & Dong, S. 1999. Guanyu yiliao baoxian feiyong kongzhi wenti de yanjiu (Research on the issue of controlling expenditure for medical care). In Zhang, D., Liu, D., & Zhang, B. (Eds.), *Shehui baozhang zhidu gaige zinan* (*The Guide for the Reform of the Social Security System*). Beijing: Gaige chubanshe. 391–401.

Du, L. 2007. Jianli jiben weisheng baojian zhidu, goujian duoyuanhua banyi xingeju (Establishing a basic health care system and constructing the new situation with multiple ways of managing medical care). In Du, L. et al. (Eds.), *Zhongguo yiliao weisheng baogao, No. 3* (*The Report on Medical and Health Care, No. 3*). Beijing: Shehui kexue wenxian chubanshe.

Du, L., & Ding, Z. 2008. Zhetongguo tese weisheng fuwu de linian zhengce he Shijian (The ideal policy and implementation of health care services with Chinese characteristics). In Du, L. et al. (Eds.), *Zhonguo yiliao weisheng fazhan baogao, No. 4* (*The Report on the Development of Medical and Health Care in China, No. 4*), Beijing: Shehui kexue wenxian chubanshe. 13–8.

Ferlie, E. 1992. The creation and evolution of quasi markets in the public sector: a problem for strategic management. *Strategic Management Journal* 13: 79–97.

Ferlie, E. et al. 1997. *The New Public Management in Action.* Oxford & New York: Oxford University Press.

Gao, R. 1999. Tansuo geren zhangfu yu gongji zhangfu fenbie yunzuo moshi, gongzhi yiliao feiyong guokai zenzhang de youxiao jizhi (Exploring the operational model of the separation of the individual account and collective account and building an effective control mechanism over the rapid increase of medical care expenditure). In Zheng, D., Liu, D., & Zhang, B (Eds.), *Shehui baozhang zhidu gaige zhinan* (*The Guide for the Reform of the Social Security System*). Beijing: Gaige chubanshe. 382–90.

Gu, X. 2008. *Zouxian quanmian yibao: Zhongguo xinyigai de zhanlue yu zhanshu* (*Toward Comprehensive Medical Care Insurance: Strategy and Tactic in China's New Medical Care Reform*). Beijing: Zhongguo laodong chubanshe.

Gu, X. 2010. *Quanmin yiliao de xintansuo* (*The New Exploration of National Health Insurance*). Beijing: Shehui kexue wenxian chubanshe.

Guan, Z. et al. 2007. Zhongguo weisheng gaige yu yiliao baozhang tixi jianshe de zongsilu (Overall considerations on health care reform as well as constructing a medical care security system in China). In Chen, J., & Wang, Y. (Eds.), *Zhongguo shehui baoxian fazhan baogao* (*The Report on the Development of Social Insurance*). Beijing: Shehui kexue wenxian chubanshe.

Guan, Z., Chui, B. & Dong, C. 2007. Chengchen zhigong jiben yiliao baoxian zhidu de fazhan (The development of the basic medical care insurance system for staff and workers in cities and towns). In Chen, J., & Wang, Y. *Zhonguo shehui baozhang zhidu fazhan baogao, No. 7* (*The Report on the Development of the Social Security System in China, No. 7*). Beijing: Shehui kexue wenxian chubanshe. 37–63.

Guangzhoushi renmin zhengfu 2001. Guangzhou chengzhen zhigong jiben yiliao baoxian shixin banfa (The measures for the trial-implementation of basic medical care insurance for staff and workers in cities and towns). November 1.

Guojia Tigaiwei et al. 1999a. Guanyu zhigong yiliao zhidu gaige de shidian yijian (Opinions concerning the reform of the medical care system for staff and workers). In Zheng, D., Liu, D., & Zhang, B. (Eds.), *Shehui baozhang zhidu gaige zhinan* (*The Guide for the Reform of the Social Security System*). Beijing: Gaige chubanshe. 100–3.

Guojia Tigaiwei et al. 1999b. Guanyu zhigong yiliao zhidu gaige kuoda shidian de yijian (Opinions concerning the expansion of pilot programs for the reform of medical care system for staff and workers). In Zheng, D., Liu, D., & Zhang, B. (Eds.), *Shehui baozhang zhidu gaige zhinan* (*The Guide for the Reform of the Social Security System*). Beijing: Gaige chubanshe. 104–8.

Guowuyuan 1998. Guowuyuan guanyu jianli chengzhen zhigong jiben yiliao baoxian zhidu de jueding (The decision of the State Council concerning the establishment of a basic medical care insurance system for staff and workers in cities and towns). *Guanwuyuan gaobao* (*The Bulletin of the State Council*) 33: 1250–4.

Hong, W. 1995a. Jianli geren yiliao zhanghui yu shehui tongchou xiangjiehe moshi de xingchangshi (New adventure in establishing a model for combining personal accounts with social unified funding). *Zhongguo weisheng shiye guanli* (*The Management of China's Health Care Enterprises*): 8.

Hong, W. 1995b. Shenzhenshi yiliao baoxian gaige de nandian yu chulu (The difficulties and solutions for medical care insurance reform in Shenzhen municipality). *Zhongguo weisheng shiye guanli* (*The Management of China's Medical Care Enterprises*): 1.

Huang, H. 2020. *Social Protection under Authoritarianism, Health Politics and Policy in China.* New York: Oxford University Press.

Interview (one interviewee) April 28, 2000.

Interview (one interviewee) May 12, 2000.

Interview (two interviewees) May 11, 2000.

Interview (two interviewees) morning May 11, 2000.

Interview (two interviewees) January 23, 2002

Lee, P. 2013. China's health care reform in perspective. In Cheung, F., Woo, J., & Law, C. (Eds.), *Health Systems: Challenges, Visions, and Reforms from A Comparative-global Perspective.* Hong Kong: HKIAPS, Chinese University of Hong Kong. 331–58.

Lee, P. 2019. *Re-engineering Affordable Care Policy in China, Is Marketization A Solution?* London & New York: Routledge.

Liu, S. 2004. *Zhongguo yiliao gaige de zhidu fenxi* (*Systems Analysis of China's Medical Care Insurance*). Taipei: National Cheng Chi University.

Peng, P. 1996. Zai quanguo zhigong yiliao baozhang zhidu gaige kuada shidian huiyi kaimushi de jianghua (The speech at the opening of national conference regarding the expansion of pilot programs in the reform of the medical care security system for staff and workers). In Guojia tigaiwei fenpei he shehui baozhang si (Ed.), *Zhigong yiliao baozhang zhidu gaige* (*The Reform of the Medical Care Security System for Staff and Workers*). Beijing: Gaige chubanshe. 3–21.

Pollit, C., & Bouchaert, G. 2004. *Public Management Reform: A Comparative Analysis.* Oxford & New York: Oxford University Press.

Savas, E. S. 1987. *Privatization, The Key to Better Government.* Chatham, NJ: Chatham House Publishers, Inc.

Shanghaishi caizhengju 2001. Guanyu zai benshi yiliao jigou zhankai yaopin jizhong zhao-biao caigou shidian gongzuo de rougan yijian (Several opinions concerning the task of pilot programs in the procurement of pharmaceutical products through unified collective bidding in the municipality). In Liu, J. (Ed.), *Shanghai weisheng nianjian 2001* (*Shanghai Yearbook of Health Care 2001*). Shanghai: Shanghai kexue jishu wenxian chubanshe.

Shanghaishi weishengju & Shanghaishi caizhengju 2001. Shanghai yiyuan yaopin shouzhi liantiaoxian guanli zanxin banfa (Provisional measures for the two-line management of revenue and expenditure for pharmaceutical products in hospitals in Shanghai). In Liu, J. (Ed.), *Shanghai weisheng nianjian 2001* (*Shanghai Yearbook of Health Care 2001*). Shanghai: Shanghai kexue jishu wenxian chubanshe.

Shanghaishi yiliao baoxianju et al. 2002. Shanghaishi jiben yiliao baoxian zhenliao xianmu fanwei guanli zanxin banfa (Provisional measures for managing the scope of medical treatment items allowed by basic medical insurance in Shanghai municipality). In Liu, J. (Ed.), *Shanghai weisheng nianjian 2001* (*Shanghai Yearbook of Health Care 2002*). Shanghai: Shanghai kexue jishu wenxian chubanshe.

Shanghaishi yiliao baoxianju et al. 2003. Shanghaishi chengzhen zhigong baoxian ding-dian lingshou yaodian guanli zanxin baofa (Provisional measures for the manage-ment of designated retail drug stores for the basic insurance of staff and workers in *the* cities and towns in Shanghai). In Liu, J. (Ed.), *Shanghai weisheng nianjian 2004* (*Shanghai Yearbook of Health Care 2003*). Shanghai: Shanghai kexue jishu wenxian chubanshe.

Shenzhenshi renmin zhengfu 2013. Shenzhenshi shehui yiliao baoxian banfa (Measures for the social medical care insurance of Shenzhen Municipality).

Song, X., & Liu, H. 2001. Yiliao baoxian peitao cuoshi (Complementary measures for medi-cal care reform). In Song, X. (Ed.),2 *Zhongguo shehui baozhang tizhi gaige yu fazhan baogao* (*Report on the Reform and Development of Social Security System in China*). Beijing: Zhongguo remin daxue chubanshe. 84–106.

Wu, R. 1999. Tan yiliao baoxian zhidu gaige (On medical care reform). *Renmin daxue fuyin baokan ziliao* (*References for Reprinted Newspapers and Magazines of People's Univer-sity*) 2: 5–7.

Wu, R., & Chen, J. 1999. Jianli chengzhen zhigong baoxian zhidu, quanmian tujin woguo baoxian zhidu gaige (Building the insurance system for staff and workers in cities and towns and propelling insurance reform on all fronts in China). In Zheng, D., Liu, D., &

Zhang, B. (Eds.), *Shehui baozhang zhidu zinan* (*A Guide for the Reform of the Social Security System*). Beijing: Gaige chuban she. 358–74.

Zhu, R. 2002. Guanyu zhigong yiliao baozhang zhidu gaige wenti (Issues regarding the reform medical care security system of staff and workers) in Laodong he shehui baozhangbu & zhonggong zhongyang wenxian yanjiushi (Eds.), *Xinshiqi laodong he shehui baozhang zhongyao wenxian xuanbian* (*Selected Important Documents of Labor and Social Security during the New Era*). Beijing: Zhongguo shehui baozhang chubanshe & zhong yang wenxian chubanshe. 266–74.

7 Financing Basic Medical Care

This chapter will tackle the issue of funding, as the foregoing analysis has already dealt with spending coupled with program specificity including produce/service specificity in the case of BMCI.

Here the study will address several key issues of the financial management of BMCI—the entirely new managerial and financial vehicle to manage, control and regulate the financial flow from premium contributions at the funding end to the payments of medical care services at the spending end. The study will start to examine BMCI first on the issue of the PA-USFA scheme considering marketization of public funding. Then it will proceed to tackle the alternative procedural linkages of PA to USFA based on pilot programs. Moreover, the study will discuss how BMCI was introduced in territorial jurisdictions in two cases, Shanghai and Guangzhou, focusing on the exercise of program specificity and dealing with the alienation of entitlement from funding of the past.

Marketization of Funding Functions

To build the BMCI program in each jurisdiction, the principal task was concerned with the installment of a novel financial management that consists of the two account schemes, namely, personal account (PA) combined with unified social funding account (USFA). A the design of BMCI, some analysts tend to suggest that it mainly follows the German model of mandatory plans of health care insurance (Chapter 2 & 6). According to Professor Gu Xin, it is more precise to take the BMCI program as a mixture of German model and Singaporean model. Following the Singaporean model, for instance, PA is taken as a form of compulsory saving that relies on the premium contribution from each enrollee, coupled with a share by the work unit. Legally speaking, it is treated as a form of personal property, belonging to each enrollee. And it can pass onto heirs as inheritance. Like the German model, USFA operates as a risk pooling reservoir that is sustained by premium contributions of all enrollees, covering claims from the insured in accordance with the plan (Gu 2008: 161–6).

In financial terms, the PA-USFA accounting scheme served as a building block not only for an independent funding source relying upon a sizable scale of risk-pooling in each jurisdiction, but also for the transaction-centered management of

DOI: 10.4324/9781003389934-9

insurance funding. The PA-USFA scheme played important roles in the financial management of BMCI, ensuring the reliability of funding sources for basic medical care, and maintaining the effective operation of funding programs. According to the 1994 Opinion, the BMCI programs would be able to overcome the waste of healthcare resources and lessen the mounting financial burden on the party-state, work units and individuals alike (Guojia Tigaiwei et al. 1999).

Theoretically speaking, the PA-USFA scheme laid the foundation of management and operation relying on the inward-resource-flow (IRF) system. Payment for service is tied to premium collection through mechanisms of transactions. Each item of services was accountable in the transaction that would be handled in strict budgetary and accounting terms. To put it in another way, no medical care service was to be rendered unless the enrollee had made a premium contribution of equal value, coupled with the share shouldered by the work unit in a co-insurance system. The 1994 Opinion states that the PA-USFA scheme was built upon the principle of "revenue to match expenditure" (*yizhi dingsou*) (Guojia Tigaiwei et al. 1999). In fact, the said principle did not remain as empty promise, for it became operationalized through market mechanisms in terms of the quid pro quo exchange of equal values.

The PA-USFA scheme differed from the accounting scheme under conventional funding of social security in general and medical care. The PA-USFA scheme was intended to maintain budgetary balance and operate with an independent funding source. And it was separate from the public financial management of the party-state hierarchy (including the government and public enterprises) under the CPE. By design, a NDPE (often called executive agency, medical care insurance institute, or social security institute interchangeably) was installed in each jurisdiction, serving as the custodian of the BMCI foundation operating with the PA-USFA scheme, and acting as an intermediary between the insurer and insured (including the employer and employees).

While BMCI maintained its managerial and financial independence operating through the IRF system, its main financial source still relied on the existing budgetary channels of these public organizations embracing the government units, service units and public enterprises. Premium contributions were charged to *either* the state budget for the personnel who had enjoyed PFMC in case of the government units and service units *or* the enterprise budget for staff and workers who had used to subscribe in LIMC. There were four financial channels. First, in the case of government units (taken as fully quota state-budgeted work units), premium contributions to the PA-USFA scheme are to be charged to the state-budgeted fund of the administrative work unit concerned. Second, for partially state-budgeted work units (also called "differential quota budgeted work units"), for example, service work units such as publishing companies, hospitals etc., and those self-financed and entrepreneurially oriented service units, premium contributions to the PA-USFA scheme normally came from the medical care fund of the service work unit concerned. Third, in those public enterprises, premium contributions of staff and workers to the PA-USFA scheme had to be charged to the welfare fund (often derived from retained revenue or production costs); and fourth in the case of retirees, their premium contributions have to be charged to the labor insurance expenditure account at the enterprise level (Guojia Tigaiwei et al. 1999: 101).

From the perspective of public financial management, BMCI remained in co-existence with, but distinctly separate from the conventional financial system embedded in the CPE. During the economic reform, the linkage of public finance and BMCI was mediated through market transactions. Working within the IRF system, in other words, the BMCI foundation dealt with its counterparts, for example, the work unit and enrollee, through market transactions in the sense that medical care entitlements needed to be matched with premium contributions, supposedly through an exchange of equal values. Both the work unit (i.e., the employer) and enrollee (i.e., the employee) had to pay for medical care entitlements in a co-insurance system according to the scheme for the calculation of premium contributions. In accordance with the 1994 Opinion, for example, the amount of funding for BMCI (meaning premium contribution to the PA-USFA scheme) should not exceed 10 percent of the average annual total of wage bill, beyond which an approval from the finance department of the government would be required (Guojia Tigaiwei et al. 1999). Considering the funding sources as well as the method of calculation, it is noteworthy that premium contributions to either the USFA or the PA (in part) were to be derived from a portion of the "supplementary wage" at the public enterprise level. It is apparent that BMCI is taken as a form of non-wage compensation.

Conceptually speaking, medical care, together with retirement pension, is considered as part of non-wage compensation introduced in connection with the low wage policy under the CPE. As a matter of the historically rooted obligations made during the early period of CPE, not only was the work unit obligated to shoulder a share of premium contribution, but also public finance (at the local level) needed to meet its portion of financial responsibility. For example, in the event that work units encountered financial difficulties, the 1994 Opinion recommended for further consideration of additional funding sources to lend needed assistance as follows: First, public revenue, for example, taxation, for BMCI benefits for civil servants in the government and members of other public organizations such as the personnel of service units, political parties and associations, and second, retained revenue (part of which was often converted into a "welfare fund") to support insurance for staff and workers employed by public enterprises (Guojia Tigaiwei et al. 1999).

BMCI represented a co-insurance system, meaning that by design, the work unit was no longer solely responsible for funding medical care, and instead, the enrollee was required to assume a role as a buyer in the health care insurance markets. For the implementation of the PA-USFA scheme, the enrollee and the work unit (i.e., employee and employer), in principle, had to pay for their respective share of premium contributions. As just noted in the cases of the municipalities of Jiujiang and Zhenjiang, for example, while the work unit was required to pay up to 10 percent of the average annual total wages for its premium contribution, 1 percent of an employee's wage entered into the PA (Guowuyuan 1995: 4–12; Guojia Tigaiwei et al. 1999: 101).

The Options of Funding in BMCI Package

Emerging from the pilot programs in Jiujiang and Zhenjiang during the BMCI reform in 1994, some preliminary thoughts were articulated on the functional division of labor between the PA and the USFA. Trying to analyze the PA-USFA scheme, Wu Bangguo proposed three conceptual alternatives to separate the PA from the USFA as follows: The level of expenditure, types of services, and medical conditions. First, regarding the amount of expenditure, PA was to cover small expenditures and USFA, larger ones; second, the clinical visits of outpatients were to be covered by the PA while hospital care for the inpatient by the USFA; and third, concerning types of illness, minor ones were to be covered by PA and serious ones by USFA (Wu 1999). In comparable terms, Lee has proposed to adopt the classification of medical care services into three zones: Clinical care in Zone I, hospital care in Zone II and HESI in Zone III (normally covering the expenditure exceeding the payment-ceiling of the BMCI plan). It appears that PA matched the financial needs of clinical care in Zone I and USFA covered funding of hospital care in Zone II (Chapter 4; Lee 2019). However, the early designs of funding did not cover HESI in Zone III, which was subsequently tackled in the later period of policymaking when policy actors were confronted with policy issues of SMCI in 1998 and onward (Chapters 5 and 8).

The PA-USFA scheme consisted of an essential component of the BMCI design, the introduction of which marked a significant change from "proto-insurance" at the work unit level during the pre-reform era to a full-fledged public insurance system at the provincial/local level in mixed economy. From the vantage point of the policymaking circles, BMCI, armed with PA-USFA, were comparable with what the conventional funding modes (LIMC and PFMC) had provided, for example, in terms of both clinical care and hospital care. It is evident that the BMCI was intended to address the issue of alienation of entitlements from funding. For example, Wu Mutu and Chen Jinpu pointed to the institutionalized funding through BMCI, explaining that the new design of BMCI aimed at lessening the financial burden of the state and enterprises through risk pooling (i.e., through USFA) mechanisms and "socialized [macro] management" while ensuring the provision of basic medical care for staff and workers. Also, it could promote awareness of self-paid insurance and cost consciousness among employees in view of the features of co-payment, deductible etc. Moreover, PA worked as a built-in saving mechanism incorporated into BMCI in anticipation of the further aging of the population (Wu & Chen 1999: 358–74). Falling into Zone I and Zone II, the PA-USFA scheme covered the full range of basic medical care services equivalent to what had previously been made available only to employees in the public sector in the pre-reform framework of the CPE.

Premier Zhu Rongji's view carried considerable weight in the exercise of program specificity pertaining to the thrifty version of BMCI in conjunction with the briefing session on pilot programs of the medical care reform presented by the leadership team (led by Peng Peiyun) on October 27, 1997. Upon his insistence, the enrollee had to shoulder some percentage of premium contributions to

PA, although the work unit was chiefly responsible for premiums contributions to USFA. Also, he underscored that the thrifty version of BMCI did not cover the expenditure exceeding the payment-ceiling. In the said briefing session, Zhu made several salient points that merit further discussion. First, according to Zhu, BMCI only provided the "lowest standards of medical care security," meaning the essential types of curative care services (including examinations, diagnosis, treatments, and medicine) and the lowest possible funding level in absolute terms. Second, the BMCI needed to have "broad coverage," referring to all jurisdictions, all work units, all employees, and all residents. Third, in principle, the BMCI ought to match the funding level of conventional funding programs (PFMC and LIMC) that included clinical care in Zone 1 and hospital care in Zone II, but not serious illness and HESI beyond the payment-ceiling. Fourth, in the utmost consideration of the state financial capacity, BMCI did not exclude the scenario where its funding level might not match entirely that of the conventional funding packages, even though it assumed the same standards and types of the services as the pre-reform packages. Fifth, there was a residual category of medical care beyond the BMCI, to be financed by supplementary medical care insurance, commercial insurance, social relief, and public revenue. And some better-performing enterprises with surplus were allowed to top up the funding level of the thrifty version of BMCI. Sixth, the two sectors of public employees (i.e., public personnel of the government and other public organizations and the staff and workers in public enterprises) ought to be made comparable in the types of services and standards of benefits but allow the former to enjoy a slightly higher funding level. Seventh, retirees who ought to enjoy privileged retirement benefits (i.e., so-called "leave for recuperation," *liuxiu*) *ought* to be subsidized by public finance considering "historical debts" that the society owed them (Zhu 2002: 266–79).

Overall, the provincial/local jurisdictions had no escape from financial responsibility for the implementation of the BMCI program, regardless of which plans were adopted. And they were confronted with three options as follows: (1) the social unified funding package for major illness only, (2) a thrifty version embracing clinical care and hospital care (likely at a very modest funding level as being adopted for flexibly employed personnel and agricultural laborer, see Chapter 9), and (3) an enriched version including SMCI. The provincial/local government, not the central government, had to shoulder all the financial responsibility for the introduction of social security policy, (including medical care), operating with the "financial undertaking system" (*caizheng baogan* or FUS) introduced in 1980 and modified as "revenue sharing system" (*fenshuizhi* or RSS) in 1994 respectively (Chapter 5; Ge & Gong 2007: 28–31: Gu 2008: 229–42; Lee 2019). Of course, the provincial/local governments could assume a lighter burden if only an insurance plan focusing on HESI (in case of NRCMCI and URMCI introduced later) only or even a thrifty version of BMCI matching the funding level of the conventional funding program (or perhaps, at a further reduced funding level). It appeared at the end of the day, however, that the central government had to convince the provincial/local government to accept the last alternative—a version of BMCI matching the funding level of the conventional funding programs but not exceeding the payment-ceiling. By doing so, the1998 Opinion reflected a concern to minimize, if not entirely avoid, infringement upon the vested interests of staff and workers the entitlement package of basic medical care as previously articulated in the conventional PFMC and LIMC programs without program specificity regarding funding prior to economic reform (Guojia Tigaiwei et al. 1999). Above all, the BMCI may be considered a better alternative to the conventional funding programs on two counts: First, it operated as a larger and effective scale of risk pooling beyond the work unit level, and second, BMCI demonstrated its strength in building an institutionalized funding run by the NDPE, and handling financial management of medical care in a consistent, coherent, systematic and stable fashion (Chapter 3).

However, BMCI left several issues unanswered during the early phases of drafting and packaging endeavors, mainly funding gaps on two counts. First, the central policymakers appeared to respond to the drastic increase of expenditure and financial burden of social security including medical excessively by lowering overall level of expenditure of BMCI in visible way, albeit they did insist to maintain the same categories of medical care entitlements in clinical care in Zone I and hospital care in Zone II. Second, it took time in responding to the demands for financing HESI cases, while policy actors were keen to answer the demands of the workforce for social security, which were exacerbated by cases of difficult and bankrupted SOEs. Moving from the thrifty version to the enriched version that was armed with SCMI starting in 1998, the BMCI surpassed a higher funding hurdle, coupled with more and better services in terms of product/service specificity. These issues will be saved for further discussion in the next chapter.

The Three-passage Model

Given that provincial/local governments finally accepted the proposed PA-USFA scheme, there was an issue surrounding the linkage between the PA and the USFA to be straightened out in the twists and turns of policy formation from 1994 to 1996. During the early period of policy experiments and pilot programs, when policymakers dwelled on the matter of segregating clinical care in Zone I from hospital care in Zone II about the packaging of services and measures of funding and spending, they finally found ways to build procedural steps to connect the PA with the USFA, given the chain of cost-incurring episodes in each process of curative care.

Both the PA and the USFA were given well-defined roles, and each addressed different demands of basic medical care. In accordance with the 1994 Opinion, the PA-USFA scheme covered medical care services to both outpatients and inpatients (Guojia Tigaiwei et al. 1999). In this early design of the medical care insurance program as just noted, the PA was to fund clinical visits and minor illnesses normally involving a modest sum of expenditure, while USFA was intended to cover serious illnesses and other defined benefits, likely involving hospital care that is costly in most cases (Zhang 1999: 6). In addition, the deposit into the PA was treated as a form of personal savings derived partly from one's take-home pay (e.g., the 1 percent mentioned above) and partly from a certain percentage of the supplementary wage (the share of 5 percent set aside by the work unit as noted). Thus, the deposit into the PA represents a kind of risk-pooling mechanism, whereby saving accumulates over a certain length of time to cover expenses of a medical event in the future. That is to say, the funds deposited in a PA could only be used by the enrollee himself/herself for defined medical care purposes. Taken as a form of personal property owned by the enrollee, the said deposit could be passed onto inheriting family members under current laws (Guowuyuan 1995; Guojia Tigaiwei et al. 1999).

It is entirely plausible that many jurisdictions would find it preferable not to include the PA option in their early policy experiments for the following reasoning: Enrollees (e.g., especially the new recruits) could eventually afford absorbing the cost of their premium contributions into the PA through out-of-pocket payment (OPP), as the compensation package was restructured to keep tempo with the increase of take-home pay in the midst of economic growth (Zhu 2002: 268). In managerial and financial terms, the OPP was considered superior to the PA in that the former entailed the saving of substantial administrative costs while more choices were given to enrollees. USFA could therefore play a better and effective role in funding, considering the main purpose of BMCI was to provide risk pooling mechanisms to absorb the less affordable medical bills of major illness, for example, HESI cases.

As shown in the earlier pilot programs in Jiujiang and Zhenjiang, the PA-USFA scheme offered a managerial and financial linkage of the PA to the USFA by making the payment out of PA account a prerequisite for submitting a charge to the USFA (Guojia Tigaiwei et al. 1999). Accordingly, the PA-USFA design divided three interconnected passages in its payment scheme. In operational terms, as stipulated in the 1994 Opinion and tested in pilot programs in Jiujiang and Zhenjiang, an enrollee had to pay for medical care services by charging to one's PA in the first passage; as soon as the PA was exhausted, one could enter into the second passage by paying a deductible up to an amount of 5 percent of the average annual wage of the jurisdiction from the preceding year. After the deductible had been met, the enrollee entered into the third passage, in which the remaining sum was to be covered by the USFA according to a schedule of co-payment: For instance, 10–20 percent for a sum of less than 5,000 RMB, 8–10 percent for an amount exceeding 5,000 RMB but less than 10,000 RMB, and 2 percent for an amount exceeding 10,000 RMB (Guojia Tigaiwei et al. 1999). By design, the risk pooling mechanisms enabled the BMCI to cover the greater and greater amount of funding demands, as moving to the higher classes of HESI in terms of both expenditure and seriousness of illness.

It is argued that the three-passage model made better use of the PA by first exhausting the deposits in PA. Moreover, it is conceivable that the direct linkage of the PA to the USFA might help avoid disputes over the operational definition of basic medical care, without entering into the issue of what kinds of services should be provided within the financial coverage of either the PA or the USFA. It is up to each enrollee to decide to make use of which account procedurally depending on one's plan of treatment. Theoretically it appears that the three-passage model tends to minimize unnecessary micro-management. However, the model inadvertently created an incentive for the enrollee to exhaust the deposits in PA in Zone I quickly and unnecessarily to hasten entry into payment under the USFA in Zone II, as demonstrated by the results of the pilot programs in Jiujiang and Zhenjiang (Wu & Chen 1999: 360–1; Zheng 2002: 140–3). According to Wang Dongjin, the problem of overspending was found not only in Jiujiang and Zhenjiang starting in 1994 but also invariably in all other jurisdictions that took part in expanded experiments from 1996 onward because of their having adopted the three-passage model (Wang 2008: 64).

As for remedies for the three-passage model, there were two alternatives, as follows: (1) the combined-blocks model (*bankuai jiehe moshi*) in Hainan Province and Shenzhen Municipality and (2) the three-fund management model (*sanjin moshi*) in Qingdao and Tanggu Municipality (Zheng 2002: 140–3). In the case of Hainan Province, the combined-blocks model provided some effective measures for segregating the functions of the PA and the USFA from each other. While the PA was, in principle, responsible for expenditures for clinical visits and minor illnesses, the USFA covered only hospitalization and major diseases (Wu & Chen 1999: 361). The Hainan case took one step forward by compiling a list of major illnesses to be incorporated into the USFA, which was strictly responsible for mutual help among enrollees by relying on risk-pooling mechanisms, as well as by listing six categories of illnesses that were not to be covered by the USFA. In the Hainan case, the use of the PA was separable, namely not related to eligibility for entry into USFA payments, and enrollees were given a clear and unambiguous area of responsibility for co-payment. Enrollees were fully aware that they had to shoulder any responsibility exceeding PA limits, which consisted of 50–60 percent of the total of the insurance fund, a ratio established based on observed regularity and calculation (Song & Liu 2001: 95; Zheng 2002: 141–3).

The three-fund management model was introduced in another group of municipalities, such as Qingdao, Tianjian, and Yantai, and in cities in Zhijiang, among others (Song & Liu 2001). This model demonstrated considerable merits by creating a new social insurance institute (or executive agency) to enact a set of financial and risk-pooling mechanisms while still allowing the work unit to play some useful role (Zheng 2002). The model comprised three funds that were managed separately: The social unified fund (*shehui tongchou jin*; hereafter, SUF), the enterprise adjustment fund (*qiye tiaoji jin*; hereafter, EAF), and the personal account fund (*geren zhangfu jin*; hereafter, PAF). Falling into Zone II, the SUF was entrusted to and managed by the social insurance institute, covering major illnesses (i.e., anything less than catastrophic in nature) of staff and workers. The enterprise management handled EAF in Zone III, subject to supervision by the labor union and the CRSW, and provided financial aid to those staff and workers who were considered financially overburdened in selected cases. Regarding the management of PAF in Zone I, the enterprise management acted on behalf of staff and workers. A deposit into PAF was considered the personal property of each employee but designated for a well-defined category of common medical events. Although enterprises took part in the pilot program of the three-fund model, for example, 93 percent of enterprise units in Qingdao and 96 percent in Yantai respectively, some enterprises in hardship still could not fulfill the obligation of making contributions to ESF and PAF (Song & Liu 2001; Zheng 2002). In addition, enterprises still found themselves entangled in the heavy workload of the day-to-day management of medical social insurance. Taken as an adverse effect of the administrative overload, the enterprise management often denied access to medical care services in enterprise medical care facilities for residents of the community, resulting in under-utilization of health care resources, and so forth (Song & Liu 2001: 97–8).

It is evident that the three-passage model became a main controversy among various provincial/local jurisdictions during policy experiments from 1994 onwards, and the consensus that emerged subsequently tended to move away from the said model and was oriented toward an option to allow a clear separation of the PA and the USFA. In the process of implementation starting in 1998 on an experimental basis and in 2001 formally, various jurisdictions endeavored to find alternative funding sources for their respective PA-USFA. To identify a general pattern, it is pertinent to choose two empirical cases for comparison in the next section.

The Case of Guangzhou

Focusing on the issue of installation, there existed commonalities in BMCI, coupled with differences, across various jurisdictions throughout the country. To avoid unnecessary repetition, this study will choose two cases to illustrate the common features of BMCI, and then proceed to identify the differences as much as possible. Among others, the PA-USFA schemes were invariably adopted in Guangzhou and Shanghai, two cosmopolitan scale municipalities with considerable concentration of public enterprises built under the CPE prior to economic reform. Both municipalities finally accepted the recommendation of the State Council regarding the package combining clinical care with hospital care, that was taken comparable to the types and standards of medical care services covered by LIMC and PFMC, despite their original preference for a narrow and less expensive option, for example, hospital care in Zone II only.

The inauguration of BMCI in Guangzhou was preoccupied with the concern of vested interests of the cohorts of senior employees and retirees. In the case of Guangzhou, moreover, BMCI was introduced to roughly two-thirds of the residents (or about 64 percent of the total of workforce), who were relatively senior, while other packages of medical care insurance were saved for the remaining 36 percent, most of whom were young of age, including "flexibly employed personnel" (often taken as outside personnel, temporary workers and contractual workers) and agricultural laborers (Chapter 9).

The Guangzhou BMCI program operated with the PA-USFA scheme in accordance with the 2001 Measures and, subsequently, the 2010 Measures (as amended in 2012). Like all other jurisdictions, the Guangzhou policymaking team had to face the issues of setting up a charging scheme for collecting premium contributions in the BMCI program and securing the funding source for the risk-pooling mechanisms based upon the scale of the economy. Guangzhou's BMCI program had two versions. The thrifty version of the earlier phase was focused on the operation of the PA-USFA scheme to be examined here, and the enriched version embraced an additional component of supplementary medical care insurance (SMCI) to be discussed in the next chapter.

To determine how high a premium contribution each enrollee had to make, the Guangzhou policymaking team worked with the so-called "basic figure," the formula of calculation pertaining to each enrollee's share of premium contribution to the PA-USFA. In the BMCI of Guangzhou, the basic figure was based on the average annual income in the municipality. According to the basic figure, each enrollee was required to make a premium contribution in the range of between 300 percent and 60 percent of the average annual income in a given jurisdiction. An enrollee whose average annual income exceeded 300 percent of the annual average was to make a premium contribution based on 300 percent (but no more than 300 percent), and the one whose average annual income fell below 60 percent of the average, was to make premium contribution based on 60 percent (and no less than 60 percent).

The basic figure formula was intended to accommodate both high-income bracket and low-income bracket enrollees. On the one hand, the high-income bracket enrollees whose annual average income exceeded 300 percent did not have to make the portion of premium contribution higher than 300 percent. That is to say, the employees of a high-income bracket beyond 300 percent of average annual wage were incentivized to join the BMCI as a 300 percent premium contribution ceiling was in effect. On the other hand, low-income bracket employees' average annual income below 60 percent was not to be denied subscription in BMCI, considering their essential medical care demands. From a policy perspective, the basic figure (calculated within the range from 300 percent to 60 percent range) ensured all members of the workforce were to be given equal access to the same basic medical care entitlement. By doing so those enrollees who belonged to a high-income bracket (exceeding 300 percent) would not be put in the disadvantageous position of paying more than what they received. Meanwhile, the low-income bracket enrollees would not be deprived of basic medical care regardless of their low income.

From a financial and managerial perspective, moreover, the PA-USFA scheme divided the work unit's expenditure on medical basic care into two portions: One portion was credited to PA to cover clinical treatments, and the other portion entered the risk-pooling of the USFA to cover ordinary hospital care (Chen 1994). By design, PA represented the funding mechanism for the transfer of financial resources saved by each enrollee from one point in time to another in the future. It was taken as a form of "vertical relationship," meaning to take advantage of saving one's own income at an earlier period for a needed use by the same enrollee at a later time. On the other hand, the USFA relied on a mechanism of transferring financial resources among enrollees in a reciprocal relationship, that is, a "horizontal" relationship, by which they shared the large financial pool created by the deposit of premium contributions made by all enrollees. The USFA was associated with large expenditures toward hospital care for each enrollee below the stipulated payment-ceiling (Mo 1996).

In Guangzhou, the PA-USFA scheme followed the co-insurance system where both enrollee and work unit were held responsible for making their own shares of the premium contributions. For the PA, each enrollee was required to make a premium contribution, assuming a share of financial responsibility for one's own medical care expenses. Such policy change was indicative of the transformation from a free-ride mentality of "work-unit collectivism" under CPE to a culture of choice-making and consumer responsibility in the marketplace (Chen 1994).

In addition, the Guangzhou BMCI program endeavored to make the more attractive to the enrollee by adopting an "enriched" version of the PA to the extent that not only was it recognized as the enrollee's personal property, which could be inherited by one's offspring, but it could also be used by family members, similar to the case of Shenzhen (Guanzhoushi zhengfu 2012: Article 20). In addition, the PA allowed coverage for some non-basic services and drug prescriptions (Guanzhoushi zhengfu 2012: Article 24).

In the case of Guangzhou, the use of the USFA, which was not related to the PA operationally, had to follow a set of explicit criteria to fit into well-defined categories, and had to be served by designated providers due to considerations of cost containment and other managerial purposes (Guanzhoushi zhengfu 2012). In Guangzhou, the boundary between the PA and the USFA was clearly drawn, separating each other rigorously for the most part, albeit there was some overlap in certain exceptional cases that were handled through the listing and categorizing methods.[1] By and large, Guangzhou learned to provide remedies against overspending inherent in "the three-passage model" of the earlier PA-USFA design in Jiujiang and Zhenjiang. To discourage enrollees from jumping from the PA to the USFA, the Guangzhou program accordingly adopted a brand of "combined blocks model" so that the PA and the USFA components remained operationally segregated, similar to like the case of Hainan (Zheng 2002: 141; Guanzhoushi zhengfu 2012: Article 22–30).

The Guangzhou BMCI package operated strictly within the IRF system with few exceptions in that all enrollees had to fulfill their obligation of premium contributions before they were allowed to enjoy their entitlements. This BMCI program catered to two distinct groups of residents with household registration in Guangzhou: Currently employed personnel and retirees. Both were required to fulfill 15 years of premium contributions, but they differed from each other in terms of the ways and means to do so. In the Guangzhou program, enrollees of the ordinary type were required to set aside from their supplementary wage, that is, 10 percent of the basic figure calculated on the basis of the average annual wage for a premium contribution, that is, 2 percent from each enrollee and 8 percent from the work unit (Guanzhoushi zhengfu 2012).

The case of retirees was complicated, however. They were treated differently in the BMCI program in that a "transition fund" was established to help them meet the obligation of making premium contributions in full for a period of 15 years. In parallel to the transition fund, additionally, the work unit was required to create a "special fund" at the respective level. Besides, the special fund was intended to help retirees fulfill the obligation of making contributions to the BMCI transition fund.[2] The BMCI program of Guangzhou tried to maintain some measure of flexibility, if not generosity, toward retirees. For instance, although those retired fewer than 20 years had to pay by themselves in full the charges to the transition fund, they were qualified to enjoy hospital care and "special clinical treatment" once they had paid 50 percent of the charges to the transition fund (Guanzhoushi zhengfu 2012: Article 10). Moreover, those retirees who had not met the required length of 15 years of employment in Guangzhou were still allowed to join the program, provided they continued to make their contributions to the transition fund in full (Guanzhoushi zhengfu 2012: Article 8–10). In addition, the design of the transition fund took into consideration the obligation of the work unit regarding senior personnel and retirees considering their past contributions and actual needs. For example, a portion of the contribution of the work unit to the transition fund entered directly the PA depending on age.[3]

According to Mo, a policy analyst in Guangzhou, the fact that government could intervene in funding BMCI was inseparable from the wealth (assets) that government at various levels had collected, built, and withheld during the CPE period, especially with reference to the alienation of social security entitlements from funding in the case of earlier cohort of the workforce employed under the low wage policy during the CPE period. Mo argues,

> In state assets contain an accumulation of residual value from the labor of currently employed staff, workers, and retirees. Therefore, part of the appreciation from state assets should be appropriated to cover a portion of the medical care insurance fund. (Translation provided.)
>
> (Mo 1996)

Above all, in the implementation of BMCI, the Guangzhou policy leadership did try their best to heed the vested interests of the workforce who made sacrifices under the low wage policy of the pre-reform era.

Financing BMCI in Shanghai

Shanghai played a leading role in forced modernization with a sizable group of public enterprises under the CPE. The social security concerns, including retirement benefits and basic medical care, emerged as a salient policy priority there. In place of the PFMI and LIMI programs built during the era of the CPE, Shanghai Municipality inaugurated an urban insurance program (UIP), an equivalent version of BMCI, in October 2000, but with a series of amendments based on feedback from trial-implementation conducted up to 2010 when the final version was completed (Hu 2001: 267–9; Wu, Li & Li 2008: 70–71). The urban insurance program (UIP) was ready for implementation to the full extent, anchored in the 2010 Measures.[4]

UIP was focused on the workforce conventionally employed within the perimeter of the CPE, including civil servants in the government, the personnel of service units, and staff and workers in public enterprises.[5] Comparable to Guangzhou, the Shanghai municipal leadership team endeavored to compensate the senior employees and retirees for the fact that they had received less in the remuneration package (including both wage and non-wage compensation) under the low wage policy from the 1950s to the early periods of the economic reform in the late 1970s and 1980s. Shanghai was one of the earliest industrial bases in China, meaning that it had to work with a higher proportion of senior employees and retirees than the latecomers in industrialization during the CPE. As it turns out, Shanghai's approach placed emphasis on financial "compensation" for both senior employees and retirees by helping make premium contributions as well as by offering better terms to retirees in the exceedingly elaborated payment schemes.

In Shanghai, the thrifty version of UIP adopted the early design of BMCI recommended by the State Council. And the enriched version of UIP was subsequently produced by adding a new layer of the local supplementary medical care insurance (abbreviated as LSMCI) (Wu, Li & Li 2008). The UIP fund worked with its own accounts, namely, the PA-USFA scheme. Although the LSMCI program worked with a separate account, it operated in close collaboration with the UIP fund, normally covering large sums of expenditure exceeding the payment-ceiling. In terms of financial management, UIP corresponded with clinical care in Zone I and hospital care in Zone II, while the enriched version of UIP embraced an additional LSMCI that fell into Zone III. It is noteworthy in the Shanghai situation where the use of LSMCI increased and was often not limited to financing the demands of HESI (including catastrophic medical care events). In fact, LSMCI was often used to satisfy some additional demands of retirees to maintain the same standards of medical care equivalent to those of LIMC and PFMC in accordance with relevant laws and regulations.

In the UIP package, the PA-USFA scheme was adopted in line with the pilot programs of Jiujiang and Zhenjiang, as previously endorsed by the State Council. That is to say, the premium contribution to the PA-USFA scheme was calculated according to the so-called "basic figure" just noted. However, the operational definition of "basic figure" differed slightly from that of Guangzhou. In Shanghai, the basic figure referred to a range between 60 percent and 300 percent of the average wage of the working population in Shanghai from the previous *month* (Shanghai renmin zhengfu 2010: Article 5), whereas in the Guangzhou case comparatively, the basic figure was calculated based on an average *annual* wage. In Shanghai, the PA-USFA scheme was given greater procedural flexibility to apply the previous month's wage of the enrollee for calculating the basic figure, and to account for those enrollees needing to move in or out of the BMCI fund.

The UIP fund required the work unit to contribute 10 percent of the basic figure based on the previous month's average wage while each enrollee was to contribute 2 percent of the basic figure. In the additional layer, the LSMCI fund required the work unit to contribute 2 percent of the basic figure, along with another 2 percent from each enrollee, where both contributions were to be credited to the LSMCI fund (Shanghai renmin zhengfu 2010).

Through the UIP, premium contributions by enrollees and work units were credited to the PA and the USFA respectively to pay for various kinds of basic medical care services. In principle, the use of either the PA or the USFA did not hinge on use of the other. That is to say, the use of the PA was not a prerequisite to charging to the USFA. In congruence with the case of Guangzhou, the UIP was characterized as the "combined blocks model" rather than the "three passage model" of Jiujiang and Zhenjiang. With its elaborated and complex schemes, the UIP program lent considerable recognition to senior employees and retirees who had been employed with tenure in the public sector under the CPE, reflecting the weight of the idea of "historical debts" in conferring the entitlements of basic medical care to senior members and retirees of public organizations. Not only were these senior employees and retirees required to pay less, but they were also given a share of medical care insurance benefits which was larger than that given to ordinary job-holding enrollees. In UIP, for example, premium contribution by each enrollee (i.e., 2 percent of the basic figure) was to be credited to the PA in the full amount. Moreover, approximately 30 percent of the premium contribution by the work unit (i.e., out of 10 percent of the basic figure) was to be credited to the PA on the basis of the age brackets of currently employed personnel and retirees, while the remaining was to be credited to the USFA.[6] Here seniority carried weight in awards of entitlements mostly depending on how long an employee worked under the low wage policy. Moreover, taking actual healthcare needs into consideration, those who were in higher age brackets are more prone to sickness and need more financial help from the USFA to cover hospital care and serious illness (Shanghai renmin zhengfu 2010: Article 11).

As a general principle, employed staff, workers and retirees enjoyed clinical services and emergency care that were chargeable to the PA when the enrollees had made a deductible payment (or fulfilling the "payment starting criterion," abbreviated as PSC) (Shanghai renmin zhengfu 2010: Article 25). No sooner than the PA had been exhausted and the deductible paid, an enrollee was entitled to payments made by the LSMCI program which was specifically tied to the seniority accumulated according to the schemes as enacted.[7]

In the case of hospital care and observation room services during clinical visits, both employees and retirees had to make a deductible payment (e.g., a given percentage calculated based on the average income from the previous month) before they were to be entitled to benefits chargeable to the USFA under a co-payment scheme established according to the status of employment and times of retirement. Once the deductible had been paid, for example, the employees were eligible to claim 85 percent of payment (with a co-payment of 15 percent) from the USFA and retirees 92 percent (with a co-payment of 8 percent) (Shanghai renmin zhengfu 2010: Article 24 & 5). However, when the retiree had exhausted his/her share of the USFA, the remaining portion of the payment was to be charged to the accumulated savings of the PA and/or to be covered by his/her co-payment (Shanghai renmin zhengfu 2010: Article 26). Furthermore, there were schemes pertaining to USFA for both current employees and retirees covering the clinical care for major illness and for family care services (Shanghai renmin zhengfu 2010: Article 24).

The payment-ceiling of the USFA was explicitly set at 700,000 RMB in accordance with the 2010 Measures. Any amount below the payment-ceiling was to be absorbed by the USFA based on given ratios for various categories of hospital care, serious illness in clinical visits, emergency observation room services, and home care services for both currently employees and retirees (Shanghai renmin zhengfu 2010: 24–26). Suffice it to say, the Shanghai's UIP demonstrated how the municipal policymakers endeavored not only to build a BMCI system to meet the demands of enrollees for basic medical care services but also to compensate the senior employees and retirees for their sacrifices under the low wage policy during the pre-reform era.

It is evident in both cases of Shanghai and Guangzhou that senior employees and retirees were given favorable terms in premium contributions and payment schemes (i.e., deductibles, co-payments, and supplementary insurances). For implementation, these favorable terms made the BMCI reforms more attractive than the conventional fund programs such as PFMC and LMCI, and tended to facilite implementation.

Concluding Remarks

In the foregoing analysis, the study is focused on the financial management (including especially the PA-USFA scheme)—one of the core features of the risk pooling mechanisms and transaction-centered management that characterize BMCI. It is argued that the new public management of BMCI constitutes an integral part of the IRF system that is market oriented. Accordingly, financial resources are handled and held by a brand of NDPE (consisting of executive agency, insurance management committee and supervisory committee) that operates independent of the government. From political perspective, the study has tried to demonstrate that in the process of designing and building BMCI, how sovereign planners tackled these non-funded or under-funded claims of social security entitlements—unsolved issues left by forced modernization through the CPE developmental strategy during the pre-reform era (Chapters 3 and 4). The study has also made use of two cases, Guangzhou and Shanghai, to illustrate how the provincial/local governments endeavored to find means and ways to ensure that the medical care entitlements of all senior employees and retirees were to be honored and funded properly through BMCI.

Notes

1 The USFA may still financially cover some specific types of clinical visits regarding cases of major illness which are explicitly defined in the 2008 Provisional Measures (as amended in 2011) (Guanzhoushi zhengfu 2012: Article 22–4).

2 For example, the amount of assistance from the transition fund depended on the number of years the retiree was employed under the CPE. For those retired 25 years before the introduction of the BMCI program, for example, the special fund was to cover all

charges to the transition fund on behalf of those retirees. For those retired at least 20 years but less than 25 years before the introduction of BMCI, the special fund was to pay 50 percent of charges to the transition fund while the retiree had to pay the remaining 50 percent.

3 For example, 1 percent for those who are 35 years of age or younger, 2 percent for those between 35 and 45, 2.8 percent for those 45 to retirement age, and 5.1 percent for retirees (Guanzhoushi zhengfu 2012: Article 6–15).

4 The full title of the 2010 Measures is "The Measures for Basic Medical Care Insurance in Cities and Towns of Shanghai," put forth on December 20, 2010 (abbreviated as the "2010 Measures" hereafter) (Shanghai renmin zhengfu 2010).

5 As prescribed in Article 2 of the 2010 Measures, the UIP caters to all personnel employed by so-called "employing units" (yongren danwei) or employers in the public sector, namely, all of those working in "enterprises, apparatus, service units, civil associations, and civilian-managed non-enterprise units." These public personnel include both the currently employed staff and workers and retirees, but it is the retirees who appear to enjoy considerable privileges (Shanghai renmin zhengfu 2010: Article 2).

6 For the currently employed staff and workers, three brackets are established: Those who are 34 years of age and below, those from 35 to 44 years of age, and those from 45 of age to retirement age. For the retirees, two brackets are adopted: The age group from retirement age to 74 and those who are 75 years of age and above (Shanghai renmin zhengfu 2010: Article 25).

7 These who started their employment before December 31, 2000, and have crossed the hurdle of the deductible payment equivalent to 10 percent of the annual average wage of the municipality become entitled to assistance from the LSMCI as follows: 70 percent (or co-payment of 30 percent) for those who were born before December 31, 1955; 60 percent (or co-payment of 40 percent) for those who were born between January 1, 1956, and December 31, 1965; and 50 percent (co-payment of 50 percent) for those who were born on or after January 1, 1966 (Shanghai renmin zhengfu 2010: Article 25). Those who began their employment after January 1, 2001 are to be responsible for any amount in full after crossing the hurdle of deductible payment, when their PA has been exhausted. There is also an elaborate payment scheme for retirees to cover expenditures for clinical and emergency cases, which takes into consideration different classes of providing units which have been chosen in order to avoid congesting higher echelon public hospitals (Shanghai renmin zhengfu 2010: Article 23).

References

Ge, Y., & Gong, S. 2007. *Zhongguo yigai: wenti, gengyuan, chulu* (*China's Healthcare Reform: Problems, Roots & Solutions*). Beijing: Zhongguo fazhan chubanshe.

Gu, X. 2008. *Zuoxian quanmin yibao: Zhongguo xinyigai de zhannue yu zhanxu (Towards National Healthcare Insurance: Strategy and Tactics for New Healthcare Reform in China)*. Beijing: Zhongguo laodong shehui baozhang chubanshe.

Guanzhoushi zhengfu 2012. Guanyu zhigong jiben yiliao baoxian shixing banfa (Measures for implementation of basic medical care insurance for workers and staff in the cities and towns of Guanzhou Municipality). Directive No. 80.

Guojia Tigaiwei et al. 1999. Guanyu zhigong yiliao zhidu gaige de shidian yijian (Opinions concerning the pilot experiment for reforming the medical care system for staff and workers). In Zheng, D., Liu, D., & Zhang, B. (Eds.), *Shehui baozhang zhidu gaige zhinan* (*Guideline for the Reform of the Social Security System*). Beijing: Gaige chubanshe. 100–2

Guowuyuan 1995. Guanyu Jiangsusheng Zhenjiangshi Jiangxisheng Jiujiangshi zhigong yiliao baozhang zhidu gaige shidian fangan de pifu (Reply to the proposal for a pilot experiment of the reform of the medical care security system for staff and workers in Zhenjiang Municipality, Jiangsu Province and Jiujinag Municipality, Jiangxi Province). *Renshi zhengce fagui zhuankan (Journal of Regulations of Personnel Policy)*: 6. 84–106.

Hu, S. 2001. *Yiliao baoxian he fuwu zhidu* (*The Medical Care Insurance and System of Services*). Chengdu: Sichuan renmin chubanshe.

Lee, P. N. 2019. *Re-engineering Affordable Care Policy in China, Is Marketization A Solution?* London & New York: Routledge.

Mo, D. 1996. Guanzhou yiliao baoxian zhidu gaige de zongti silu (An overall consideration of the medical insurance reform in Guangzhou), *Guandong laodongbao* (*Labor Journal of Guangdong*) March 28.

Shanghaishi renmin zhengfu 2010. Shanghaishi chengzhen zhigong jiben yiliao baoxian banfa (The measures for the basic medical care insurance for staff and workers in cities and towns of Shanghai Municipality). www.shanghai.gov.cn/shanghai/node2314/node3125/node3127/suerobject6a1269.him

Song, X., & Liu, H. 2001. Yiliao baoxian zhidu gaige ji peitao cushi (Reform of as well as complementary measures for medical care insurance). In Song, X. (Ed.), *Zhongguo shehui baozhang tizhi gaige yu fazhan baogao* (*Report on the Reform and Development of the Social Security System in China*). Beijing: Zhonguo renmin chubanshe. 358–74.

Wang, D. 2008. *Huigu yu qianzhan: Zhongguo yiliao zhidu gaige* (*Restropect and Prospect: The Reform of the Medical Care Insurance System*). Beijing: Zhongguo shehui kexue chubanshe.

Wu, R., & Chen, J. 1999. Jianli chengzhen zhigong yiliao baoxian zhidu quanmian tuijin woguo yiliao zhidu gaige (Constructing a medical care insurance system for staff and workers in cities and town and propelling the reform of the medical care insurance system in China). In Zheng, D., Liu, D., & Zhang, B. (Eds.), *Shehui baozhang zhidu gaige zhinan* (*Guideline for the Reform of the Social Security System*). Beijing: Gaige chubanshe. 358–74.

Wu, Z., Li, Y., & Li, X. 2008. Shanghai yiliao baozhang zhidu gaige yu fazhan bao (Report on the reform and development of medical care security in Shanghai). In Wang, H. (Ed.), *Shanghai shehui baozhang gaige yu fazhan baogao* (*Report on the Reform and Development of Social Security in Shanghai*). Beijing: Shehui kexue wenxian chubanshe. 70–1.

Wu, B., 1999. Wu Bangguo fuzhongli zai quanguo chengzhen zhigong yiliao baoxian zhidu gaige gongzuo huiyi shang de jianghua (The speech of Vice-Premier Wu B., in the national conference on the task of reforming the medical care insurance in cities and towns in China). In Zheng, D., Liu, D., & Zhang, B. (Eds.), *Shehui baozhang zhidu gaige zhinan* (*Guidelines for the Reform of the Social Security System*). Beijing: Gaige chubanshe. 22–32.

Zheng, G. 2002. Zhongguo zhigong yiliao baozhang zhidu bianqian yu pinggu (The transformation and assessment of the medical care security for staff and workers in China). In Zheng G. et al. (Eds.), *Zhonguo shehui baozhang zhidu bianqian yu pinggu* (*The Transformation and Assessment of the Social Security System in China*). Beijing: Renmin chubanshe. 119–59.

Zheng G. et al. (Eds.), 2002. *Zhonguo shehui baozhang zhidu bianqian yu pinggu* (*The Transformation and Assessment of the Social Security System in China*). Beijing: Renmin chubanshe.

Zhu, R. 2002. Guanyu zhigong yiliao baozhang zhidu gaige wenti (Issues regarding the reform medical care security system of staff and workers). In Laodong he shehui baozhangbu & zhonggong zhongyang wenxian yanjiushi (Eds.), *Xinshiqi laodong he shehui baozhang zhongyao wenxian xuanbian* (*Selected Important Documents of Labor and Social Security during the New Era*). Beijing: Zhongguo shehui baozhang chubanshe & zhong yang wenxian chubanshe. 266–74.

8 Supplementary Medical Care Insurances

In the policymaking process, there was the transformation from a thrifty version of BMCI in 1994 to an enriched version in 1998. Characteristic of "low level and broad coverage," the former intended to make essential medical care available to the largest possible size of enrollees in all jurisdictions, all work units and all residents throughout the country. As advocated by Premier Zhu Rongji, the thrifty version of packaging lent the topmost priority to considering the financial strain of the country during the early period of economic reform (Zhu 2002: 266–79; Huang 2020: 88–90). The thrifty version only covered the medical bill for a fixed amount under the payment-ceiling, amounts above which were to be handled through work unit funding subject to the approval of the head of the work unit and/or the bureau level (Lee 2019). The enriched version was required for an addition—so-called supplementary medical care insurance (SMCI). By design, SMCI meant not only to bridge the funding gaps between thrifty version and the conventional funding programs (e.g., PFMC and LIMC), but also to deal with the case of high expenditure and serious illness (HESI), representing an upgrade in terms of program specificity. Trying to tackle the issue of HESI, for sure, the enriched version marked an unprecedented and innovative landmark in the public funding of healthcare in China.

Inaugurating supplementary medical care insurances (SCMI) can be taken as purely policy-oriented regarding the choice of options based on merits, and it also involved the tensions of political interests, coupled with the challenges of maintaining a balance of interests between echelons of government, between the government and work units (including enrollees), and between work units and enrollees. The study here will first discuss the evolution of various types of SMCI at the central and provincial/local level. To assess the concrete situation of policymaking and implementation at the provincial/local level, the study will then conduct a comparative analysis of the three cases of Guangzhou, Shenzhen, and Shanghai. Also, the study will proceed to identify their common characteristics, discern their differences, and examine the subjective perceptions of policy actors and contextual considerations.

Quasi-Collective Goods and Risk-Pooling Mechanisms

Marking the first phase of policy formation, the BMCI reform commenced in 1994 when the State Council formally authorized pilot programs to be conducted in

DOI: 10.4324/9781003389934-10

Jiujiang Municipality, Jiangxi Province and Zhenjiang, Jiangsu Province as previously mentioned. In this early period of policymaking, the BMCI reform was intended to provide basic (or essential) medical care to the workforce employed in the planned sector at a low funding level. In the interpretative scheme among the circle of policymakers and analysts, priority ought to be given to providing medical care to "common and frequent cases of illness" (*changjianbing, changfabing*) for the largest possible number of patients, given the limited budget for medical care expenditure. Besides, these common and frequent cases were taken as involving least expenditure among various medical care options, and therefore it was deemed the most feasible level of funding (Wu & Chen 1999: 364–7).

As proposed originally in 1994, the early BMCI package only covered clinical care in Zone I and hospital care in Zone II and did not include HESI (including catastrophic medical care) in Zone III, an issue that the provincial/local governments had devoted considerable attention to, as being demonstrated by the pilot programs that they had sponsored (Chapter 4; Lee 2019). Not only did the low funding level of medical care here make good financial sense from the perspective of financial management, but also it was in congruence with the expectation of the people who had just moved from the austerity during the early years of economic reform after Mao. The principle of "low level" was justifiable considering the rapid and uncontrollable increase of spending for medical care at the onset of economic reform. Besides, the "low level" of funding and expenditure appeared to be an answer to the financial shortage caused by the pro-growth policy tending to squeeze funding for social security available to public enterprises and local governments (Ge & Gong 2007; Duckett 2013; Huang 2014; Lee 2019).

In the early BMCI design, although policy designers identified a category of cases where expenditure exceeded the payment-ceiling of BMCI, it was left untreated within the BMCI scheme in the pilot programs of Jiujiang and Zhenjiang in 1994. In 1998, however, when sovereign planners needed to work on the final drafts of BMCI, they were able to accommodate a residual and undefined category above the payment-ceiling. According to Premier Zhu, policymakers ought to insist on two principles: First, to decide on the funding level of basic medical care and payment-ceiling of the unified funding foundation and control expenditure for medical care and second, to handle the medical care expenditure that exceeded the payment-ceiling through commercial insurance, enterprise supplementary insurances, and social relief (Zhu 2002: 273). As illustrated in one of the earliest BMCI programs, the expenditure of medical care above payment-ceiling was left to commercial insurance in Xiamen (Lee 2019).

For some valid considerations, the early BMCI package did not include the most expensive cases of HESI: After all, HESI (including catastrophic medical care events) had not been covered by either PFMC or LIMC in the first place, as they were entirely new to the BMCI design. Contrary to the central ministries' view, many provincial/local jurisdictions considered the experimental insurance programs for HESI as one of the most favorite alternatives to be incorporated into a new public funding program such as BMCI. They had found risk-pooling mechanisms through an insurance scheme dealing with HESI quite effective based on the preceding pilot programs and policy experiments prior to the BMCI reform (Chapter 4; Lee 2019: 101–3).

Although HESI (including catastrophic medical care cases) involve very high expenditure, they are still considered manageable through some forms of risk-pooling mechanism. During the deliberation over the final drafts of BMCI in the late 1990s, available statistical data indicated that the expenditure for HESI cases consisted only of a small fraction of the total expenditure of co-payments that exceeded payment-ceiling. Under the circumstance where no risk-pooling mechanism was available, some enterprises would face financial ruin as they encountered even a very small number of HESI involving a few staff and workers. According to Wang Dongjin, the policymakers should still address the issue of HESI cases in statistical terms, namely, the most expensive but least frequent cases, to implement medical care insurance reform. Although each HESI case is exceedingly costly, the probability of its occurrence is relatively low, representing an ideal case to be tackled through risk-pooling mechanisms relying on some form of actuarial and financial scheme often found in the design of a BMCI program, as argued by Wang (2000: 132).

During the early phases of policy formation pertaining to BMCI, no actuarial and financial calculation was available to lend a precise assessment as to how much funding ought to be set aside for catastrophic medical care events under a thrifty BMCI package. Would additional funding be required? Would it be adequate, for the purpose of providing funding for HESI cases, just to work within the existing financial pool formed by premium contributions within a thrifty BMCI package? During the early phase of policymaking prior to the 1998 Decision, available data merely lent a general profile of the issue concerned, but not a laser-sharp assessment. Nonetheless, it suggested in the exercise of program specificity that the application of risk pooling mechanisms was entirely feasible in tackling the HESI issue. As noted by Wang Dongjin, a survey from the late 1990s era indicates that there were 696,000 users whose expenditures on medical care insurance exceeded the payment-ceiling of pilot programs in various jurisdictions, and this was 0.5 percent of the total number of patients in the sample. He further made mention that, on average, the expenditure for medical care services exceeding the payment-ceiling amounted to 10 percent of the total expenditure, ranging between 6 and 16 percent across jurisdictions (Wang 2000: 132). It appears that the then existing risk-pooling mechanisms of the program could effectively meet the funding requirement for these HESI cases.

To address political concerns, a proposal dealing with HESI cases by introducing SMCI was important to rally the support of provincial/local governments and enrollees at large. As Wu and Chen have argued, adequate coverage of HESI events through SMCI was a prerequisite, in a political sense, for extending and consolidating BMCI bases throughout the country (Wu & Chen 1999: 369–74).

In conceptual and theoretical terms, the BMCI policymaking circle made a breakthrough in articulating an explicit policy stand on HESI in the process of implementing BMCI later in 2012. As put forth in the landmark policy paper, the 2012 Advisory Opinion, central policymakers began to be confronted explicitly with several theoretical issues relating to HESI in conjunction with the implementation of URMCI and NRCMCI (Guojia fazhanwei et al. 2012). In line with the 2012 Advisory Opinion, it was argued that in operational terms, a well-designed risk pooling scheme would be able to deal with HESI once for all and render the control measure based on payment-ceiling unnecessary. It is entirely feasible to make HESI the core concern not only of BMCI but also URMCI and NRCMCI (Cong 2006). Conceptually speaking, the boundary between BMCI and SMCI is not necessary regarding HESI. The notion "basic" needs to be redefined and a new formulation of BMCI for a broader scope is in demand (Sun 2013a, 2013b; Wu 2013). For the purpose of implementation, however, it is up to the central government and a provincial/local jurisdiction to incorporate HESI into the discrete insurance plans in respective jurisdictions in the process of implementation in China, a policy issue to be discussed further (Chapters 9–12).

The Issue of Historically Rooted Obligations

The second phase of policymaking of the BMCI reform commenced in conjunction with one salient issue in 1996: Namely, the overall funding level of BMCI was too low. In the thrifty version of the BMCI package, there existed the obvious gaps of the funding level in the public funding for medical care between the BMCI design on the one hand and the conventional funding of health care in PFCI and LIMC on the other (Zhang 1999). According to Wu Ritu and Chen Jinpu, it is estimated that, on the basis of statistical data relating to the funding and payment of basic medical care insurance in 1996, the total payment of BMCI consisted of only 70 percent of the total expenditure of the PFMC and LIMC programs, meaning that the level of the PFMC and LIMC exceeded the level of BMCI by 30 percent, equivalent to 20 billion RMB (Wu & Chen 1999: 372).

Why was it imperative to fill up the shortfall of 30 percent in the thrifty version of the early BMCI package? Since social security policy is taken as an integral part of the remuneration package for the workforce employed under the low wage policy within the CPE framework, the party-state entity assumed obligations to make funding available to honor non-wage compensation, that is, payments covering social security entitlements for workers and staff so employed and retirees in public enterprises and public personnel of the government and other public organizations. From a political perspective, it was reasonable to make good on the "historical debts" to the workforce in the planned sector by addressing the issue of the alienation of entitlements from funding.

Regarding the issue of non-wage compensation, theoretically speaking, the workers and staff who had been employed under the CPE ought to enjoy the room of choice between the conventional public funding of social security and the new packages proposed during the reforms. It would become arguable for the current generation of public employees under the PFMC and LIMC programs to be forced to accept new packages of basic medical care at obviously lower standards without honoring the rightful claims to non-wage compensation (so-called "historical debts") to employees in the public sector (Wu & Chen 1999: 369; Wang 2000:

132–5). The government's obligation to answer the claims of social entitlement was not absolved Despite new packages of social security offered during economic reform. Nor was financial responsibility to be diluted by new social security programs replacing outdated programs in any proposed reform. In the matter of social security reforms, theoretically speaking, entitlements as well as the funding level of new programs should remain commensurate with those of the comparable packages provided for in the past.

In fact, sovereign planners did not start to address the said "gaps" until after the early phases of BMCI packages took shape from the mid-1990s onwards, while employees in the planned sector, such as public personnel in government and other public organizations, and staff and workers made their claims known. As just noted, Premier Zhu Rongji made his statement about the social security reform and specially mentioned SMCI on October 27, 1997 (Zhu 2002: 266–74) Meanwhile, the top leaders further articulated their positions on "historical debts" as previously mentioned during a series of meetings and conferences leading to the 1998 Decision that authorized the full-scale implementation of BMCI. In his speech at the commencement of the working conference on the reform of basic medical care insurance for staff and workers in November 1998, Vice-Premier Wu Bangguo conveyed the consensus of the top leadership team about closing the gaps between the conventional funding of medical care and the new BMCI, by authorizing the establishment of enterprise supplementary medical care insurance (ESMCI) for staff and workers at the enterprise level (Wu 1998). Vice-Premier Wu's view on SMCI for staff and workers was spelled out in written form in the 1998 Decision, stating that 4 percent of the total annual wage would be set aside for financing ESMCI for staff and workers at the public enterprise level (Guowuyuan 1998). According to Wu, moreover, the fund for ESMCI (i.e., 4 percent of the total annual wage) would be chargeable to the welfare fund, and/or to production costs subject to approval of the financial bureau at the respective echelons of the local governments (Wu 1998).

With Wu's announcements about the ESMCI, the BMCI reform was thereby launched after the 1998 Advisory Opinion on an experimental basis and then formally in 2001. In fact, the central government lost no time in promulgating the 2000 Opinion to establish the subsidy for SMCI to ensure that civil servants and public personnel in other public organizations would not suffer from low standards of medical benefits because of the inauguration of BMCI (Laodong baozhangbu & caizhengbu 2000).

Since the thrifty BMCI package was funded at a comparatively lower level, it was justified to propose the SMCI to address the said shortfall as noted. By and large, SMCI covered large expenditures above the BMCI payment-ceiling, that normally fell into Zones II and III, that is, expenditures for hospital care and other HESI events as just noted, in addition to the diverse requests and different preferences among enrollees (Wang 2000: 132–3; Song & Liu 2001: 100–1; Zheng et al. 2002: 155–7). In other words, the SMCI "kills two birds with one stone": It would make funding available to fill both the said "gaps" and HESI cases. Provincial/local leaders paid close attention to the issue of HESI (including catastrophic medical care events) because of their policy experiments dealing with the same issue prior to the BMCI reform during the late 1980s and early 1990s.

In view of rising expectations, the new cohorts of workforce would not be content with a basic medical care at a "low level" of expenditure either, as what the thrifty BMCI package offered while being focused on providing "essential" medical care services, short of covering HESI cases (Wu & Chen 1999: 369–74; Wang 2000: 132–5). As a result of the cultural change in the healthcare sector since 1979, moreover, enrollees sought both better quality and more choices of medical care services beyond the overly simple and thrifty packages of the pre-reform decades. The rise of medical care consumerism called for a major overhaul, besides, promising better quality and more choices of medical care. Proposals for healthcare and public insurances with "multiple levels" were therefore put on the policy agenda to answer the diverse healthcare demands accompanying the further improvement of living standards and continuing economic growth. No less than BMCI, SMCIs were taken as a major policy innovation in the public funding of medical care ever since the beginning of PRC in 1949 (Sun 2013).

Program Specificity of SCMI

As the healthcare policy circle reached consensus on the SCMI policy in the late 1990s, it is pertinent here to analyze how the various echelons of government and work units took further steps to introduce this policy. Like the early version of BMCI, SMCI represented another layer of medical care insurance to be incorporated into the proper of BMCI in the process of marketization. Echoing the policy position of the central government, some jurisdictions explicitly treated SMCI as "transitional policy," targeting the cohorts of senior employees and retirees of the work unit, who had taken part in "forced modernization" under the CPE before economic reform (Guowuyuan 1998; Wu 1998).

Still working with the IRF system, the SMCI was often integrated with BMCI in operational and managerial terms. The exercise of program specificity was focused on the endeavors of government units and work units at respective levels to make funding available and inject it into the SMCI system operating with risk-pooling mechanisms. Conceptually speaking, policymakers adopted three categories of SMCI programs that were financed mainly by the enrollee, work unit and government unit at the respective levels. The first category of SMCI is concerned with the so-called "large medical care expenditure subsidy" (*daer yiliao feiyong buzhu*; hereafter, LMCES), which targeted catastrophic medical care events, often covering those expensive items which exceeded the USFA payment-ceiling. By and large, the work unit was responsible for making the LMCES available, coupled with a share contributed by staff and workers regarding supplementary medical care insurance (SMCI).

It appeared that the various echelons of government took "large medical care expenditure subsidy" (LMCES) seriously in the process of implementation. According to a survey in various jurisdictions in early 2002, cited in a set of internal references, for example, the LMCES was introduced to 76.67 percent of the 30 municipalities. And indicated in the same survey, each enrollee's share of annual contribution, on average, was about 60 RMB in full and was either paid by the enrollee himself/herself or by the employing work unit or both. Thus, the enrollee and work unit each contributed a share of the premium for the chosen LMCES scheme. Accordingly, this same scheme absorbed about 85 percent of the "large amount expenditure" that exceeded the payment-ceiling of BMCI (meaning 15 percent of co-payment by the enrollee) (Deng & Liu 2008).

According to Wang Dongjin, overall, various jurisdictions adopted two options to handle the funding of LMCES as follows. First, in the case of Xiamen, which the author visited personally, LMCES is entrusted to a commercial insurance company on a contractual basis. Second, in Zhenjiang, representing the majority of jurisdictions across the nation, LMCES is managed by a social insurance institute, a non-departmental public entity (Wang 2000: 129).

In the field investigation conducted by the author's research team in 2002, Xiamen's BMCI represents one of the earlier cases of LMCES among the expanding pilot programs in 1996, making use of commercial insurance to deal with the issue of catastrophic medical care events. Xiamen's LMCES arrangement requires each enrollee to make a contribution of 18 RMB out of PA, coupled with 6 RMB by the work unit, chargeable to USFA annually; and if the payment-ceiling is exceeded, the insurance company, namely, China-Pacific Life Insurance Corporation, pays 90 percent (or 10 percent of co-payment by the enrollee) to the stipulated amount exceeded (Anonymous 2002a, 2002b).

The second category of SMCI schemes is offered to those personnel employed in the public sector, embracing two sub-categories: Sub-category I, so-called "public personnel medical care subsidy" (*gongwu renyuan yiliao buzhu*; hereafter, PPMCS) included all public personnel such as civil servants, personnel affiliated with political parties, service units, and other public organizations, and Sub-category II covers staff and workers of public enterprises. On the eve of the full-scale implementation of medical care insurance throughout China in 2000, the Office of State Council issued a policy paper, the 2000 Opinion, detailing a guiding principle for maintaining medical care entitlements to public personnel at the existing level and suggesting ways to afford a level of subsidy compatible with economic development and financial capacity in the respective jurisdictions (Laodong Baozhangbu & Caizhengbu 2000). It was shown that the PPMCS policy answered the demands of public personnel throughout China in a timely fashion. For example, 43.3 percent adopted and implemented PPMCS as of the year 2002, according to the statistics of 30 municipalities. As noted by the same survey, various jurisdictions tried to make better use of PPMCS creatively to stretch it to cover some defined benefits. In Hunan Province, for example, the PPMCS covered clinical treatments for a category of selected diseases, part of the co-payment for prescriptions, and special treatments regarding uses of medical devices (Deng & Liu 2008).

As a general principle, the 2000 Opinion tries to elaborate the conditions of implementation of PPMCS, underscoring the issue of HESI events with an explicit purpose to cover those items of expenditure exceeding the payment-ceiling in USFA for public personnel. It was intended to cover only those public personnel at the central and provincial level according to the measures and criteria of subsidy to be worked out by respective departments and jurisdictions considering their financial conditions. In operational terms, moreover, each item of expenditure needed to be explicitly listed and included in the relevant catalogs for the application of medicine, lists of medical care services, and criteria for use of medical devices. In addition, it fell under the scope of payments for BMCI coupled with a required portion of co-payment by the patient (Laodon Baozhangbu & Caizhengbu 2000).

Sub-category II pertains to enterprise supplementary medical care insurance (*qiye buchong yiliao baoxian*; hereafter, ESMCI), which aims at filling the gap between lower standards of BMCI and existing, higher standards of enterprise-managed medical care of well-to-do enterprises. ESMCI follows the same consideration as PPMCS since the existing level of medical care insurance for public employees ought to be consistently maintained regardless of the lower level of the thrifty BMCI package as prescribed. In accordance with the 1998 Decision, ESMCI is allowed to charge to the welfare fund account up to 4 percent of the supplementary wage. However, if 4 percent of the supplementary wage is found to be inadequate, the remaining amount is chargeable to production costs upon approval by the bureau of finance at the respective administrative level within the jurisdiction With reference to the nature of ESMCI, it is, in the 1998 Decision, explicitly stated: as a transitional measure, enterprises are permitted to establish ESMCI in order *not* to lower the level of consumption of medical care by staff and workers in some specific trades in the case of BMCI (Guowuyuan 1998).

The third category is concerned with SMCI policies of a commercial nature. By and large, commercial health care insurance (hereafter, CHCI) addresses non-basic medical care services, but it can still fill gaps left by BMCI. As just noted, Xiamen Municipality has made use of CHCI to cover so-called "large medical care expenditure subsidy" (LMCES), but HESI involves an even larger sum of expenditure than that of LMCES. CHCI offers, in fact, a wider scope of health care insurance services, and it is not confined to the sort of insurance services provided for Xiamen case (Anonymous 2002a; Liu 2004: 160–86). It was and is taken, fittingly, as part of the "tertiary industry" that has been promoted due to its expanding market share and great potential for investment ventures during the reform era. For example, there were 42 life insurance companies and 35 real estate insurance companies that offered nearly a thousand healthcare insurance products, including supplements to hospitalization, life insurance, long-term care, and insurance for invalids in the 2000s (Deng & Liu 2008: 120).

From the foregoing analysis, SMCI took shape not only for bridging the funding gap between BMCI and conventional funding programs, but also answering the demands of HESI cases that represented an entirely new dimension of public funding of health. The former dealt with the issue of alienation of entitlements from funding, namely, concerning claims to entitlements for employees in the public sector, that had been enacted by the laws and regulations. In the latter, furthermore, it was concerned with the matter of product/service specificity—choices among better actuarial and financial alternatives, and how to upgrade the use of available insurance funds for better protection of the enrollee. And it was added to BMCI as an integral part, answering multiple demands of residents in a growing economy. Has it taken root in all jurisdictions throughout China? It is pertinent to review some selected cases below and to shed light on the patterns and variations of policy implementation across jurisdictions in China.

SMCI Policy in Municipal Jurisdictions: Guangzhou and Shenzhen Compared

In the evolution from the thrifty BMCI package to the enriched version, policy-makers began to work toward a new healthcare developmental strategy aimed at answering the "multiple tiers" (*duocengci*) of healthcare demands. In the case of Guangzhou, not only did the multiple tiers of healthcare demand referred to the range of options between BMCI and SMCI, but also to several tiers within SMCI in accordance with the 2012 Measures (Guangzhoushi zhengfu 2012).[1] Beyond the thrifty BMCI package introduced in the initial period of healthcare insurance reform, three categories were inaugurated in Guangzhou, representing a replica of what the central government had recommended as noted above, and suggesting that Guangzhou would toe the policy line of the central government and provincial government closely. These three categories are taken as three tiers of insurance demands as well.

The first tier pertained to the SMCI targeting large expenditure illness, an insurance package funded by the so-called "subsidy for major illness" (*zhongda jibing buzhu*; hereafter, SMI). It was designed to operate with a set of risk-sharing mechanisms to meet the funding demands brought about by HESI, a gap left in the thrifty BMCI package. The Labor and Social Insurance Administration (LSIA) managed SMI in collaboration with the Department of Finance at the municipal level. Falling into Zone III, SMI worked to absorb costs for medical care beyond the payment-ceiling of what could normally be covered by BMCI. For SMI-related entitlements, the work unit had to contribute on behalf of the enrollee an amount of 0.29 percent of the average monthly pay of each enrollee from the previous year. SMI covered up to 95 percent of the expenses for hospital care and defined items of clinical services exceeding the payment-ceiling that was determined according to the accumulated annual total payment by the BMCI foundation. However, the total expenditure of SMI for each enrollee was limited to 150,000 RMB within a budgetary year. The SMI also paid for defined items for the special clinical treatment of chronic illness in accordance with mandated standards (Guangzhoushi zhengfu 2012: Article 40–1).

The second tier encompassed two sub-tiers: tier I and Sub-tier II. The former was to fund supplementary insurance to civil servants and other personnel in public organizations while the latter was to finance insurance to staff and workers in public enterprises. Targeted at two different groups of employees in the planned sector, both were designed to make up for the shortfall in medical care insurance benefits between the newly introduced BMCI and the conventional funding programs (PFMC and LIMC) of the pre-reform era (Guangzhoushi zhengfu 2012: Article 42).

These two sub-tiers of SMCI schemes were funded through their respective financial sources as they were during the pre-reform era. Although one may consider both as being in Zone III, in fact they also covered some other types of benefits in Zone II and to a lesser extent, Zone I. For instance, Sub-tier I, namely the Public Personnel Medical Care Subsidy (*gongwu renyuan yiliao buzhu*; hereafter, PP-MCS) was financed through public funding, amounting to 4 percent of a total wage bill, from the municipal jurisdiction. And Sub-tier II, that is, the supplementary medical care insurance for staff and workers (hereafter, SMCISW) was likewise calculated at 4 percent of the total wage bill for the work unit, and was chargeable to the business account of the enterprise unit in accordance with the 2012 Measures (Guangzhoushi zhengfu 2012: Article 42). In principle, the Guangzhou medical care insurance policy lent support to SMCISW, which was managed and financed by the work unit. For example, SMCISW was to cover 70 percent of three types of payment made by the BMCI foundation: The sum of payment before paying the deductible (likely Zone I), the part of the co-payment after the deductible payment but below the stipulated payment-ceiling (Zone II), and the part of the co-payment above the payment-ceiling (i.e., in Zone III) (Guangzhoushi zhengfu 2012: Article 42). Beyond the first and second tiers that operated entirely within public finance management as noted above, the third tier, related to commercial medical care insurance (CMCI), the enrollment into which was at the discretion of the enrollee, and subject to the enrollee's own needs and financial ability (Guangzhoushi zhengfu 2012: Article 39).

Shenzhen and Guangzhou are in close geographical proximity, but they remain separate from each other in terms of institutional affiliation. Each enjoys its full administrative and financial autonomy. Shenzhen did not offer a form of SMCI when it first started its pilot experiment in 1996, but the municipality added it to the BMCI package from 2003 onward. The SMCIs were finalized in 2013, coupled with adjustments and amendments. The Shenzhen municipal government also introduced three categories of SMCI, bearing close resemblance to those of Guangzhou. Conceptually speaking, the three categories can be treated in terms of a three-tiered structure for public medical care insurance: HESI (including catastrophic illness) in the first tier, SMCI for employees in the planned sector in the second tier, and enrollees in commercial medical care insurance (CMCI) in the third tier.

In accordance with the 2013 Measures, there was a cluster of SCMI programs with three tiers, on top of the BMCI (embracing Scheme I, II and III) in Shenzhen municipality (Shenzhen renmin zhengfu 2013: Article 17). The first tier of SCMI package pertained to the so-called local supplementary medical care insurance (LSMCI) program, working with a set of risk-sharing mechanisms to fill the gaps in expensive HESI cases (i.e., in Zone III) which were not previously covered by the earlier design of BMCI. Furthermore, the second tier of SMCI was designed to bridge funding gaps between the early version of BMCI and the conventional funding programs of PFMC and LIMC that had been built during the CPE period. Like Guangzhou's design, the second tier consisted of two schemes (or comparable with two sub-tiers in Guangzhou's package): Namely the public personnel medical care subsidy (abbreviated as PPMCS) and work unit supplementary medical care insurance (abbreviated as WUSMCI). And in the third tier, the commercial medical care insurance (abbreviated as COMCI) provided additional choices of commercial medical care insurance to enrollees depending on their preferences and economic status (Shenzhen renmin zhengfu 2012: Article 2).

Among the several SCMI packages, LSMCI in the first tier by nature differed from WUSMCI and PPMCS in the second tier. With regard to program specificity, in the first tier, LSMCI, was designed to absorb any big spending beyond the payment-ceiling set by the BMCI, most of which falls into HESI cases in Zone III. As noted in the Zhenjiang and Xiamen pilot programs, the remedies of similar SMCIs were provided by making use of financial risk-pooling mechanisms and by creating additional funding sources to fill any shortfalls in the BMCI basic design in Shenzhen. Like the policy and practice of other jurisdictions, Shenzhen adopted the standard design to integrate LSMCI into BMCI in accordance with the 2013 Measures (Shenzhen renmin zhengfu 2013).

In the second tier, WUSMCI and PPMCS are personnel-centered, catering to specific medical care services for some kinds of personnel who had been employed in the public sector in the CPE system. As previously noted, they were meant to fill gaps created by the early, thrifty BMCI design and, taken together, were supposed to supersede the PFMC and LIMC programs, the level of which was higher than the "basic," or "low-level" funding. To enforce the idea of low-level benefits as mentioned, the early, thrifty BMCI design established a payment-ceiling for medical care services, beyond which the insurance did not cover, for example, often high-cost cases or less frequent cases of a HESI nature, as previously mentioned.

In legislative terms, WUSMCI and PPMCS were taken to top off the early, thrifty BMCI design in accordance with the "2013 Measures," and included some privileges beyond the basic medical care categories—privileges justified in terms of non-wage compensation to sacrifices made under the low wage policy prior to the economic reform. They were colored heavily with corporatism in order to accommodate the vested interests of the workforce who worked under the old CPE regime, and were intended to maintain the then-existing level of consumption by beneficiaries of the previous PFMI and LIMC programs. They meant to maintain the vested interest of those who worked in the public sector under CPE. Furthermore, PPMCS provided coverage of benefits to public servants and members of public organizations whose medical bills went beyond the funding limits of BMCI.

In the second tier, PPMCS worked with a kind of risk-pooling mechanism, but it did not rely on premium contributions made by an ordinary insurance scheme of BMCI through the IRF system. Instead, it was supported in part or in full by public revenue and is handled directly through the state budget through the ORF system (Shenzhenshi renmin zhengfu 2012). However, WUSMCI followed the common practice of the insurance system by relying financially on the retained revenue of public enterprises (i.e., up to 4 percent of the total wage bill), in consistency with the design of the BMCI system in general (Shenzhen renmin zhengfu 2013: Article 110). This meant that better-performing and revenue-earning enterprises were likely to shoulder the financial burden for WUSMCI for their own units more than their poorly performing counterparts, albeit the government attempted to set limits on what better-performing units were permitted to spend, with a view toward egalitarianism.

Through the foregoing comparative analysis, above all, Shenzhen and Guangzhou are found surprisingly similar to each other concerning the core features of an enhanced BMCI, for example, the three-tier structure of SMCI. Would Shanghai's policy experience produce a different pattern from Shenzhen and Guangzhou? This study needs to go into the Shanghai case to reach a conclusion.

SMCI Programs made in Shanghai

It appears that the establishment of a SMCI package was as much as politically motivated as the other policy options pertaining to funding, insurance, and provision of medical care in the case of Shanghai. In the introduction of SMCI, three issues enjoyed considerable salience, deserving further discussion. First, SMCI was intertwined with the redistribution of interests among various groups of personnel who were entrenched in the structure of the CPE, resulting in a new configuration of interests in which personnel in governmental and quasi-governmental units were able to retain vested interests more than other groups in the case of Shanghai. For example, relative to the government officials and personnel of quasi-government apparatus, the staff and workers of public enterprises seemed to have been among the losers who could only fetch whatever was left during economic reform. The redistribution of interests did not rely upon market-mechanisms but on the exercise of mandatory power by the party-state, especially involving the issues of so-called "historical debts".

The introduction of SMCI meant who were more entitled than others about the claims for additional benefits. For example, SMCI addressed the issue of gaps between the conventional funding of basic medical care and the newly proposed UIP (i.e., BMCI equivalent in Shanghai) design in addition to the benefits of HESI. With reference to the claims derived from the "gaps," Shanghai's policymaking team was confronted with controversies about who was better off than the others. As they argued, for example, that within the municipal jurisdiction, employees of a small number of public enterprises had already enjoyed a relatively high standard of medical care and spent considerably more on medical care than the other sister work units. Besides, the privileges of these high standard medical care benefits were even not shared equally among all public personnel of government departments and other public organizations (presumably in those service work units, differential-quota budgeted work units, and/or revenue-oriented work units).

Second, Shanghai municipal leadership was reluctant to tackle SMCI considering that the municipal finance had already been overly strained by the social security reforms. For instance, Shanghai faced some challenges in drafting a policy of UIP (or BMCI) for the workforce in the planned sector in view of the very high percentage of wage funds that had gone into funding medical care entitlements prior to the healthcare reform. As claimed, the Shanghai municipal government would be overburdened with even more funding to be set aside for UIP, and SMCI meant to add even more financial responsibility to the jurisdiction. According to

Standing Vice Mayor Zuo Huanchen, it was proposed in the UIP reform design of the earlier vintage put forth by the State Council that the total funding would be calculated at 8 percent of the average wage of staff and workers (6 percent for USFA and 2 percent for PA), but in the case of Shanghai, each enrollee actually enjoyed a much higher standard of medical care benefits, say, 17 percent of the average wage for the LIMC program, while for the PFMC program it was even higher, reaching 23–24 percent of the average wage for each enrollee (Zuo 2000: 4). The phenomenon of large spending in social security in general and medical care might be taken as the attempts made by work units to circumscribe the strict wage control and improve non-wage compensation of employees in the name of collective welfare at the work unit level during economic reform. In the perception among the members of the workforce, they needed to seek an improvement of non-wage compensation if wage compensation is denied.

Third, the municipal leadership team felt considerable difficulties in undertaking the task of building up consensus among personnel in the public sector in the medical care reform. And SMCI simply complicated the thorny problem in the process of implementation as being attested in a long story told by Vice Mayor Chen LIanyu. When the 2000 Measures were being implemented in early 2001, for example, Vice Mayor Chen gave a briefing related to the merging of the PFMC with the proposed programs of UIP (equivalent to BMCI) as recommended by the State Council. Chen argued for his recommendation of upgrading the UIP benefits to civil servants and party cadres in the government and public personnel of other public organizations by claiming that they were not necessarily better off than staff and workers in public enterprises. Chen cited co-payments of the PFMC of current personnel and retirees as 10 percent and 5 percent for clinical visits, and 8 percent and 4 percent for hospital care, respectively. He further pointed out that disparities still existed in the PFMC programs at the municipal, district, and work unit levels, and these were further complicated by different modes of management within the three levels. During the 9th Five Year Plan period from 1995 to 1999, moreover, the spending on the PFMC program registered a dramatic increase of about 54 percent from 220 million RMB to 410 million RMB during the same period (Chen 2002: 4–6). To sweeten the deal and persuade public personnel covered by the PFMC program to join the municipal UIP package, Chen proposed, as a first step, a 2 percent pay increase in the name of a "supplementary wage" to all PFMC enrollees to offset the reduction of medical care funding from the preceding PFMC program. The same wage increase was also applicable to staff and workers in public enterprises (Chen 2002: 6). As the second step, Chen recommended the installment of subsidy schemes for SMCI. While 4 percent of the average wage was to be set aside for establishing the subsidy scheme to SMCI for staff and workers in public enterprises, he recommended a comparable scheme for public personnel in government units, quasi-government units, and other public organizations accordingly, in line with the policy paper issued by the central government.[2]

At the end of the day, Shanghai municipal leadership did follow the policy guidelines of the central government, addressing the issue of SMCI, and adopting a three tier structure in the exercise of program specificity. In the first tier, for instance, the SMCI scheme embraced HESI (including catastrophic medical care events), just like what was done in Guangzhou and Shenzhen. High priority was given to particularly expensive illnesses, such as cancer, mental illness, dialysis, etc., for those public personnel in PFMC and staff and workers in LIMC, respectively.

In the second tier, Shanghai municipal leadership also adopted a public personnel supplementary medical care insurance (*gongwu renyuan buzhu yiliao baoxian*; abbreviated as PPSMCI) program for civil servants in the government and public personnel in service work units and other public organizations in order to bridge the discrepancy between the conventional funding programs (i.e., PFMC and BMCI) in accordance with the 2001 Opinion.[3] The 2001 Opinion authorized setting aside 4 percent of the total wage to cover PPSMCI for civil servants and other public personnel—2 percent to be appropriated through public revenue and the other 2 percent to be contributed by the work unit, with 2 percent out of 4 percent to be entered into a pool for the USFA to absorb 50 percent of the portion of OPP made by the enrollee in the case of hospital care and emergency observation room services (Wu, Li & Li 2008: 91–2). Shanghai Municipality, moreover, established the supplementary fund (*fujia jijin;* abbreviated SP), representing a package of SMCI for staff and workers in public enterprises to top off the BMCI package. The SP was focused on the discrepancies between LMCI and UIP (Shanghai version of BMCI) regarding the medical care for employees of public enterprises. For example, it was explicitly stipulated in the 2000 Measures that the SP should pay up to 80 percent of medical care expenses when they exceeded the payment-ceiling of the early version of UIP program, that is, the limit of 70,000 RMB in accordance with the 2010 Measures (Shanghaishi renmin zhengfu 2010: Article 27).

In the third tier, room for optional, commercial medical care insurances (CMCIs), did exist for various SMCIs in Shanghai. For example, there was a variety of group-centered arrangements of SMCI schemes available to tackle the risks of illness and help alleviate the financial burden of enrollees at the enterprise level. In practice, these were managed typically by non-governmental entities such as the Shanghai Federation of Labor Union. For instance, the Shanghai Federation of Labor Unions took charge of the establishment and management of so-called "medical care mutual help security plans" (*yiliao huzu baozhang jihua*; abbreviated as MCMHSP) in four schemes, all of which adopted mechanisms of pooling of financial resources among enrollees at the enterprise level.[4] In line with the tradition of Union activism in Shanghai, by and large, the labor unions made the drafting and introduction of these four insurance schemes possible at the enterprise level, featuring a special brand of SMCI policy made in Shanghai.

Concluding Remarks

In the foregoing analysis, this study endeavored to document how policymakers at the central and provincial/local levels tried to deal with the funding of basic medical care that exceeded the payment-ceiling in the BMCI packages, demonstrating the process of defining, articulating, and packaging SCMI at both the central level and provincial/local level. In fact, the BMCI reform was not complete until the policy issues of SCMIs had been properly addressed. SCMI was intended to cover a "residual," ill-defined category of medical care in the early BMCI designs and was gradually incorporated into an enhanced BMCI. It is evident that sovereign planners were confronted with the task to bridge the gaps of conventional funding of medical care and the thrifty version of BMCI, that stemmed from the alienation of entitlements from funding and historically rooted obligations of the party-state entity.

This study further suggests that the difference between the central leadership and provincial/local policymakers was a matter of perception and sensitivity as well as policy experience. For example, Vice-Premier Wu Bangguo began with the view that the gaps between the conventional funding packages (i.e., PFMC and LIMC) and the BMCI designs needed to be dealt with, but without addressing specifically the issue of HESI, including catastrophic medical care events (Wu 1999). By contrast, the study shows that in all three cases, Guangzhou, Shenzhen and Shanghai, policymakers lost no time in addressing the said issue directly and worked out respective insurance plans to resolve the issue at hand. While provincial/local policymakers worked on the first front, sustaining the brunt of the consequences pertaining to each important decision, they lent HESI high priority, attributing not only to political pressure from the rank and file of bureaucrats and employees of public enterprises, but also to the intrinsic logic and reasoning of the insurance scheme regarding the provision of quasi-collective goods through risk-pooling mechanisms.

Notes

1 The full title of the policy paper is "Measures for Trial Implementation of Basic Medical Care Insurance for Staff and Workers in Cities and Towns in Guangzhou Municipality," first issued in 2001, subsequently reissued July 30, 2008, and amended and implemented September 1, 2012 (known as the 2008 Measures amended in 2012) (Guangzhoushi zhenfu 2012).

2 See "the Opinion of the Ministry of Labor and Social Security and Ministry of Finance Regarding the Implementation of Medical Care Subsidy for State Public Personnel" (Laodong shehui baozhanbu, caizhengbu 2000; Chen 2002: 6).

3 The full title of the policy paper reads as follows: The Opinion Regarding the Trial Implementation of Supplementary Medical Car Insurance in Shanghai (abbreviated as the 2001 Opinion), as promulgated in 2001 (Wu, Li & Li 2008: 91–2).

4 The first scheme was targeted at nine specific types of "particularly serious illnesses" of catastrophic nature. Each enrollee was required to contribute a fixed sum, say 60 RMB (not to be refunded upon the expiry of the term) or 1,180 RMB (to be refunded in full upon expiry of the term) for a fixed period of insurance. The second scheme catered to the demands of currently employed staff and workers with regard to the benefits of hospital care, clinical care for major illness, family care services, and emergency observation room services. For a fixed period of insurance, the user had to pay a fixed charge, say 50 RMB (not to be refunded to the enrollee upon the expiry of the term of insurance) or 2,050 RMB (to be refunded to the user upon the expiry of the term). Like the second scheme in terms of defined categories of services with slightly adjusted schedules of charges, the third scheme catered to the demands of retirees from the work unit. The fourth scheme has to do with the specific types of illness afflicting women employees

(e.g., breast cancer and ovarian cancer). These schemes were sponsored by labor unions in public enterprises and were funded by the premium contributions of enrollees, and it adopted a managerial system like the third scheme (Wu, Li & Li 2008: 94–8).

References

Chen, L. 2002. Shanghai changwu fushichang Chen Lianyu zai Shanghai jiguan shiye gong-fei yiliao naru yiliao shishi qidong gongzuo huiyi shang de jianghua (Speech of Standing Vice Mayor Chen Liaoyu at the work conference to initiate the implementation of incorporating enrollees of PFMC into the apparatus and service units of medical care insurance). In Liu, J. (Ed.), *Shanghai weisheng nianjian 2002 (Shanghai Yearbook of Health Care 2000)*. Shanghai: Shanghai kexue jishu wenxian chubanshe.

Cong, S. 2006. Lun goujian yi dabing baozhang wei heixin de yiliao baozhang zhidu (On the building of a medical care security system centering on major illness security). *Shehui baozhang zhidu (Social Security System)* 6.

Deng, D., & Liu, C. 2008. *Zhongguo shehui baozhang gaige yu fazhan baogao, 2006–2007 nian (The Report of Reform and Development of Social Security in China Year, 2006–2007)*. Beijing: Remin chubanshe.

Duckett, J. 2013. *The Chinese State's Retreat from Health*. London & New York: Routledge.

Ge, Y., & Gong, S. 2007. *Zhongguo yigai: wenti, genyuan, chulu (China's Medical Care Reform: Problem, Roots and Solution)*. Beijing: Zhongguo fazhan chubanshe.

Guangzhoushi zhengfu 2012. Guangzhoushi chengzhen zhigong jiben baoxian shixing banfa (Measures for the trial-implementation of basic medical care insurance for staff and workers in cities and towns in Guangzhou Municipality). *Guangzhoushi zhengfu mingling No. 80 (Guangzhoushi zhengfu directive No 80)*.

Guojia fazhan gaigewei et al. (2012). Guanyu kaizhan chengxiang jumin dabing baoxiang gongzou de zhidao yijian (The advisory opinion regarding the launching of the task of major illness insurance for residents in cities and countryside). In Guojia weisheng jishenwei (Eds.) *2012 nian shenhua yigai wenjian huibian (The 2012 Collected Documents of Further Health Care Reform)*. Beijing: Guojia weisheng jishenwei. 126–3.

Guowuyuan 1998. Guowuyuan guanyu jianli chengzhen zhigong jiben yiliao baoxian zhidu de jueding (The decision by State Council concerning the establishment of a basic medical care insurance system for staff and workers in cities and towns). *Guowuyuan gongbao (Bulletin of State Council)* 33.

Huang, Y. 2014. *Governing Health in Contemporary China*. London & New York: Routledge.

Huang, X. 2020. *Social Protection under Authoritarianism, Health Politics and Policy in China*. New York: Oxford University Press.

Laodong Baozhangbu, Caizhengbu 2000. Guanyu shixing guojia gongwuyuan buzhu de yigpjian (Opinion concerning the implementation of medical care subsidy for public personnel). *Guowuyuan gongbao (Bulletin of State Council)* 21.

Lee, P. N. 2019. *Re-engineering Affordable Care Policy in China, Is Marketization A Solution?* London & New York: Routledge.

Shenzhenshi renmin zhengfu 2012. Shenzhenshi shihui yiliao baoxian banfa (Measures for the social insurance of Shenzhen Municipality. bsz.sz.bao.com. (Retrieval date: October 10, 2013).

Shenzhenshi renmin zhengfu 2013. Shenzhenshi shehui yiliao baoxian banfa (Measures for the social medical care insurance of Shenzhen Municipality).

Song, X., & Liu, H. 2001. Yiliao gaige zhidu gaige ji peitao cuoshi (The reform of the medical care system and its complementary measures). In Song, X. (Ed.), *Zhongguo shehui baozhang tizhi gaige yu fanzhan baogao* (*The Report on the Reform and Development of the Social Security System in China*). Beijing: Zhongguo remin daxue chubanshe.

Sun, Z. 2013a. Shishi dabing baoxian shi jianqin renmin jiuyifudan de guanjian (The key link to lessening the people's burden is through big expenditure insurance). *Shehui baozhang zhidu* (*Social Security System*) 3.

Sun, Z. 2013b. Shishi dabing baoxian shi jianqin renmin jiuyi fudang de guanjian (The implementation of a major illness insurance as a crucial link for lessening the medical care burden). *Shehui baozhang zhidu* (*Social Security System*) 3.

Wang, D. 2000. *Zhonguo shehui baoxian zhidu de gaige yu fazhan* (*The Reform and Development of Social Insurance in China*). Beijing: Falu chubanshe.

Wu, B. 1998. Wu bangguo fuzongli zai quanguo chengzhen zhigong yiliao baoxian zhidu gaige gongzuo huiyi kaimushi de jianghua (Vice-Premier Wu Bangguo's speech at the commencement of the national work conference on the reform of the medical care insurance system for staff and workers in cities and towns in China). In Zhongguo weisheng nianjian bianji weiyuan bianji weiyuanhui (Ed.), *Zhongguo weisheng nianjian 1999* (*Yearbook of China's Health Care 1999*). Beijing: Renmin weisheng chubanshe.

Wu, R. 2013. Guanyu dabing baoxian de sikao (Considerations on the reform of major illness insurance). *Shehui baozhang zhidu* (*Social Security System*) 5.

Wu, R., & Chen, J. 1999. Jianli chengzhen yiliao baoxian zhidu, quanmian tuijin woguo jiben yiliao baoxian zhidu gaige (Build a basic medical care insurance system for staff and workers in cities and towns, and push forward the reform of the medical care insurance system in China). In Zheng, D., Liu, D., & Zhang, B. (Eds.), *Shehui baoxian gaige zhinan* (*Guidelines for Social Insurance Reform*). Beijing: Gaige Chubanshe.

Zhang, Z. 1999. Zai quanguo chengzhen zhigong yiliao baoxian zhidu gaige gongzuo huiyi shang de Jianhua (Speech at the national work conference concerning the reform of medical care insurance for staff and workers in cities and towns). In Laodong yu shehui baozhang bu yiliao baoxiansi (Ed.), *Zhongguo yiliao baoxian gaige zhengce yu guanli* (*The Policy and Management of Medical Care Reform in China*). Beijing: Zhonguo laodong shehui baozhang chubanshe.

Zheng, G. et al. 2002. *Zhongguo shehui baozhang zhidu biange yu pinggu* (*The Change and Assessment of the Social Security System in China*). Beijing: Remin daxue chubanshe.

Zhu, R. 2002. Guanyu zhigong yiliao baozhang zhidu gaige wenti (Issues regarding the reform medical care security system of staff and workers). In Laodong he shehui baozhangbu & zhonggong zhongyang wenxian yanjiushi (Eds.) *Xinshiqi laodong he shehui baozhang zhongyao wenxian xuanbian* (*Selected Important Documents of Labor and Social Security during the New Era*). Beijing: Zhongguo shehui baozhang chubanshe & zhong yang wenxian chubanshe. 266–74.

Zou, H. 2000. Zai 1999 nian Shanghai weisheng gongzuo huiyi shang de jianghua (Speech at the 1999 work conference on health care). In Liu, J. (Ed.), *Shanghai weisheng nianjian 2000* (*Yearbook of Health Care in Shanghai 2000*). Shanghai: Shanghai kexue jishu wenxian chubanshe.

Part III

Medical Care Insurances in the Non-planned Sector

9 Urban Resident Medical Care Insurance and Beyond

This chapter is devoted to an analysis of the urban resident medical care insurance (*chengshi jumin baoxian* or URMCI), coupled with a discussion on other two medical care insurance packages (e.g., one for agricultural laborers and the other for flexibly employed personnel) in urban China. These three packages, along with BMCI, are supposed to cover nearly all populations in cities and towns throughout China, representing further steps toward the completion of the basic medical care reform in urban China for a time span for more than three decades from the early 1990s. The reform of the public funding of medical care faced two sectors of the population in China: The planned sector and non-planned sector. Falling into the planned sector, BMCI was formally launched in 2001. NRCMCI and URMCI commenced in 2003 and 2007 respectively, and they represented the reform effort to cover the population in the non-planned sector. Moreover, the programs for the agricultural laborers and flexibly employed personnel were targeted at the workforce in the non-planned sector too.

Moving toward modernization and rapid economic growth since 1979, moreover, agricultural laborers and flexibly employed personnel (or temporary workers) started to assume visible role in the labor markets in urban China, but these two groups were neither included in the net of social security nor in medical care until the later phase of the healthcare reform (Guo 2006; Zheng & Lu 2007; Hua 2010; Zheng 2011). But they represent a substantial and expanding portion of the workforce in the urban sector. There were different estimates for the numbers of agricultural laborers and flexibly employed workers, for example, taken together, from 226 million in 2007 to 273.95 million in 2014, indicating a salient tendency of continuous growth (Hua 2010: 191; Jiang 2016; 19). The study will try to examine and assess alternative insurance plans for these two major groups of the workforce based on selected empirical cases in Guangzhou and Shenzhen.

In the policymaking process, the case of BMCI differs from the cases of URMCI and NRCMCI in reference to the weight of policy priority for HESI chosen by policy actors. In the former case, provincial/local jurisdictions were originally inclined to focus on HESI only but later on, they conceded to the central policy actors by accepting a package that combined both expensive services (such as hospital care and HESI) with less expensive clinical care, to maintain the established remuneration policy of the CPE vintage (Chapters 3, 7 and 8). In the latter two

DOI: 10.4324/9781003389934-12

cases, the central actors started with the priority of HESI, but they subsequently made concessions to provincial/local jurisdictions by incorporating the less expensive and more popular components such as clinical care into the insurance package (Chapters 10 and 11).

Here the study will begin with a review of the origin and background of URMCI. To be followed, the study will address the principal issues of URMCI product/ service specificity concerning cases of high expenditure and serious illness (HESI). Moreover, the study will tackle the issues of program specificity such as the funding and spending side of URMCI. Finally, an analysis will be specifically devoted to the insurance programs for the emerging workforce in economic reform in urban China—agricultural laborers and flexibly employed personnel, based on the cases of Guangzhou and Shenzhen.

Inaugurating Urban Resident Medical Care Insurance (URMCI)

During policy evolution, BMCI and URMCI was closely related. The former were offered to employees in the public sector while the latter catered to the needs of their family members. Beginning in the 1950s, sovereign planners did *not* use family as a unit for designing and organizing the public funding policy for social security (including medical care) during the onset of CPE in the 1950s. As the newly introduced BMCI did not include the employee's family member, it was necessary for policymakers to tackle medical care of the family members separately. Consequently, these family members were treated as "urban residents" (*chengshi jumin*), who were holders of household registrationin each municipal jurisdiction. During the pre-reform era, the "half insurance" of medical care for family members was concerned with a scaled down medical care benefits managed by the work unit (Guowuyuan 2007: Chapter 4). As soon as the BMCI was formally launched in 2001, it was timely to build URMCI for family members and dependents to focus mainly on the expensive and serious illness on top of the repackaged entitlement and benefit (equivalent to the old version of "half insurance") that had been offered to the same group prior to economic reform.

URMCI was formally introduced in 2007 under some favorable circumstances for implementation. As a latecomer in policy packaging and implementation, URMCI could benefit from its predecessors such as BMCI (formally beginning in 2001) and NRCMCI (introduced in 2003) regarding relevant experiences and needed information about designs, program specificity and product/specificity. In addition, URMCI represented an improvement for making better use of healthcare resources at the macro level, and the improved delivery of healthcare in the community clinics and medical care facilities at the micro level.[1] As family members and dependents of the employees fell into the net of work-unit collectivism, the introduction of URMCI could take advantage of the assistance and cooperation from the work unit as well as the local government.

In the process of drafting, policy actors were able to take advantage of two URMCI pilot programs conducted at the provincial/local level: The pilot program in Zhenjiang, Jiangsu, conducted in 2004 and another one in Fuzhou, Jiangxi in 2005. Subsequently in October 2006, it was proposed in the 6th Plenum of the 16th Party Congress of the CCP to build an urban resident medical care insurance centering on "unified funding" (namely, a set of risk-pooling mechanisms) for major illnesses. Accordingly, Premier Wen Jiabo convened the standing committee of the State Council to launch URMCI pilot programs in April 2007, and meanwhile, established the joint inter-ministerial conference for the purpose. The URMCI was formally inaugurated in May, with Vice-Premier Wu Yi acting as the team leader of the joint inter-ministerial conference (Lu 2007). The said conference consisted of representatives from eight ministries, together with the office of URMCI being organized within the Ministry of Labor and Social Security (MOLSS). It is noteworthy that the State Council made it clear that the said inter-ministerial conference, coupled with its office, was to become a permanent apparatus to coordinate the implementation and management of URMCI throughout the country thereafter (Guowuyuan 2007; Lu 2007).

Vice-Premier Wu Yi oversaw three seminars in the Eastern, Central and Western Regions at the territorial level, sponsored by the State Council, to solicit the opinions of policy actors from the provincial/local jurisdictions on June 20, 28 and July 5 in 2007, respectively. Meanwhile in July, the State Council promulgated the 2007 Advisory Opinions concerning the extension of pilot programs to more jurisdictions, marking an all-out effort to implement URMCI throughout the country. The inauguration of URMCI began with the pilot programs initiated at the provincial level, for example, two to three municipalities each chosen at the provincial level in 2007, to be extended to more than 70 municipalities further in 2008. The aim was to install pilot programs in 80 percent of the municipalities by 2009, with a full-scale of implementation by 2010 (Lu 2007).

In view of smooth implementation of URMCI, it is pertinent to examine the main characteristics and managerial and financial designs. To what extent can URMCI be taken as a case of marketization? How does it operate? In managerial terms how does it differ from the practice of public administration in general? To begin with, URMCI relied upon transactions between two sides in the marketplace: The subscribing family unit and the URMCI foundation (normally represented by the executive agency). The family unit concerned was expected to make premium contributions for the medical care insurance, while the URMCI foundation was responsible for collecting premium contributions and covering expenditures.

Characteristic of URMCI, the subscribing family was subsidized by both the employing work unit and the government. Although these public entities were not a party directly involved in the transaction, they assumed financial responsibility for subsidizing the family unit concerned. In the case of URMCI, the transaction was based on contractual relations in that the subscribing party paid a fee to URMCI foundation in exchange for insurance benefits, covering their family members. The URMCI only covered the package of medical services concerning HESI, and it was not intended to substitute for the existing medical care for dependents of the public personnel that the work unit normally subsidized.

Theoretically speaking, URMCI falls into the hybrid mode of governance from the policy-oriented formulation. On the one hand, it operates with market mechanisms, taking clues from the markets in the decision-making process. On the other hand, hierarchy-oriented concerns are incorporated into the market transactions. For instance, the exercise of program specificity (including product/service specificity) was closely associated with non-market-oriented policy goals (e.g., the emphasis on HESI, as well as the issue of externality) the enforcement of which relied on the exercise of command through a hierarchy.

As a form of insurance, URMCI represented an ingenious and innovative design of public financial management with regards to the combination of inward-resource-flow (IRF) system with the outward-resource-flow (ORF) system. URMCI relied upon the (IRF) system to the extent that each market transaction was made financially accountable, as budgetary balance was an overriding concern. Each item of a premium contribution needed to match each set of entitlements given to the enrollee in the insurance plan. The IRF system was characteristic of resource-internalization accompanying cost-externalizing effects. It is noteworthy the IRF system is not intended to handle public policy, including the issue of externality as previously noted (Chapter 3). Accordingly, by the design, URMCI was complemented by a subsidy scheme to enrollees, which worked with the ORF system that allocated financial resources through exercise of command, answerable to authorities in each hierarchy structure. And it tended to produce resource-externalizing results, for example, provision of quasi-collective goods, intended for positive spillover effects to the multitude of residents in the community. This is like NRCMCI to be tackled in the next two chapters.

The Program Specificity of URMCI Funding Schemes

The design of URMCI closely followed that of NRCMCI in several key features, for instance, the priority of HESI inter alia, but the former differed from the latter with respect to such distinct characteristics as scale, membership, funding sources, packaging of services and spending in an urban setting. As a public medical care insurance system, URMCI operated with risk-pooling mechanisms in terms of building the foundation that was sustained by premium contributions from a multitude of enrollees to help financially those who fell sick in each medical event, given that, actuarially, episodes of illness did not concentrate in one particular time period, but spread out over a considerable length of time. The scale of risk-pooling needed to be large enough to generate a reservoir of revenue source and to meet the financial demands to cover the medical care events overtime. In a theoretical sense, the larger the reservoir of funding is the better. Moreover, URMCI represented a form of investment in risks, expecting some financial return when the defined risks failed to take place.

As key to the design of URMCI, it was necessary to choose the so-called "unit of unified funding" (*tongchou danwei*), that is, the jurisdiction where the URMCI foundation operated. In accordance with the 2007 Advisory Opinion, the municipality (with county status or above) was chosen as the organizational locus of "unified funding," but it was expected by 2011 that the municipality (of prefectural status) would eventually become the chosen organizational unit for "unified funding" (Guowuyuan 2007; Zheng 2011). This was indicative of a broad policy trend toward territorial integration of insurance programs nationwide. As a result, in choosing the unit of "unified funding" for URMCI, policy actors had also to consider where the BMCI plan was located, addressing the ties of the employees with family members.

To exercise program specificity, furthermore, the issue of enrollee's membership in URMCI deserves some discussion with regards to various sectors of the population dwelling in cities and towns. In accordance with the 2007 Advisory Opinion, first, the subscribers eligible for the URMCI plan embraced either unemployed urban residents or those not employed full time, and neither were they eligible to join BMCI. Second, in some jurisdictions reported, URMCI served as "supplementary insurance" for those who were used to be the holders of LIMC and PFMC in the past and those who had previously joined a form of BMCI, as the HESI was not included in their insurance coverage (Lin 2007). Third, in most cases, subscribers eligible for URMCI were the holders of household registration in urban areas. Those without household registration were not qualified to join URMCI. Fourth, some analysts tried to underscore universalism and egalitarianism—that all citizens should enjoy basic medical care—by proposing that applicants eligible for URMCI ought to include the marginal sector among urban residents, such as dependents and minors, retirees, the low-income brackets of the urban population, as well as other deprived sectors of urban residents.

According to Zuo Huangchen (a retired official from Shanghai), insurance plans such as URMCI ought to differentiate among various social groups while some priority had to be given to the needy, such as seniors, the weak and low-income and poor groups (Liu 2007a). Adhering strictly to a rigid official policy line, questions were raised with reference to restrictiveness of BMCI eligibility, and therefore some different insurance options would be needed in conjunction with URMCI. According to policy analyst Liu Dan, it was more reasonable to broaden the operational definition of "urban residents" to include all low-income and/or unemployed people (Liu 2010: 36). As a prelude to the policy of integration between URMCI and NRCMCI announced in 2016, moreover, in some other jurisdictions, for instance, in Zhenjiang municipality, Jiangxi Province, the government had adopted a flexible policy to avoid defining urban residents too rigidly and narrowly, thereby opening door to accommodate agricultural laborers or even the peasants joining URMCI (Wang 2008). In Taicang Municipality, for example, agricultural laborers who had worked there for more than two years were eligible to join URMCI (Zheng 2011: 87).

Further to the exercise of program specificity, it is germane to examine how to set a premium contribution that was required for each enrollee in the URMCI plan. As the method of calculation, two approaches were entertained: The absolute (or fixed) sum approach and the proportional approach. The former was focused on the absolute and/or fixed sum of expenditure of medical care for each enrollee to be funded, while the latter was tied to a proportion of an enrollee's compensation package. The former was most suitable for URMCI enrollees in that enrollees might not have a fixed income as the basis for accounting, and thus it was feasible to estimate the absolute sum of the expenses for medical care services expected. In contrast, the latter was more applicable to BMCI whereas enrollees were normally employed and remunerated, and therefore, premium contributions could be conveniently calculated in proportion to wages (Xu 2007).

Accordingly, URMCI plans followed the absolute (fixed) sum approach, governed by the principle of tying revenue to expenditure, and meanwhile maintaining the budgetary balance of the total sum of the foundation's assets. The total amount of funding required was derived by working backward from the estimated amount of required spending by taking into consideration basic medical demands, the family's financial ability, and the overall level of economic development at the local level. As a rule, the sum of premium contributions was based on the percentages of funding for the various types of medical care services (e.g., hospital care or clinical care or both) (Xu 2007: 40–1). In the case of Kunshan Jiangsu, for illustration, the 2007 survey indicates that the total number of enrollees in URMCI—and thus entitled to both clinical care and hospital care within the municipality—was 350,000. The average expenditure for clinical care and emergency service for each enrollee is calculated at 60 RMB, with five visits for each annually. And the total expenditure for hospital care was 5,600 RMB for each enrollee on average and one time every year hospital care for each, as approximately 5 percent of the total number of enrollees needed hospital care annually.[2] To round up the figure, accordingly, 260 RMB was chosen as the funding requirement for each enrollee in the URMCI plan of the Kunshan municipal jurisdiction (Xu 2007).

How was the premium contribution for each enrollee made? Premium contributions came from three financial sources: Family, work unit and government (Guowuyuan 2007). In principle, an enrollee's family might act on behalf of the enrollee to make a premium contribution to a URMCI plan, since a considerable number of enrollees was not employed by the work unit and lacked income to cover premium contributions. As a residue of "work-unit collectivism," moreover, the work unit with which the family members were affiliated could chip in as well, as a smaller portion of premium contributions was derived from the work unit. Prior to economic reform, the work unit did provide some forms of medical care to dependents when neither LIMC nor PFMC was made available to family members as previously noted (Chapter 4).

Like NRCMCI, URMCI was taken as a policy initiative in which the government assumed an important role shouldering a considerable portion of each enrollee's premium contributions through the ORF system. The government followed the tradition of public finance in China by adopting two optional subsidy approaches in the public sector: "hidden subsidy" (*anbu*) to subsidize the providers, and "open subsidy" (*mingbu*) to subsidize the users directly (Lee 2019). Beginning in 2009, for instance, not only the government stepped up spending in building health care facilities at the community level (e.g., urban districts, street organizations, counties and townships) in the form of a "hidden subsidy," but also promoted insurance policy in the form of NRCMCI and URMCI through "open subsidy," namely, direct financial assistance to enrollees for a share of premium contribution. In the form of open subsidy, the government introduced a subsidy to users (enrollees) of public medical care insurance in both NRCMCI and URMCI during the 2000s (Gu 2008).

Through the subsidy to users employed both the ORF system, the government could pump funding into the health care sector, putting money directly into hands of users (enrollees) in form of subsidy to premium contribution on the one hand, and on the other hand, require users to spend their money so received through markets to buy their insurance within the IRF system, meanwhile making good use of transaction-centered management accordingly (Chapter 2).

In the case of URMCI starting in 2007, a basic pattern of the government's subsidies to premium contributions emerged from pilot programs across jurisdictions. In accordance with the 2007 Advisory Opinion, for example, the government needed to give 40 RMB to each enrollee in URMCI through the transfer of special government appropriations, including a central government's share of contribution of 20 RMB to each enrollee in the Central and Western Regions. In addition, the government assumed a role in granting 10 RMB at a minimum to children, students, the disabled and other low-rate insurance cases, and 5 RMB at a minimum to enrollees in need (such as seniors, the handicaps or disabled, and members of low-income families (Guowuyuan 2007).

The rates of premium contributions to URMCI plans increased subsequently from 2007 onward. And as of 2010, the standard of the subsidy to enrollees was raised to 120 RMB, together with upward adjustments of the share to be contributed by each enrollee. The shares from echelons of government were adjusted upward too, as the central government tried to step up spending for the regions and individuals in need. For instance, the central government's share of subsidy to the Central and Western regions, coupled with selected areas (mostly poor, backward areas) in the Eastern region, reached 60 RMB average for each enrollee. In principle, the rates varied from one group to another, such as students, children, seniors, disabled, and other enrollees in hardship. Allowances were also made available to seniors over 60 years of age in those families experiencing hardship, for example, 60 RMB at a minimum, coupled with a share of 30 RMB being contributed by the central government for enrollees in the Central and Western regions (Zheng 2011: 44).

Product/Service Specificity in URMCI

As a public medical care insurance, URMCI incorporated both the funding and spending side of its functions in market transactions. To address the kinds of services offered and funded, one needs to investigate the packages adopted, spending schemes enforced as well as actual implementation of URMCI across various jurisdictions. Like what they did with NRCMCI, sovereign planners set major illness (*dabing*) as the priority in packaging URMCI, but its operational definition of major illness remained unclear throughout the process of pilot programs and policy experiments. With reference to the official documentation of URMCI, the 2007 Advisory Opinion remains silent about the issues of payment-ceiling criteria, although it did prescribe deductibles and co-payments as spending control measures (Guowuyuan 2007). Nonetheless, in the pilot programs conducted, the payment-ceiling was fixed at six times the average annual wage of the ordinary employed residents in each jurisdiction. For practical considerations, policy actors needed to enforce the payment-ceiling criteria because they did not want to see the URMCI foundation being overly exposed to the risks of uncontrollable costs of major illness caused by some medical events in the future.

Conceptually speaking, it is pertinent to try to provide an operational definition of "major illness" and thus to clarify what kinds of services are to be funded and provided for. "Major illness," referring to high expenditure, serious illnesses (*gaoe zhongbing*; or HESI), remained a key policy controversy in healthcare in China throughout economic reform. The notion of serious illness (*zhongbing*) is concerned with the medical-scientific aspect of the case whereas high expenditure (*gaoe*) points to the financial-economic implications of a cure. The term "catastrophic medical care events" represents a sub-category of HESI, placing emphasis on the extreme financial impact on individual patients, families and sometimes the work unit with which they are affiliated. HESI was made the core feature of NRCMCI and URMCI, since BMCI had been formally inaugurated (Sun 2013a, 2013b). This meant that only hospital care was covered in most cases while the real HESI was often left out.

As soon as URMCI was put on the policy agenda for implementation, the choice of major illness versus minor illness was cast into the limelight of policy debates over the exercise of product/service specificity. For proponents advocating for the priority of major illness over minor illness in the packaging of services in URMCI, it was argued that major illness involved high expenditure, and most enrollees could not bear the enormous costs, albeit it was true that most families might afford to pay for clinical care that was less expensive. Those who argued for adding minor illness to the packages reasoned that the thinking of a great majority of enrollees (or prospective enrollees) tended to shy away from insurance against major illness because it rarely occurred anyway. As most enrollees took cues from markets, they could not see their interest at stake tangibly and immediately, for example, in HESI cases. Treating a HESI episode as less noticeable and remote, many of them were willing to take a chance of not falling ill in any serious way and thus not having to shoulder any high expenditure.

In conjunction with making of URMCI, most enrollees (and/or prospective enrollees) tended to focus less on HESI in their conceptualization of market transactions, but more on common and frequent illnesses that would occur often in appreciable ways and could be handled through clinical care. The tension between sovereign planners and most residents was often manifested in policy debates over, and implementation of URMCI and NRCMCI.

Like NRCMCI, the issue of HESI in URMCI was concerned with the "extent of benefit (*shouyimian*)" versus the "sum of expenditure (*shouyie*)," representing the conceptualization by actors in policy circle (Zhang 2009; Zheng 2011). The former referred to the number of enrollees who benefited from the insurance plan, while the latter was concerned with the absolute amount of funds that each enrollee enjoyed. Out of a sense of ownership, most enrollees were willing to join an insurance plan when they saw themselves benefiting noticeably from a plan, paying less attention to how expensive and/or how serious each case was. Contrary to the policymakers' policy priority, as a result, most enrollees did not lend much weight to the package for HESI (Zhang 2009).

In accordance with the 2007 Advisory Opinion, the URMCI foundation was intended mainly to cover hospital care and special cases of clinical care, although most enrollees preferred an insurance package covering clinical care of minor illness (including mostly common and frequent cases) at least (Guowuyuan 2007). As a matter of the consumer's sovereignty, policy actors concerned had to take cues from the markets and heed the demands of enrollees in their exercise of product/service specificity and program specificity. Like the packaging of NRCMCI in which consumer's preference carried considerable weight, three URMCI packages of services emerged in the actual choices in the process implementation:

- Package I: unified funding of major illness only, covering hospital care and special cases of clinical care (cancers, dialysis, chronic illness, etc.)
- Package II: hospital care plus clinical care
- Package III: unified funding of major illness plus a family account for minor illness (Zhang 2009).

In all three packages, the major illness account and the minor illness account remained separated in accounting and managerial terms. For example, in Package I, the major illness account was reserved only for cases of hospital care plus part of HESI, as minor illness care was paid for through OPP. In Package II, major illness was covered by the unified funding account while minor illness was taken care of through a separate risk-pooling account. In Package III, the family account was focused on clinical care, operating independently from the unified funding account for major illness.

While Package I dealt with a small number of cases and each case is costly, commanding a large "sum of expenditure" (*shouyie*), i.e., high expenditure average in each case, Packages II & III were effective to cover many less expensive cases concerning the issue of large "extent of benefit" (*shouyie*), the large number of cases treated. At the end of the day, it appeared that Package I could lend priority to highly expensive cases (including HESI) and that was what the central government originally endorsed. Packages III & II were found preferable to local jurisdictions, and they were merited for being able to maintain a large market share through the provision of clinical care services and thus ensure a steady revenue flow to the URMCI foundation.

Some critical voices were raised against an overemphasis on HESI at the expense of minor illness with regard to the packaging of URMCI. Policy analyst Zhang Yong argued that the model of "major illness first" was bound to have a limited effect on improving accessibility to healthcare. In the case of Wuhan, cited by Zhang, an unemployed adult resident paid 340 RMB annually for URMCI but was only given a co-payment of 30 RMB for clinical care in each incident. Such a small co-payment would inevitably affect residents' enthusiasm for enrolling in URMCI. Moreover, low-income residents tended to have limited purchasing power to match medical bills, and often fell through the URMCI net, resulting in a "reverse choice" scenario. Co-payment benefited high-income residents more than low-income ones—defeating the ideal of egalitarianism and the principle of income transfer to the poor. With reference to the healthcare resource input, it was argued that the efficiency of intervening in the case of major illness was far inferior to the efficiency of intervening in the case of frequent and common diseases, as argued by some analysts (Zhang 2009: 30).

As a compromise, it was generally accepted among policy actors at the provincial/local level that while funding needed to concentrate on major illness (mainly hospital care), minor illness (mostly clinical care) also ought to be entertained in order to sustain residents' motivation to join URMCI (Wang 2008). As just mentioned above, Package II and III represent just such a compromise. For example, in Zhenjiang municipality, policymakers adopted the principle of "ensuring [the priority of] major illness and yet accommodating minor illness" (*baoda, guxiao*). As the former represented a tendency of what was taken as Adaptation (C) to be dictated by "relations" (by command/politics), the latter was concerned with Adaptation (A), namely, taking clues from markets, in Williamson's formulation (Chapter 2).

As a theoretical observation, over emphasis of HESI created strains in the process of implementation of URMCI, comparable to NRCMCI. First, it could not resolve the inner conflict in each enrollee regarding the relative weight of preferring healthcare for serious illnesses versus common and frequent diseases, and between HESI versus minor illness, given the scarcity of health care resources. The controversy was concerned with the relative weight of different preference mixes within each consumer (i.e., enrollee), and it was not often a choice of either one or the other, but a proper mix between the two. Second, it provided no solution to the frictions between those enrollees who tended to prefer clinical care (e.g., common, and frequent diseases) and those policymakers who gave priority to HESI. Third, the government could not dictate the choice made by the enrollees. By the design of URMCI, the government did not assume the role as one party in transactions with the insurer, albeit it provided a subsidy to the enrollee to purchase insurance plans. Consequently, these tensions were manifested in the compromise regarding the mixture of major and minor illnesses in the exercise of product/service specificity pertaining to the packaging of URMCI.

Financial Management and Spending Control Measures

Introduced after BMCI and NRCMCI, URMCI was well positioned to learn from its predecessors about program specificity, product/service specificity, organizational models, and managerial instruments. In accordance with the 2007 Advisory Opinion, it was recommended that URMCI ought to make use of the experience of managerial systems of BMCI, trying to improve its managerial methods and enhance efficiency. Where appropriate, it was suggested for URMCI to learn from

NRCMCI too, for instance, to explore feasible approaches to integrate with the latter in some regions considering the trend of rapid urbanization and the relatively smaller financial gaps between the two. The trend of urbanization appears very rapid, as the percentage of urban residents in the total population increased from 17.9 percent in 1978 to 43.9 percent in 2006 as cited by Gu (2008: 122).

Overall, the URMCI represents an entirely new system of public financial management that differs from its counterpart operating in the government. By design, it was supposed to work with together with the IRF system, coupled with transaction-centered management, to control resource leakage in the transactional triad as mentioned previously, and to enhance the accountability of the insurer, enrollee, and provider alike regarding each item of funding and spending in the marketplace. In the interpretative frame of reference among policy actors, URMCI was expected to operate in full adherence to the principle of fixing funding to match spending, striking a balance between spending and revenue with a reasonable margin of saving (Guowuyuan 2007).

The newly established URMCI foundation served as the risk pooling reservoir sustained by the collection of premium contributions. It was anchored to a special account that housed social security funds and was listed separately from all other items of public finance. And it performed core functions of financial management, for instance, collecting premium contributions and remitting insurance payments through market transactions. Also, it covered the main spending functions for hospital care and special cases of clinical care in accordance with the 2007 Advisory Opinion, attesting the significant growth of hierarchies amid marketization. It was also recommended by the 2007 Advisory Opinion that whenever feasible, risk-pooling mechanisms (in the form of unified funding) for clinical care expenditure were to be introduced gradually.

Copying from BMCI and NRCMCI, URMCI relied on an executive agent to handle the entire range of functions within the hybrid mode of governance. Connected by a network of market transactions, the executive agent signed service agreements with designated providers, such as hospitals, clinics, and drug stores. It also operated with transaction-centered management. Accounting exercises were well linked with incentives and penalties, technical and medical standards, and the conventional mode of regulatory control, etc. (Renli ziyuan shehui baozhangbu 2009). The introduction of URMCI began to be interfaced with some of the main themes of the healthcare reforms propelled by several rounds of policy debate since the early 2000s, culminating in the new healthcare reforms of 2009.

Regarding spending control measures pertaining to URMCI, some salient features of spending schemes about financial irregularities as well as the improvement of efficiency deserved further analysis. First, URMCI was introduced in conjunction with a variety of managerial reforms affecting payment methods and addressing such matters as the enforcement of quality criteria, the control of irregular medical behaviors, the reduction of induced medical demands, the efficient and effective allocation of health care resources, as well as the concerns of deprived and underprivileged urban residents among others. To control abuses and unreasonable costs, URMCI borrowed from BMCI by making use of standard schemes such as deductibles, co-payments and payment-ceilings. Second, the scheme of deductibles and co-payments were widely used to encourage the larger number of visits to medical care facilities in lower echelons of health care hierarchy. Third, the scheme of a payment-ceiling was fixed at six times the annual average income of all residents each jurisdiction to protect the URMCI foundation against the risk of unexpectedly large claims (Renli ziyuan shehui baozhangbu 2010). It is a matter of an actuarial exercise and the practical experience for policymakers to determine whether payment-ceiling mechanisms ought to stay or be abolished, an issue raised in the 2012 Advisory Opinion to be dealt with in Chapter 12, the concluding chapter.

To control spending, furthermore, a component of accountability was incorporated into the family account and the personal account; and, in some cases, a sort of undertaking responsibility system (the so-called *chenbaozhi*; URS) was adopted in URMCI, like NRCMCI. Going beyond conventional payment methods according to listing and catalogs of services, new payment methods, such as payment using a global budget, clinical visit quota, and diagnosis-related-groups (DRG), were put into use on an experimental basis amid introducing URMCI plans across jurisdictions.

Agricultural Laborers and Flexibly Employed Personnel

It is germane here to examine two "residual categories" of personnel namely, agricultural laborers and flexibly employed personnel, who were neither included in BMCI nor in URMCI even after the new healthcare reform starting in 2009. One category concerned "flexibly employed personnel," namely, residents who were holders of household registration but lost their permanent jobs for one reason or another: For example, previous employees of enterprises that were downsized or bankrupt for pure business and managerial reasons; those employees displaced by technological upgrading; and those fallen victim to closure of employing enterprises because of market fluctuations. Without a permanent job, they lost the footing for enrolling in BMCI, but it was well taken in the public policy circle that they still were entitled to basic medical care under the affordable care policy.

Since the central government had been slow in putting the public medical care insurance of flexibly employed personnel on agenda, some jurisdictions started to take initiatives to find some alternatives other than formal, well-defined programs especially for them, for example, allowing them to join existing insurance packages. In one pilot program conducted in Huzhou, Jiangxi in 2007, it was proposed that flexibly employed personnel ought to be given the choice to join either BMCI or URMCI, in order to overcome procedural rigidity and create room to secure needed basic medical care insurance for them. In Keshan County, Beijing Municipality, for instance, the local government made use of URMCI to fill the gap for flexibly employed personnel who enjoyed the status of household registration but were not permanently employed, before a separate program was to be created (Xia 2007). Furthermore, for private-owned enterprises, URMCI appeared more attractive than BMCI for flexibly employed personnel considering the lower income level of their employees and the smaller financial resources commanded by the respective work units (Liu 2007a).

Another category comprised agricultural laborers hired as manual labor—construction and industrial workers, employees in the service sector, and domestic helpers—together with their family members, minors, and other dependents. Such agricultural laborers contributed to the economy in the urban sector significantly (Dai & Mao 2010). In fact, they were products of a worldwide trend of urbanization and modernization, but they were caught in a dilemma between the employment status and the household registration system. They were needed in the job markets in cities, but encountered many restrictions associated with the household registration system—the system that had been established in the aftermath of the Great Leap Forward to restrict the entry of peasants into urban areas, control the growth of urban populations, and to cope with too high a tax burden due to expenditure for welfare facilities and infrastructure. Consequently, they were not entitled to resident-based rights and privileges in education, welfare and services provided by the municipality in question (Guo 2006). They were often called "outside laborers" or "employees from outside," meaning implicitly that in a way, they were marginalized and treated as outsiders to benefits and entitlements normally made available to employees in the urban sector (Hua 2010).

Agricultural laborers were recruited by various sectors of the urban economy during economic reform, and they were among the largest groups that were not included in any public medical care insurance until the later phase of the healthcare reform as just noted. Agricultural laborers are taken as peasants who engage in non-agricultural employment in urban settings for short or long term. According to existing surveys and investigations, agricultural laborers are characterized as a very young and productive workforce in China as follows: High job mobility, young age (mostly 35 years of age or younger), middle school education (junior and senior high schools) and often married, but they are considered as underdogs in the mixed economy, for instance, being employed in labor intensive jobs, and normally lacking of representation in industrial relations (Zheng & Lu 2007; Hua 2010; Jiang 2016).

Agricultural laborers were treated as second class residents in the urban sector, but they were still given some forms of benefits, coupled with other social security entitlements, albeit at a modest level as compared with the regular staff and workers who were employed in public enterprises (Zheng & Lu 2007). Focusing on basic medical care insurances only, a survey, with a large sample of 15,509 individuals, was conducted in 2014, to examine distinct policy orientations toward agricultural laborers in four municipalities of metropolitan scale, such as Beijing, Shanghai, Guangzhou and Shenzhen (Jiang 2016). According to the survey, most agricultural workers were allowed overlapping subscriptions in a variety of medical care insurance plans, promising the introduction of a policy of integration in the future (Chapter 12). For instance, they were formally given an option to enroll in NRCMCI in their hometown. In practice, however, it was subject to personal considerations, conveniences and accessibility for them to take full advantage of it. Regarding the samples of enrollment in NRCMCI, the highest figure, nearly 80 percent, was registered among agricultural laborers in Beijing, with the lowest, less than 50 percent, being recorded among agricultural laborers in Shenzhen. Shanghai and Guangzhou were ranked in between, that is, above 60 percent (Jiang 2016).

It is warranted to examine the feasibility for each of four cities was willing and able to incorporate agricultural laborers into the insurance plans of its own jurisdictions. The survey indicates that, insofar as the subscription of either BMCI or URMCI was concerned, one municipal jurisdiction was more open than another to embracing agricultural laborers in varying degrees, but they were considered restrictive overall. In the case of BMCI, Shanghai and Shenzhen scored high by allowing overlapping enrollment of agricultural laborers, for instance, 32.2 percent and 29.9 percent, respectively, with Beijing and Guangzhou scoring lower than the preceding two, for example, 13.96 percent and 18.11 percent respectively. Regarding enrollment in URMCI, Shenzhen appeared markedly more accommodating, for example, 12.86 percent, visibly higher than the other three jurisdictions: 1.93 percent in Beijing, 2.11 in Shanghai, and 2.71 percent in Guangzhou (Jiang 2016).

Agricultural laborers were not denied treatment for illness in four municipal jurisdictions, but not all of them were able to be treated for illnesses. For example, among those who were treated were registered as follows: 61.09 percent in Beijing, 72.8 percent in Shanghai, 65.2 percent in Guangzhou, and 67.8 percent in Shenzhen. Besides, not many of them were able to take advantage of community health facilities. For instance, only about 16 percent of the agricultural laborers were able to make use of community health care service centers/stations in Beijing while more than 30 percent were able to do so in the other three jurisdictions. The varying percentages of treatment were attributed to the availability of medical facilities at the community level (Jiang 2016).

As the focus of this study, another crucial issue has to do with how much each agricultural laborer could benefit from public funding in health care. The percentage of expenses of medical care *not* covered by any public funding was high overall. As indicated in the survey, percentages for OPP were registered as high as follows: 78.9 percent in Beijing, 66.34 percent in Shanghai, 84.76 percent in hand 60.63 percent in Shenzhen (Jiang 2016). A substantial increase of insurance funding for basic medical care for agricultural laborers remained much to be desired, given the enormous efforts in this direction made in the past.

The Cases of Guangzhou and Shenzhen

It is germane to go in depth, based on field investigations by the author, into some selected cases in to know more precisely what considerations were at play in designing and implementing policy regarding social security issues of the workforce left unprotected by BMCI and URMCI. Guangzhou and Shenzhen, two empirical cases chosen, rely heavily on agricultural laborers and flexibly employed personnel for their modernization and economic growth during economic reform. And they addressed some issues that were in common, and others dissimilar and unique. Nonetheless, both were equally innovative in public medical care insurance in their own way.

As one of the earliest municipalities that took the lead in economic reform, the Guangzhou municipal government established in 2009 a basic medical care insurance program for so-called "outside personnel" (*wailai gongzuo renyuan*), mostly agricultural laborers, in accordance with the policy described by the 2009 Circular.[3] In fact, "outside personnel" constituted a significant portion of the workforce, about 36 percent of the total population in Guangzhou, but they had not been treated as a priority in terms of insurance and social security until 2009.

Following policy endorsed by the State Council and the Guangdong provincial government, Guangzhou municipality issued the 2009 Circular, offering to "outside personnel" (mostly agricultural laborers) for the first time a relatively generous package of medical care insurance, which included ordinary clinical care in Zone I, hospital care in Zone II, and even HESI (including catastrophic medical events) in Zone III.[4] Accordingly, the outside personnel medical care insurance (hereafter, OPMCI) program was allied to the ordinary BMCI in operational and managerial terms. It adopted a funding plan that included SMCI, explicitly addressing the need for HESI in Zone III.

However, the municipal government did not treat outside personnel equally on par with regular employees in public enterprises. It instead endeavored to adjust the payment scheme by differentiating outside personnel from the regular employees of public enterprises. It set a deductible (or payment starting criterion, PSC) lower, that is, at 50 percent of the corresponding requirement for BMCI, and meanwhile outside personnel were given medical care benefits at a modest standard relative to the regular workers in public enterprises. Besides, it struck a balance by scaling down the level of benefits which they could receive by setting the payment-ceiling of insurance at 80 percent of the comparable BMCI standard for regular staff and workers (Guangzhoushi laodong yu shehui ju 2009).

Working on the forefront of healthcare reform, Guangzhou was active in making some form of public medical care insurance to the group of flexibly employed personnel too. The Guangzhou Municipality took three years to work out a policy to extend, in 2005, basic medical care insurance benefits to flexibly employed personnel. In accordance with the policy paper 2005 Provisional Measures, medical care insurance benefits were given to the flexibly employed personnel who already had household registration in Guangzhou but lost their footing in the planned sector of the economy for one reason or another, including "post-transfer" workers (taken as full-time, part-time, or flexibly hired employees); employers in private business and their hired personnel; and freelance professionals, among others. The 2005 Provisional Measures mainly covered hospital care, financed through the funding sources of the hospital care insurance (HCI). Through the work unit, or enrollee by oneself, or both, each enrollee had to make contributions to the HCI fund at a rate of 4 percent of the average monthly wages. Each enrollee could start to enjoy medical care benefits as soon as obligatory contributions had been made for six full months.

It is worthwhile to dwell on the case of Shenzhen as well to analyze how the municipal policymakers tackled the issue of medical care insurance for agricultural laborers and "temporary personnel" (namely, flexibly employed personnel), neither of whom were regular staff and workers in public enterprises and were, therefore, not included in BMCI. Highlighting major changes and significant improvements in healthcare reform, the second generation of medical care insurance was not put forth until 2013 when the Shenzhen government promulgated in September 2013 its policy paper, 2013 Measures.[5] Of the second generation, three packages named Scheme I, Scheme II, and Scheme III were offered, and the last two addressed basic medical care insurance of "temporary workers" (i.e., flexibly employed personnel) and agricultural laborers respectively as previously mentioned (Chapter 4).

The two schemes, Scheme II & III, overlapping with hospital care insurance (HCI) for the first-generation prior to 2013, were mainly designed, among other reasons, to meet the demands of personnel who were not employed as regular staff and workers in the jurisdiction. However, temporary workers were given slightly better terms than agricultural laborers. In a formal sense, the former were *not* excluded from enrolling in Scheme I, and it was subject to negotiation between the work unit and its employees if they were allowed to join Scheme I, meaning that the work unit was given an option to hire temporary workers by offering an attractive remuneration package including Scheme I, depending on the market situation.

Scheme II was designed for temporary workers, covering not only clinical care and cases of minor illness but also hospital care and/or major and expensive cases of illness (equivalent to the low-cost versions of Zones I and II).[6] Scheme III was devoted to agricultural laborers, covering both clinical visits and minor illness too, but only to a limit (say, no more than 1,000 RMB) (Shenzhen renmin zhengfu 2013: Article 54).

In accordance with the 2013 Measures, legally speaking, the Shenzhen government allowed all residents, whether permanent or temporary, to subscribe to *any* of the available schemes found to be most suitable and affordable. Moreover, the second-generation harbored policy intent in making full use of allocating healthcare resources to alleviate over-congestion in high-tier public hospitals and making better use of community health care facilities. For example, the 2013 Measures required the work unit to designate a community clinic managed by a chosen hospital for each insured laborer pertaining to either Scheme II or III. That is to say, each insured enrollee was to be "tied down to" (*bangding*) a community clinic under the supervision and management of one designated hospital. However, this resulted in a more restrictive range of choice than otherwise.[7] Highlighting the brilliant aspect of Shenzhen experience, nevertheless, the implementation of Scheme II and III led to more and better use of community clinics, and it represented an integral part of China's healthcare strategy to alter the top-heavy reverse pyramid shape of the allocation pattern of health care resources, which overly relied on large and modern hospitals.

Of the second generation of healthcare reform in Shenzhen, Schemes II and III made considerable improvement on policy as well. In contrast to previous packages of the first generation, both schemes broadened their coverage to include not only hospital care but also clinical care and minor illness. In this way, the Shenzhen government was able to narrow the gap of medical care benefits between two classes of medical insurance beneficiaries, namely regularly employed personnel in the planned sector and temporarily hired personnel (including agricultural laborers).

Improving the chance of success considerably, moreover, it was effective managerially to implement Scheme II and III by adopting a "workfare" model through which the work unit was able to slice off a portion of wages and set it aside for insurance funding for an often marginalized and socially vulnerable lower class.

Concluding Analysis

To sum up, the foregoing analysis argues that URMCI was intended to fill the gap left by BCMI by covering the dependents of regular staff and workers in public enterprises and public personnel in the government and quasi-government units in timely fashion in 2007, coupled with two other insurance plans were focused on agricultural laborers and flexibly employed workers who represented an emerging sector of workforce during economic reform. Differing from BMCI, all three insurance plans just examined above were more future-oriented and had less concern with vested interests in the policymaking process.

In all three packages, moreover, sovereign planners chose the HESI as the top priority in the exercise of product/service specificity, highlighting the policy concern of spillover effects to the community. Taking exception to sovereign planners' policy stand, however, majority of enrollees tended to focus on clinical care to deal with common and frequent illnesses, resulting in what is taken as Adaptation (A), an adjustment to users' preference in the marketplace (Chapter 2). It is nonetheless evident that sovereign planners adopted an unprecedented innovative policy design to fuse markets into hierarchies to build a risk pooling reservoir operating independently from the government, marking a fundamental shift from the pure ORF system of conventional funding modes in direction to an IRF system in the case of public insurances, as argued in this study. For what were left uncovered by the basic medical care insurance were the peasants who represented the largest sector of the Chinese economy, a topic to be examined accordingly in the next chapter.

Notes

1 Like NRCMCI, in fact, URMCI bolsters up the purchasing power of users, sustains basic medical care markets, and provides funding sources *through* markets to public providers at the lowest reaches of the health care hierarchy. Moreover, URMCI represents one of the two-prong approaches to upgrade primary care services to the people at the community level (e.g., public funding to the users; and, low-price primary care through subsidized public providers). And it was launched complementary with a major effort of the government to build and strengthen entirely new community medical care facilities from the county level (or urban district) down to the neighborhood level, placing emphasis on primary care, public and preventive care, and gatekeeping and referral procedures starting in the 2000s (Lin 2007; Wu 2008).

2 Working backward for the standard of funding for each enrollee, therefore, the calculation according to formula is as follows:
The funding requirement for hospital care: 5,600 RMB × 5% × 60% × 35,000 = 5,880,000 RMB
The funding requirement for clinical care: 60 × 5 × 30% × 35,000= 3,150,000 RMB
The total of funding required: 5,880,000 + 3,150,000 = 9,030, 000 RMB
Average funding requirement for each enrollee: 9030,000/35,000 = 258 RMB (to round up, at 260 RMB) (Xu 2007).

3 The full title is "Circular Regarding Relevant Issues in Basic Medical Insurance Involving Participation of Employees Without Household Registration" (hereafter, "2009 Circular"); it was put forth on July 9, 2009 (Guangzhoushi laodong yu shehui ju 2009).

4 The 2009 Circular was issued on the basis of the policy espoused by the State Council in 2006 and 2009, and the Guangdong provincial government in 2009 (Guangzhoushi laodong yu shehui ju 2009).

5 The full title reads as "Measures for Social Medical Care Insurance for Shenzhen Municipality, Issued by the Shenzhen Government on September 29, 2013," abbreviated here as 2013 Measures) (Shenzhenshi renmin zhengfu 2013).

6 The "unified funding medical care insurance" (*tongchou yiliao baoxian*, or USMCI) can be traced to the early version of "hospital care insurance" (zhuyuan baoxian, or HCI) as first adopted in 1996, but subsequently amended in 2003 and 2008) was offered to those "outside personnel" who held only temporary household registration in Shenzhen (Guangdongsheng yiliao baozhang zhidu gaige yanjiu xianmu bangongshi 1999: 40–1, 202–3; Song 2001: 95–6; Shenzhenshi remin zhengfu 2012).

7 The idea of designating community clinics for temporary workers, including agricultural laborers, was first presented in the draft of "Measures for Social Medical Care Insurance for Shenzhen Municipality" in 2012 and was subsequently incorporated into the present policy paper under the same title in 2013. Accordingly, each temporary worker is tied to a community clinic under a designated hospital (Shenzhenshi remin zhengfu 2012; Shenzhenshi renmin zhengfu 2013: Article 32, 33 & 34).

References

Cai, R. 2007. Renren budengyu renren pinjun xiangyou (All men are equal does not mean that all men enjoy equal benefits). *Zhongguo shehui baozhang (China's Social Security)* 9: 35.

Dai, B., & Mao, Z. 2010. Chengzhenghua Jincheng Zhong chengzhen jumin jiben yiliao baoxian kechixu fazhan celue yanjiu (Research on the strategy of sustainable development of basic medical care insurance for residents in urbanized areas). *Zhongguo weisheng jingji (China's Health Care Economy)* 29.2: 23–5.

Gu, X. 2007a. Jumin yibao: chouzi zhidaoshao (Residents' medical care insurance: How much funding is required?) *Zhongguo shehui baozhang (China's Social Security)* 8: 46–7.

Gu, X. 2007b. *Zuoxian quanmin yibao: Zhongguo xinyigai de zhanlue yu zhanshu (Moving toward National Health Insurance: Strategy and Tactics for China's New Health Care Reform)*. Beijing: Zhongguo laodong shehui baozhang chubanshe.

Gu, X. 2008. Zuoxiang quanmin yibao: *Zhongguo xinyigai de zhannue yu zhanshu (Towards National Healthcare Insurance: Strategy and Tactics for China's New Healthcare Reform)*. Beijing: Zhongguo laodong shehui baozhang chubanshe.

Gu, X., Gao, M., & Yao, Y. (2006). *Zhengduan yu chufang, zhimian Zhongguo yiliao tizhi gaige [Diagnosis and treatment, confronting institutional reform in China's health care]*. Beijing: Shehui kexue wenxian chubanshe.

Guo, J. 2006. *Chengshi nongmin gongren shehui baozhang zhidu yanjiu (A Study on the Social Security System of Agricultural Laborers in Cities)*. Beijing: Zhongguo shehui kexue chubanshe.

Guangzhoushi laodong yu shehui baozhang ju. 2005. Guangzhoushi chengzhen linhuo jiuye renyuan yiliao baoxian banfa (The measures of medical care insurance for flexibly employed personnel in cities and towns in Guangzhou Municipality). Retrieved from www.baike/wiki/guangzhoushichengzhenlinhuojiuyerenyuanyiliaobanfa. April 15, 2015 7:35:52 Local Timezone (GMT. 8hr)

Guangzhoushi laodong yu shehui ju 2009. Guanyu feiguangzhoushi chengzhen congye renyuan canjia canjia jiben yiliao baoxian yaoguan wenti de tongzhi (The circular with regards to the issues of enrollment of non-municipal personnel in basic medical care insurance). Retrieved from *Huilal sheyi (Social labor insurance in Guangzhou)* 7 April 15, 2015 7:49:19 AM Local Timezone (GMT. 8hr)

Guowuyuan 2007. Guowuyuan guanyu kaizhan chengxiang jumin jiben yiliao baoxian shidian de zhidao yijian (Advisory opinion of the state council regarding the launching of pilot programs of basic medical care insurance for residents in cities and towns).

Hua, Y. 2010. Nongmingong shehui baozhang wenti (The issue of social security regarding agricultural laborers). In Chen J., & Wang, W. (Eds.), *Zhongguo shehui baozhang fazhan baogao No. 4. 2000: Rang renren xiangyou gongping de shehui baozhang (Report on the Development of China's Social Security No.4. 2000: All People Enjoy Equal Social Security)*. Beijing: Shehui kexue wenxian chubanshe. 190–216.

Jiang, H. 2016. Nongmingong canjia chengzhen zhigong yiliao baoxian zhuangkuang de bijiao fenxi (Comparative analysis of the participation of agricultural laborers in the medical care insurance for staff and workers). *Weisheng jingji yanjiu (Research on Health Care Economics)* 12: 29–33.

Lee, P. N. 2019. *Re-engineering Affordable Care Policy in China*. London & New York: Routledge.

Lin, F. 2007. Rang shequ weisheng fuwu chengwei jumin yibao de yitou (Making community health services support resident medical care insurance). *Zhongguo shehui baozhang (China's Social Security)* 7: 46–7.

Liu, D. 2010. Wanshan woguo chengzhen jumin jiben baoxian zhidu de tantao (Discussion on perfecting basic medical care insurance for urban residents in China). *Zhongguo weisheng jingji (China's Health Care Economy)* 29.8: 35–6.

Liu, H. 2007a. Disanzhang baowang (The third net of insurance). *Zhongguo shehui baozhang (China's Social Security)* 8: 38–40.

Liu, H. 2007b. Jumin yibao: Jinluo migu zaishengwen (Residents' medical care insurance: Warming up with earnest preparation). *Zhongguo shehui baozhang (China's Social Security)* 9: 1.

Liu, H., Wu, S., & Chu, G. 2007. Jumin yibao zoujin xiaoxian shenchu (Residents' medical care insurance walks deeply into the neighborhood). *Zhongguo shehui baozhang (China's Social Security)* 8: 42–3.

Liu, Y. 2010. Zhuhaishi chengzhen jumin yiliao baoxian xingshi dui jiuyi xinwei de yinxian diaocha (Investigation into residents' curative behavior in Zhuhai municipality under the influence of basic medical care insurance). *Zhongguo weisheng jingji (China's Health Care Economy)* 29.5: 30–2.

Lu, T. 2007. Chengshi jumin yibao "gaodiao" shidian (Conducting pilot programs for medical care insurance for residents in cities and towns on a "high profile" basis). *Zhongguo shehui baozhang (China's Social Security)* 8: 16–7.

Renli ziyuan shehui baozhangbu 2009. Guanyu quanmian kaizhan chengzhen jumin jiben yiliao baoxian gongzuo de tongzhi (The circular regarding the task for wholesale expansion of basic medical care insurance for urban residents). In Guojia weisheng jishang wei (Ed.), *2009 nian shenghua yigai wenjian huibian (The 2009 Collection of Documents of the Further Health Care Reform)*. n.p.: Guojia weisheng shengjiwei. 43–5.

Renli ziyuan shehui baozhangbu 2010. Guanyu zuohao 2010 nian chengzhen jumin jiben baoxian gongzuo de tongzhi (The circular regarding the better work of basic medical care insurance for urban residents for the year of 2010). In Guojia weisheng jishang wei (Ed.), *2009 nian shenghua yigai wenjian huibian (The 2009 Collection of Documents of the Further Health Care Reform)*. n.p.: Guojia weisheng shengjiwei. 41–4.

Shenzhenshi remin zhengfu 2012. Shenzhen shehui yiliao baoxian banfa (The measures of social medical care insurance in Shenzhen Municipality). Retrieve from bsy. sz. Bend. Bao.com October 10. 2013. 10/10/2013 10:21:29 AM Local Timezone (GMR-8hr)

Shenzhenshi renmin zhengfu 2013. Shenzhen shehui yiliao baoxian banfa (The measures of social medical care insurance in Shenzhen Municipality). Retrieved from Shenzhen baoxian shijan (Practice of Insurance in Shenzhen). December 8, 2013 10:21:50 AM Local Timezone (GMT-8hr)

Song 2001: 95–6; Guangdongsheng yiliao baozhang zhidu gaige yanjiu xianmu bangongshi 1999: 40–1, 202–3.

Sun, Z. 2013a. Shishi dabing baoxian shi jianqin renmin jiuyifudan de guanjian (The key link to lessening the people's burden is through big expenditure insurance). *Shehui baozhang zhidu* (*Social Security System*) 3: 49–52.

Sun, Z. 2013b. Shishi dabing baoxian shi jianqin renmin jiuyi fudang de guanjian (The implementation of a major illness insurance as a crucial link for lessening the medical care burden). *Shehui baozhang zhidu* (*Social Security System*) 3: 44–8.

Wang, L., Jiang, Z., & Wang, L. (2011). Chengzhen jumin jiben yiliao baoxian yu xinxing nongcun hezuo yiliao zhidu xiangxian jie de yiliao feiyong kongzhi tanxi baogao (Analysis of spending control for medical care in conjunction with an interfacing of basic medical care insurance for urban residents with the new rural cooperative medical care system). *Zhongguo weisheng jingji* (*China's Health Care Economy*) 30.7: 52–5.

Wang, X. 2008. Chengzhen jumin yiliao baoxian fufei zhidu yanjiu (Study of the payment system for the medical care insurance of urban residents). *Zhongguo weisheng jingji* (*China's Health Care Economy*) 27.12: 23–6.

Wu, Y. 2006. Tongyi sixiang chuangxin jizhi, jiji tuijin chengshi shequ weisheng fuwu fazhan (Unifying thought, creating new mechanisms, and positively pushing developing community health services in municipalities). In Guojia weisheng jiankang weiyuanhui (Ed.), *Zhongguo weisheng nianjian 2007* (*China's Yearbook of Health Care 2007*). Beijing: Renmin weisheng chubanshe. 3–7.

Xia, B. (2007). Yibaozhimen xiang chengzhen jumin dakai (The door of medical care insurance open to urban residents). *Zhongguo shehui baoxian* (*China's Social Security*) 5: 7–9.

Xiong, X. 2007. Zhidao yijian pojian erchu (Birth of the advisory opinion). *Zhongguo shehui baozhang* (*China's Social Security*) 9: 34–5.

Xu, J. 2007. Jumin yibao zhongzai zhidu sheji (Designing as key to resident medical care insurance). *Zhongguo shehui baozhang* (*China's Social Security*) 9: 40–1.

Zeng, C., & Wei, J. 2008. Nongmingong yiliao baozhang de kunjing yu chulu tanjiu (Exploring the difficulties in and solutions for medical care security for agricultural laborers). *Zhongguo weisheng jingji* (*China's Health Care Economics*) 27.4: 79–80.

Zhang, Y. 2009. Wuhanshi chengzhen jumin jiben yiliao baoxian zhidu de tantao (Discussion on the basic medical care insurance of residents of Wuhan municipality). *Zhongguo weisheng jingji* (*China's Health Care Economy*) 28.12: 29–31.

Zheng, G. 2011. *Zhongguo shehui baozhang gaige yu fazhan zhanlue* (*China's Social Security Reform and Developmental Strategy*). Beijing: Renmin chubanshe.

Zheng, G., & Lu, Q. 2007. Nongmingong jibing yu yiliao baozhang (Disease among agricultural laborers and medical care security). In Chen, J. & Wang, W. (Eds.), *Zhongguo shehui baozhang fazhan baogao (2007) No. 3: Zhuangxingzhong de weisheng fuwu yu yiaoliao baozhang* (*Report of the development of China's social security (2007) No.3: Health care services and medical care security in transformation*). 138–57. Beijing: Shehui kexue wenxian chubanshe.

10 Origins and Evolution of NRCMCI

Starting formally in 2007, new rural cooperative medical care insurance (NRC-MCI) represents an entirely new system of healthcare funding, that differs from the so-called rural cooperative medical care (RCMC)—the conventional funding mode that was embedded in the collective economy prior to economic reform. This chapter will examine NRCMCI that covers the peasantry, representing the largest sector of population in China. On the eve of introducing NRCMCI, for example, the size of rural population still consisted of more than one half of the total population in China, despite a salient trend of continuous decrease from 82.1 percent in 1978 to 56.1 percent in 2006 (Gu 2008: 122). It appears that for a long time to come, China's peasantry ought not to be left behind from the considerations of public policy, as other sectors of the population have been covered by some forms of public funding in health care.

As theorectically claimed, peasants had experience with "communal" funding of medical care under RCMC that was institutionally and managerially rooted in the collective economy at the sub-county level (e.g., commune, production brigade and/or production team level) from the 1960s to the1970s. RCMC was dismantled by the end of the 1980s in conjunction with the transformation of the collective economy into a joint-family-production-undertaking responsibility system (or JFPURS) centering on peasant households (Duckett 2013; Huang 2014). In the policy circle in China, it is well taken that NRCMCI was historically rooted in RCMC, featuring cooperative (or communal) mode of medical care. Is such a view appropriate? It is warranted here to have a close look at the official view of RCMC, and then examine continuity and discontinuity as well as similarity and difference between the two.

Furthermore, NRCMCI and RCMC, taken together, are distinguishable from the public funding of medical care in the planned sector. Both RCMC and NRC-MCI are taken as "cooperative" forms of medical care, and they differ from the work-unit-managed type of medical care (i.e., in public enterprises, government units and service units) within the planned sector under the CPE framework (Zhongguo tongji nianjian 2007: 105).

The study will start with an analysis of RCMC—the baseline from which NRCMCI grew and evolved. Then this study will proceed to examine how NRC-MCI first entered the public sector and began at the county level—lowest reach of the party-state hierarchy. Discussion will be devoted further to a comparison

DOI: 10.4324/9781003389934-13

between NRCMCI and RMCI. Subsequently, the focus shifts to policymaking and implementation at the central, provincial level, and county level where NRC-MCI is finally nested before entering the policy of integration (Chapter 12). As the NRCMCI represents a case of hybrid mode of governance, that is, combining markets with hierarchies, it is germane to examine the new institutional framework and managerial style pertaining to NRCMCI accordingly in the last section in this chapter.

The Rise and Fall of RCMC

In conceptual terms, there are three alternatives available to characterize RCMC regarding the tripods such as interpersonal network, state, and markets (Chapter 2). Although each tripod is conceptually separable from another, the three tend to be fused at the empirical level. From the official view in China, it appears that policy-makers and analysts tend to apply the interpersonal network to highlight RCMC. Considering the scale of organization, however, it is apparent that the size of a production brigade or even a production team, on which RCMC was built, nor-mally exceeded thousands—a scale larger than what could be coordinated through interpersonal networks (e.g., face-to-face relations) to operate effectively. From a sociological perspective, it seems safe to treat RCMC as a cooperative mode of healthcare that builds on the mutually supportive tripods of interpersonal network, state hierarchy and markets in the agricultural society prior to economic reform. However, it is an empirical question as to how much weight that interpersonal net-work carried in organizing RCMC and/or even NRCMCI. Therefore, the burden of proof rests on the shoulders of those who claim that RCMC represents purely a mode of pure communal funding of healthcare in the first place.

As the study argues, the rise and fall of RCMC can be better examined consider-ing the changing role of the state organization. More likely than not at the empiri-cal level, so-called RCMC worked with higher degrees of institutionalization than the notion of "cooperative" mode of medical care would entail in pure theoretical terms. Given that both NRCMCI and RCMC were built on an interpersonal net-work, as one may claim theoretically, the study argues that the former enjoyed a significantly higher degree of institutionalization, together with a higher level of marketization, than the latter.

There are various approaches to analyzing the range as well as mode of state penetration into rural Chinese society in the case of RCMC. One may measure the range of state penetration in terms of the reach of the party-state apparatus in an institutional and hierarchical sense. In rural China, the state penetration varied from one level of the party-state hierarchy to another, for example, it first reached the production brigade and after some adjustments, it was settled at the commune level during the later period of commune movement. And the range of state penetration hinged on where an institutional boundary rested, political control was exercised, and political mobilization was organized (Gu, Gao & Yao 2006; Ge & Gong 2007).

In conceptual and theoretical terms, there have been three ranges of state penetration: Broad range, medium range, and narrow range. Among earlier studies of healthcare in China, for example, Duckett adopted a broad range of the state penetration by assuming that the state penetration had already reached the brigade level and therefore, she treated the subsequent collapse of RCMC as evidence of "state's retreat," meaning the decline of political control and mobilization, coupled with the ending of ideology at the production brigade level (Duckett 2013). Echoing Tang Tsou's concept of "totalism" in modern China to an extreme, meanwhile, some Chinese scholars also treated RCMC, in this broad range of analysis, as an example of the party-state's penetration into society (Gu, Gao & Yao 2006).

In the middle range of conceptualization, the party-state's intervention in society is often limited, resulting in a mixture of the party-state hierarchy and communal relations. To put it in another way, the party-state apparatus was only able to achieve partial penetration into the collective economy. As an integral part of a collective economy, RCMC has found a foothold in the structure of state power, but it remained separate from the party-state, enjoying some measure of autonomous existence in an agricultural society. Evidence available indicates that RCMC operated at the middle range prior to the inauguration on NRCMCI (to be demonstrated shortly after).

In a narrow range, furthermore, one may take the county level as the farthest frontier where the government apparatus can formally and effectively establish its institutional, managerial, and financial presence, for example, in the case of NRCMCI.

Conceptually speaking, state penetration also assumes various mode depending on the use of alternatives instruments, such as political and ideological means, policy and economic measures, and organizational, and managerial tools, in the process of implementation. It was suggested that the state adopted alternative instruments to organize, administer, manage, and even mobilize society and, thereby, it not only penetrated into the society, but also brought about change of different magnitudes. P. N. Lee argues that the party-state did not necessarily follow only one avenue of policymaking and implementation in China, but it adopted multiple modes to tackle the same set of policy issues shifting one period to another (Lee 1987). While policymakers abandoned one policy alternative, for example, they might shift to other equally powerful policy options (e.g., from ideology and political mobilization to central planning and economic measures). Thus, in the realm of healthcare, it is entirely plausible for them to change from one mode of state intervention to another, for example, to shift among various approaches dealing with both funding and provision of medical care as documented by Lee (2019). How did NRCMCI differ from RCMC that operated during the period from the 1960s to the 1980s and beyond? In the full title of NRCMCI (i.e., new rural cooperative medical care insurance), the word "new" is added to set it off from RCMC, albeit both are ideologically treated as a form of cooperative and communal funding for medical care. The study argues that the introduction of NRCMCI represented a fresh round in a state-building movement, and was, therefore, unprecedented, being an entirely novel attempt to establish a formal foothold for state power at the county level (Lee 2019).

To begin with, RCMC owed its early origin to the collective medical care station during the collective economy of the middle 1950s, marking the incorporation of healthcare into the collective economy for the first time. Attesting to the injection of state funding, accordingly, the collective healthcare station, that first covered work injuries and clinical care, took shape in accordance with "The Model Charter for a Higher Agricultural Production Cooperative" as passed by the Third Meeting of the First Plenum of the Congress of People's Representatives in 1956. The early form of RCMC featured mutual help and a limited scale of risk pooling (*tong chou*), largely at the production brigade level while covering at most only some thousands of members, but it already went beyond the scale where interpersonal network could operate (Gu, Gao & Yao 2006; Ge & Gong 2007).

The RCMC was subsequently endorsed by the Ministry of Health (MOH) during the National Work Conference on Rural Health Care in November 1959, and was introduced to 20–30 percent of the production brigades at the beginning of 1960. Mao Zedong endorsed the policy experience with RCMC that the Leyuan People's Commune had at Changyang County, Hubei Province, providing impetus for further extension of RCMC during the People's Commune Movement. In September 1965, the CCP put forth a policy paper, through the Party Committee of the Ministry of Health (MOH), titled "The Report concerning the Priority of Health Work Shifting to Rural Areas," propelling the policy of rural "cooperative" medical care and social security, and contributing to the extension of RCMC in more than ten provinces, autonomous regions and directly administered municipalities. It is claimed that subsequently by the end of 1976, 90 percent of the peasantry took part in RCMC throughout the country. In December 1979, MOH and another five ministerial units circulated "The Draft Charter of Rural Cooperative Medical Care" (for trial implementation), marking the formal introduction of RCMC. In fact, there were continuous efforts to "rectify" and re-organize RCMC during the early phase of economic reform, stressing the principle of voluntarism as well as further improvement of funding methods. There was a series of policy papers, at least five, either directly or indirectly addressing the policies of RCMC during economic reform from 1979 to 1997, and they stayed well within the original theme and format of RCMC, despite the drastic decline of People's Communes and the collective economy. This was indicative of the growing gap between the ideal of RCMC and its implementation (Gu, Gao & Yao 2006: 141–3). The various echelons of the local government were fighting a losing battle to maintain RCMC, in conjunction with the promotion of the JFPURS, resulting in the dwindling of public financial accumulation as well as widespread poor management at the township and village levels throughout the 1980s (Gu. Gao & Yao 2006).

Like the image of barefoot doctor, communal funding of healthcare that characterizes RCMC represents largely an unfulfilled revolutionary ideal. It remains only as a claim that RCMC owed its origin to voluntarism among the multitude of the peasants responding to Mao's ideological radicalism in the countryside, in reality, it was largely a result of Maoist ideology and political mobilization, indicative of the party-state's penetration into society down to the lowest level, that is, the production brigade level. Evidence indicates that the rise of RCMC was attributable to the forceful political mobilization initiated and arranged by the Cultural Revolution Small Group, requiring party organizations and government units in all echelons to take RCMC as a "political mission" and implementing it through exercise of command and political mobilization. The demise of RCMC resulted from the fundamental shift from radical politics to economic reform (Ge & Gong 2007: 122–3). Overall, RCMC was a medical care funding scheme, inlaid in organizational structures at the collective level, not only a product of radical ideology, but also of political mobilization during the Maoist period. In a way, the decline of RCMC was an unintended result of the drastic change in developmental strategy as well as the contracting of the boundary of the party-state hierarchy (Gu, Gao & Yao 2006; Ge & Gong 2007).

Institutional and Managerial Dimensions of RCMC

How was RCMC organized, managed, and funded? In the official line of explanation, RCMC was organized on the basis of "collective voluntarism," relying mainly on retained revenue of the production team/production brigade as well as out of pocket payments (OPP) made by the peasant. In a stabilized form after the People's Commune movement, RCMC emerged as an integral part of "the rural collective economy," centering on agricultural activities at the production brigade level (or production team level in some cases). Peasants established their claim to some form of subsidy (or financial assistance) chargeable to "the public welfare fund," by virtue of membership in the production brigade/team. A medical care subsidy from the production brigade was not a kind of free give-away, but part of the non-wage compensation deriving from labor's contribution to the collective work unit. In a broad sense, RCMC was part of non-wage compensation to peasants who worked in the production brigade/team.

There were considerable variations of managerial and financial designs of RCMC at the commune, production brigade and team levels, attesting to the absence of centralizing command over funding and management. (Lampton 1977; Gu, Gao & Yao 2006; Duckett 2013; Huang 2014). However, the study argues that the state penetration reached the middle range based on the available evidence, albeit in fragmented fashion. Centering on the RCMC station at the brigade/team level, for instance, there were six types of RCMC, depending on the combination of two components: The echelons of administrative structure and managerial/ accounting functions. It is noteworthy that among six types, Type V and VI bear resemblance with a version of NRCMCI that was introduced later. The six types are given as follows:

- Type I, village-sponsored and village-managed type: Funding from retained revenue of the collective unit, either production brigade or production team, together with contributions by rural residents.

- Type II, village-sponsored and township-managed type: Funding through village contribution, and management by the township RCMC management committee or the township medical care clinics/hospital.
- Type III, joint township-village type, co-sponsored and co-managed by both levels: Financing from retained revenue at the village level, appropriation from the township level and residents' contributions, together with entitlements enacted and handled by the township administration.
- Type IV, township-sponsored and township-managed type, with the RCMC station organized by the township, and funded by three portions each from township, village and resident, respectively; subject to unified management and accounting service at the township level, coupled with standards and scopes of entitlements established at the township level.
- Type V, multi-unit type organized at the county level, for instance, in Jinshan county in Shanghai and Jianli county in Hubei province, where a cooperative medical and health care insurance system was established; enrollment based on family unit and/or enterprise, managed by the cooperative medical and health care insurance committee, and organized by the Bureau of Health at the county level.
- Type VI, "unified funding" for major illness, targeting major illness and relying on premium contributions. For example: Gaoyou Municipality where each resident contributed 1.5 RMB annually, to be deposited in a special account at the township/town level, and to allow reimbursement of medical care payment in several brackets with a progressive scheme, that is, larger payments to be reimbursed with higher percentage up to 70 percent (Baidu 2021).

Statistical data for RCMC is thin and fragmented, but some broad trends are still discernible. It is estimated that the coverage with RCMC reached 84.6 percent of the production brigades in 1975, and more than 90 percent by the late 1970s (Ge & Gong 2007: 121). However, the RCMC's decline came unexpectedly fast. Within several years from the late 1970s to the early 1980s, for example, a survey covering 45 counties in ten provinces beginning in 1985 indicates that only 9.6 percent of the peasants took part in RCMC in 1985, and declined further to 5 percent in 1986, while self-paying (OPP) patients reached 81 percent. Cited in the Second National Health Service Survey conducted in 1998, coverage with RCMC fell drastically to 9.81 percent in terms of rural population in 1993 and to 6.57 percent in 1998. The same survey indicates that only 12.68 percent of the rural population was covered by some form of public funding/insurance (including RCMC), meaning that 87.32 percent had to rely upon OPP entirely for medical care (Ge & Gong 2007: 125).

What are the key characteristics of RCMC? To answer the above questions, it is germane to dwell on the similarities and differences between RCMC and NRCMCI as follows. First, both RCMC and NRCMCI carried the name of "cooperative" but they actually represented some forms of public organization, and only each operated at a different level of institutionalization. They could not be reduced to interpersonal networks in any Sociological sense. While the former was affiliated with the production brigade/commune level, the latter rested at the county level where the government was formally organized. Second, RCMC was mainly concerned with clinical care services, and at the best, focusing on common and frequent diseases, but it did not normally include hospital care and/or cases of large expenditure. In contrast, NRCMCI was originally intended to provide funding for hospital care and other big expenditure cases like HESI, albeit clinical care was included later in most cases. Third, RCMC was inadequate in the exercise of product/service specificity. For instance, the members of the production brigade did enjoy medical care under the RCMC, but it was less than a legally defined category of entitlement enacted by the Party-state. Fourth, through RCMC, the patients were eligible for medical care because of membership in the collective unit, normally, the production brigade, and/or production team. Funding of RCMC was inseparable from the budget of the production brigade. Moreover, RCMC relied on funding from two sources: Partly from contributions of the peasants themselves, and partly from the public welfare fund (*gongyijin*) of the work unit. The expenses of medical care, that were clinical care services, were chargeable to the account of the production brigade normally through reimbursement procedure, while expenses of hospital care were shouldered summed up" (*zongjie*) at by the peasants themselves. Above all, RCMC ran short in the exercise of program specificity, for example, lacking an independent funding entity with managerial autonomy to manage RCMC. Whereas NRCMCI operated as a full-fledged form of public insurance at the county level (Sun 2013). Based on the foregoing comparative analysis, undoubtedly NRCMCI is at an unprecedented stage of policy evolution in China, a point to be elaborated in the remaining passages.

Policymaking at the Central and Provincial Level

In the case of NRCMCI, policymaking activities took place among policy actors in a large and complex institutional setting, where written communication served principally as the vehicle of coordination with some policy papers marking major phases of policy formulation and implementation. This went far beyond the interpersonal networks at the face-to-face level. In other words, impersonality is the name of game in the legal-bureaucratic context. In addition, the entire process of policymaking and implementation bore resemblance to the "sequential decision model" characterized by an incremental policymaking guided by feedback of the previous policy results, demonstrating that policy actors had always to negotiate through unknown and uncontrollable elements in the process of making policy.

NRCMCI was built as a public medical care insurance for rural China, involving a conglomerate of policy actors from the central to the provincial, prefectural, and county level in the process of policymaking and implementation. To establish NRCMCI, the central government—often represented by the State Council and ministries—played a variety of roles, including setting the policy agenda and priorities, organizing pilot programs among provinces and localities, funding various NRCMCI packages adopted, shaping consensus among provincial and local units, giving advice and guidance, and making binding rulings for echelons of the party-state hierarchy involved, just to name a few. In so far as policymaking was concerned, it was expected that "coordination teams" (*xietiao xiaozu*) were to be organized on an ad hoc basis at the central, provincial, prefectural/municipal and county level. According to Hu Shanlian's observation, the policymaking process pertaining to NRCMCI was not only based on a series of policy papers, but also relied on a number of standard operational procedures and institutional arrangements, including inter-ministerial conferences at the State Council level, NRCMCI leadership teams in various echelons of the government, and technical-advisory teams of experts at both the central and provincial level, coupled with a management committee, supervisory committee, and executive agency (i.e., alternatively taken as the NRCMCI management office) at the county level (Hu 2008).

According to the policy agenda set by the central government, NRCMCI began in 2002. It took several distinctive phases of policy implementation to establish NRCMCI in nearly three thousand counties throughout the country. The first phase lasted from 2000 to 2003. Top policymakers explicitly proposed the establishment of NRCMCI when the State Council promulgated a policy paper titled, "The Decision of Further Strengthening Rural Health Care Work" (abbreviated as the "2000 Decision" hereafter). It is noteworthy that the defining characteristics of NRCMCI were for the first time mentioned in the "2001 Opinion for Guidance" in May 2001. Its highlights included "unified funding" (a form of risk-pooling mechanism) for major illness and a new organizational infrastructure built at the county level.

At the 2002 National Conference on Healthcare Work at the end of October, 2002, Vice-Premier Li Nanqing delivered the keynote speech, clearly expounding the policy goals of developing various forms of cooperative medical care for peasants centering on unified funding for major illnesses through multiple channels, with priority given to cases of large expenditure and/or hospital care expenditure. In addition, Li suggested that as an added cushion of social security, medical care relief would be made available to families in poverty. In October 2002 the earliest pilot programs of NRCMCI were initiated in accordance with the 2002 Decision of the Party Center, CCP and the State Council. The 2002 Decision spelled out the main objectives, priorities and key measures pertaining to NRCMCI, coupled with the rural medical care relief system (RMCRS). It was made explicit in the policy agenda that NRCMCI was to be introduced through the adoption of pilot programs in selected localities, provinces and regions, "summed up" (*zongjie*) at each stage and extended accordingly. The Ministry of Health (MOH), Ministry of Finance (MOF) and Ministry of Agriculture (MOA) jointly put forth "The Opinion for Establishing a New Rural Cooperative Medical Care System" (abbreviated as the "2003 Opinion"), on January 16, 2003, and further spelt out considerable details concerning implementation (Weishengbu, Caizhengbu & Nongyebu 2003; Gu, Gao & Yao 2006: 142–3; Xiao 2010: 216–8).

In the first phase, pilot programs in various counties in 12 provinces in the Western Region and nine provinces in the Central Region were selected for policy experimentation and information gathering. A total of 43,520,000 peasants (or 74 percent of the rural population in the provinces chosen) enrolled in the pilot programs. In a separate plan, the State Council chose another group of pilot programs at the county level in another four provinces in order to monitor and compare the results among pilot programs. The State Council drafted the 2003 Advisory Opinion based on the results of four pilot programs as well as seminars and exchanges among experts. Concluding the first phase, in December 2003, Vice-Premier Wu Yi made the keynote speech at the 2003 Work Conference on the Task of NRCMCI Policy Experiments and laid down the basic policy framework while emphasizing the installation of risk-pooling mechanisms at the county level, the principle of "voluntarism" among the peasants, and the prioritization of major and expensive medical cases.

The second phase covered the period from 2004 to 2005, being highlighted by the 2004 Work Conference on NRCMCI Pilot Programs on June 6, 2004. It was convened and devoted to an exchange of experiences and opinions based on pilot programs conducted in 310 counties in 30 provinces and provincial status jurisdictions, covering 689,900,000 enrollees (or 72.6 percent of the total population of 950,400,000 peasants) as of June 6, 2004. Pilot programs extended to 233 jurisdictions in 22 provinces in the Western and Central regions with the remaining belonging to the Eastern Region. The 2004 Work Conference pledged to expand further pilot programs to cover an additional 21 percent of the counties or 163 million peasants throughout the country by June 2005.

The third phase covered the period from 2005 to 2006. It centered on the 2005 Work Conference on Pilot Programs that was convened in Nanchang in September 2005, pledging to extend pilot programs to even more counties in the country. Meanwhile the central government decided to increase the subsidy for premium contributions for enrollees in the Central and Western regions from 10 RMB to 20 RMB considering most of counties being in hardship in the two regions. At the beginning of 2006, the State Council endorsed the recommendation of the 2005 Work Conference regarding the acceleration and expansion of NRCMCI pilot programs, and decided to encourage more counties to take part in such programs, for example, about 40 percent in 2006 and 60 percent by 2007. In view of fast progress of implementation, a pledge was made to extend NRCMCI to all counties throughout the country by 2008, ahead of the original target date of full implementation set for 2010. The implementation of NRCMCI moved steadily over more than a decade, covering 805,000,000 peasants or around 98.3 percent of the total of the rural population in 2012 (Ke & San 2014: 5). By 2012, it appeared that NRCMCI was in full operation according to available statistical data. While total expenditure reached 240,8 billion RMB in the same year, the average funding for each enrollee was 308.5 RMB while the total number of beneficiaries was 1,745 billion (Ke & San 2014: 5).

The implementation of NRCMCI moved at a surprisingly fast pace through a series of pilot programs in what Yanzhong Huang takes as a "bandwagon" phenomenon, for example, for a time span of about six years from 2002 to 2008, even two years ahead of the original target date 2010 set by the central policymakers. In the case of NRCMCI, the "bandwagon" phenomenon among provincial/local government units might be attributable to the concentration of "influential resources" in the hands of groups of policymakers in various echelons of government, rather than in the hands of a singular leader as in the case of RCMC during the period of radical politics. In the policymaking context of NRCMCI, "influential resources" appeared to provide financial incentive to participating jurisdictions mostly in the form of additional funding, differing from political and ideological incentives as found in the case of RCMC. Meanwhile the degree of "functional differentiation" in the implementation and operation of NRCMCI was considerably reduced through the accumulation of policy experiences, information through pilot programs, and extensive exchanges among policy actors in the policymaking cycle.

Overall, existing party-state hierarchies had an overwhelming impact on shaping the new institution pertaining to NRCMCI. The central leadership intervened actively through consensus-building among provinces, lent substantial financial resources, and played the role of balancer ensuring that economically backward counties, provinces, and regions would not be left behind. Nonetheless, provincial jurisdictions shouldered the major responsibility for lawmaking, coordinating, designing, packaging, and financing NRCMCI within the revenue-sharing framework established during economic reform.

As a rule, a county government was directly in charge of translating general policy into discrete programs in its jurisdiction. The top-ranking officials at the county level assumed the overall responsibility to build a new set of organizations for the provision of an entirely new, composite category of service/product. Moreover, the new form of public organization working with market mechanisms was embedded in the existing structure of the county government. To put it another way, marketization accompanied the growth of hierarchies.

Facing Policy Alternatives at the County Level

Theoretically speaking, NRCMCI represents a brand of public insurance that relies upon a set of risk pooling mechanisms, the scale of which is large enough to cushion medical care risks of enrollees. In principle, the scale is the larger the better. Regarding the introduction of NRCMCI, policymakers were confronted with the choice of either the municipality or county as the vehicle of risk pooling mechanisms during the 2000s. Although many policy actors prefer the municipality, the county was finally chosen at the end of day. However, there existed an undercurrent of opinions to move upward from the county level to municipal level and even beyond regarding the scale of operation—a policy option that surfaced one decade later in the 2010s when the policy of program integration was discussed.

In the actual implementation during the beginning of the 2000s, NRCMCI operated at the county level, providing insurance funding to the composite category of medical care services to enrollees, coupled with positive side-effects to all other residents (i.e., the third parties) in the respective jurisdiction. As noted above, NRCMCI featured a hybrid mode of governance embracing components of both hierarchies and markets. Not only did its creation involve a complex set of organizational relations with respective units in the arena of the state power, but also its operation was nested in the markets.

Further to the design of NRCMCI adopted, its creation hinged on the exercise of a super-imposing mandatory power, rather than market forces only, through a evolutionary process (Gu, Gao, & Yao 2006; Wang et al. 2007). In the case of NRCMCI, the process of implementation can be taken as an exercise by a government entity in building a public organization of a non-governmental nature to fulfill public policy purposes, although the public organization is institutionally separated from, and remains managerially independent of the government. The question arises as to whether it is appropriate and suitable, in the first place, for a government entity to build a non-government unit that works in the markets. From the available evidence, it appears that the leadership of the county government intended to install NRCMCI institutionally and managerially in the way like the creation of another department within the web of bureaucratic relations at the county level, and to a considerable extent this tended to compromise the original policy intent.

NRCMCI encountered a paradox in which the government entity created a non-governmental unit, often called non-departmental public entity (NDPE) in the midst of a tendency toward bureaucratization at the party-state level. This particular NDPE was designed to perform legally defined tasks and to be separated from the government in the functional areas of personnel and financial management. Moreover, NRCMCI made use of market mechanisms to render services of a public and/or quasi-public nature, which were shaped and heavily regulated by the government, for example, the issue of market entry, types of services/products, membership and enrollment, funding schemes, and transactions with the provider etc. Moreover, NDPE had to work with the supervising departments with regard to a host of issues, for instance, the relationship between the insurer and insured, interaction between the insurer and provider, and the management of the designated providers in curative care and pharmacy, among others.

Some interesting features of NRCMCI emerge from a series of surveys and field studies, allowing a meaningful analysis and assessment of both the process of installing this insurance and its results concerning policy (Gu, Gao, & Yao 2006: 173–265; Wang et al. 2007: 92–5). First of all, the key policy actors pertaining to NRCMCI hailed from the pool of high-ranking officials of the county government. Like the exercise at the central and provincial/prefectural level, for example, in the case of Yulong County, the county magistrate served as the team leader of the NRCMCI coordination team, and played the principal leadership role, in addition to being Vice-Magistrate in charge of health. All officials from more than one dozen bureaus in relevant functional areas actively took part in policymaking and implementation in a form of "fragmented authoritarianism (Gu, Gao, & Yao 2006: 173–216).

Policy actors played a role in the deliberation and choice of alternative proposals regarding institutional framework and managerial tools for running NRCMCI. In an effective sample of 192 counties, for example, four proposals regarding various models of institutional apparatus were put forth for consideration as given below (Wang et al. 2007: 95–6):

- Proposal I: The executive agency was to be held responsible for drafting the plan for NRCMCI under the advice of the health bureau; executive agency

was also to be in charge of management and daily routine; supervision was to be conducted by the finance bureau; and the designated bank was to be in charge of collection of premium contribution and payment out of the NRCMCI foundation;
- Proposal II: The health bureau was to be in charge of drafting the plan; the executive agency would take responsibility for management; and the designated commercial bank was to be in charge of collecting premiums and making payments on behalf of the foundation;
- Proposal III: The health bureau and commercial bank were jointly in charge of drafting the plan; the executive agency would assume responsibility for supervision; and the commercial bank would be charged with approving of and paying for insurance; and
- Proposal IV: The health bureau would take responsibility for drafting; and the management center for basic medical care insurance (BMCI) for staff and workers would be in charge of fund management regarding NRCMCI.

Among the four proposed models, an overwhelming majority of counties, namely 182 out of 192 counties, chose Proposal I, which granted the executive agency autonomy not only in drafting the plan for NRCMCI, but also in taking full charge of management. Six counties selected Proposal II, which lent the executive agency managerial autonomy but not the power to draft the plan. Two counties adopted Proposal III and IV each, respectively. Both proposals did not bestow sufficient autonomy to the executive agency, treating it only as if it were a subordinate unit within the bureaucracy, the status of which was equivalent to a so-called service work unit in the conventional sense. Moreover, Proposal IV even incorporated NRCMCI into BMCI, clearly not compatible with the spirit of NRCMCI policy, considering their differences in the kinds of enrollees, packages of services, designs of funding, sponsoring organization, and labor and economic sector (Wang et al. 2007: 95–6). How was the chosen proposal, for example, Proposal I, concerning the structure of governance to be implemented? This question is to be addressed next accordingly.

The Hybrid Mode of Governance

With regards to the hybrid mode of governance, one of the most important issues has to do with jurisdiction at the county level, which sets the stage for the operation and management of NRCMCI. As just noted, the scale of risk pooling is crucial for effective and stable funding sources to cover the insurance demands of enrollees in NRCMCI. In accordance with the 2003 Opinion, it was recommended that, in principle, NRCMCI ought to be organized at the county level. Only in exceptional cases was the township level allowed as the jurisdiction for NRCMCI (Weishengbu, Caizhengbu & Nongyebu 2007). According to Xiao, the scale of NRCMCI ranged from an estimate of 1 million residents in a large county to approximately 200,000/300,000 residents in a small county. In comparison, RCMC was built at the village (or production brigade) level, normally including an estimate of 2000 residents. In some exceptional cases, RCMC was located at the township level embracing 20,000–30,000 residents (Xiao 2010: 221). It appears that the scale of coordination went beyond a form of interpersonal network based on face-to-face relations in both NRCMCI and RCMC, and, of course, NRCMCI was significantly larger. Some kinds of hierarchy were found relevant in both cases as they operated in the context of impersonality, and neither of the two was likely to work solely as an interpersonal network as just mentioned.

It is evident that NRCMCI also operated with market mechanisms that were heavily regulated and managed not only by hierarchies that were generated by the revenue-oriented market itself, but also by the party-state apparatus for public policy considerations. To focus on major, expensive medical care cases (with emphasis on HESI and catastrophic cases), the funding source for NRCMCI relied on risk-pooling mechanisms sustained by premium contributions and mediated through market transactions.

In statistical and financial terms, there are always a small percentage of enrollees who require a reasonable scale of funding for protection against the unbearable costs of hospital care and other exceedingly big expenditure cases during a given time in any system of public insurance. In program specificity pertaining to public insurance, the risk-pooling mechanisms represent an actuarial and financial design that could operate effectively with an ideal scale, for example, at the county level, municipal level or above. This entails the idea of territorial integration of risk pooling design, promising further expansion from the scale of a county to that of prefectural/municipal jurisdiction, and even to the provincial and national level from a long-term perspective (see Chapter 12).

When NRCMCI was first introduced during the 2000s, the governing structure of NRCMCI consisted of four organizations at the county level as follows: A management committee, a supervisory committee, an executive agency and designated banks. By design, the executive agency enjoyed a unique organizational status in the structure of command of the county government. It was simply not another bureau under the command of the magistrate. It remained functionally and managerially autonomous, and therefore, institutionally independent from the county government. Theoretically speaking, the executive agency was governed by the said two committees, filling the void of command over the executive agency, as the county magistrate was not given direct charge over it (Gu, Gao, & Yao 2006).

The committee type of decision-making differed from the executive type that was represented by the command under the county magistrate. The former owed its strength to ensuring full exchanges and consultation among members, greater transparency of the decision-making process, a relatively comprehensive deliberation of alternatives, sensitivity to policy guidelines, laws and regulations, and an accommodation for diverse interests, but it also suffered from some shortcomings such as time-consuming deliberation, and not infrequently, indecisiveness. To performing executive duties, the latter merits for its secrecy, swiftness, unity, and accountability, but it came up short for its narrowness, subjectivity and arbitrariness (Gu, Gao, & Yao 2006).

A 2005 survey of 257 countie available sheds considerable light on the composition of members in the two committees. In the case surveyed, the composition of the NRCMCI management committee indicated the share of membership from bureaus of various functional arenas as follows: 243 (or 94.6 percent) from the health care department; 239 (or 93 percent) from finance, 232 (or 90.3 percent) from agriculture; 237 (or 92.2 percent) from civil affairs; 159 (61.9 percent) from development and reform; 207 (or 80.5 percent) from auditing; 109 (or 42.4 percent) from food and drug; 113 (or 44 percent) from assistance to poverty; 0 from discipline and investigation, 0 from agricultural laborers; and 163 (63.4 percent) from farmer representatives. In the case of NRCMCI supervision committee, representation was heavily concentrated in the following functional areas: 221 (86 percent) from auditing; 210 (or 81.7 percent) from discipline and investigation; 200 (77.8 percent) from farmer representatives; 130 (or 50.6 percent) from agriculture, and 48 (18.7 percent) from farmers. From the above data, it is evident that the feature of functional representation from the bureau level thickly colored the composition of the two committees (Wang et al. 2007: 95–6).

Above all, not only was NRCMCI built by, but also managed by policy actors who were concurrently government officials at the county level. However, the officials from relevant functional areas took part in policymaking and enforcement legally *not* by virtue of their bureau affiliation but rather in their capacity as members of the management committee or supervisory committee. Of course, they were also not regarded as members within the formal hierarchy of the county government despite informal relations among them (Gu, Gao, & Yao 2006: 173–265; Wang et al. 2007: 92–5). In such a case where the formal power structure was likely to be embedded on the interpersonal networks, did the dual identity of such individuals enhance liaison between the relevant bureaus and those who manage NRCMCI, or did it give rise to conflict? How likely was it for a non-departmental public entity to develop its own independent identity? These are empirical questions to be answered.

The executive agency was pivotal in the operation and management of NRCMCI. It oversaw collecting premiums from enrollees and arranging financial appropriations, and transferring funds to the special account. At the forefront of enforcement, the executive agency set up its branches or authorized the relevant units to establish themselves at the sub-county level and to administer the task of collection. At respective levels of government, the financial office/bureau established standard operating procedures of financial appropriation in order to ensure the right amount of funds would be transferred in a timely fashion to the NRCMCI foundation (Gu, Gao, & Yao 2006: 173–265; Wang et al. 2007: 92–7).

In addition, some forms of ex post managerial tools were found relevant in the context. For example, the supervisory apparatus, procedures, and mechanisms were put in place to hold the executive agency accountable to the NRCMCI management committee and the NRCMCI supervisory committee. The NRCMCI management committee was, in turn, made accountable to the supervisory committee and the Congress of People's Representatives at the respective level of jurisdiction (Weishengbu, Caizhengbu & Nongyebu 2007).

In accordance with the 2003 Opinion, furthermore, the NRCMCI foundation was established and managed by both the NRCMCI management committee and executive agency. To run the foundation, it was recommended to establish a special account in a designated bank (preferably a commercial bank) to maintain financial accountability, minimize risks of irregularity, and ensure full compliance with the rules and regulations made by respective government departments. Furthermore, all financial matters and accounts were to be subjected to periodical auditing under the auditing office/bureau in each jurisdiction (Weishengbu, Caizhengbu & Nongyebu 2007).

By and large, the local governments were expected to provide staff to help establish and manage the NRCMCI foundation in the initial phase. Often, the county government was to contribute manpower and absorb the considerable financial cost of establishing NRCMCI. For example, the government officials/ party cadres had to go to the limit in campaigns to cajole peasants to enroll in NRCMCI and even to find ways on behalf of NRCMCI to help collect premium contributions. In other words, NRCMCI did not rely on its own personnel hired by its apparatus to collect and manage its funds, but civil servants in government performed these tasks. Likely as an interim arrangement, moreover, NRCMCI was to be run directly by personnel seconded from the county government, but paid by the government (Gu, Gao, & Yao 2006; Wang et al. 2007). On the spending side, moreover, it was explicitly stated in the 2003 Opinion that the government units of county/municipal jurisdiction would be responsible for setting up the scope, amount and standards of expenditure as well as spending control measures. Again, the excessive reliance on the local government was the issue of implementation at its initial stage in the case of NRCMCI. As time is required to install new styles of financial management in the process of policy implementation, it is worthwhile to continue observation when new research material becomes available.

Concluding Remarks

The foregoing analysis has examined the evolutionary path from RCMC to NRC-MCI, highlighting the differences and similarities between the two. In this chapter, furthermore, this study argues that NRCMCI represents a case of marketization under the sponsorship of the government, but it does not go all the way to a full-fledged corporate form of organization in tandem with a free market system. Instead, it has only moved half the way from the party-state hierarchy to markets. Examples include the separation of financial management from the government and the establishment of an autonomous public body managerially independent of the government. It is better characterized as a "one arm's length" approach toward public policy, a popular recommendation advanced by NPM advocates during recent decades. However, the "one arm's length" approach only results in less bureaucracy and has yet to take a clear and explicit stand on what kind of market-oriented approach should be recommended in the realm of public policy, and how large it ought to be. NRCMCI addresses the issue of how to apply market mechanisms in funding certain categories of specific product/services to enrollees, coupled with the spill-over effects to an undifferentiated multitude of people in a given jurisdiction in a unique economic and social setting (Weishengbu, Caizhengbu & Nongyebu 2007). As the study has just examined the institutional dimension of NRCMCI, the next chapter will be devoted to a discussion of its managerial and financial issues.

References

Baidu 2021. Nongcun hezuo yiliao zhidu (Rural cooperative medical care system). https://baike.com/item/

Duckett, J. 2013. *The Chinese State's Retreat from Health.* London & New York: Routledge.

Ge, Y., & Gong, S. 2007. *Zhongguo yigai, wenti, genyuan, chulu* (*China's Medical Care Reform: Issues, Roots & Solutions*). Beijing: Zhongguo fazhan chubanshe.

Gu, X. 2008. *Zuoxian quanmin yibao: Zhongguo xinyigai de zhanlue yu zhanshu* (*The Strategy and Tactics of the New Medical Care Reform in China*). Beijing: Zhongguo laodong shehui baozhang chubanshe.

Gu, X., Gao, M., & Yao, Y. 2006. *Zhengduan yu chufang, zhimian Zhongguo yiliao tizhi gaige* (*Diagnosis and Prescription, Confronting China's Medical Care Reform*). Beijing: Shehui kexue wenxian chubanshe.

Hu, S. 2008. Woguo xinxing nongcun hezou yiliao zhidu de yunxing zhuangkuan yu pingjia enfengxi (The operation and assessment of the new rural cooperative medical care system in China). *Zhongguo weisheng jingji* (*China's Medical Care Economics*) 27: 2.

Huang, Y. 2014. *Governing Health in Contemporary China.* London & New York: Routledge.

Ke, Y., & San, D. 2014. Cong Zhongyang yihao wenjian kan nongcun weisheng shiye fazhan (To examine the development of health enterprises in the countryside in light of the center's number 1 documents). *Weisheng jingji yanjiu* (*Research of Health Care Economics*):3: 11.

Lampton, D. 1977. *The Politics of Medicine in China: The Policy Process, 1949–77.* Boulder, CO: Westview Press.

Lee, P. N. 1987. *Industrial Management and Economic Reform in China.* Hong Kong, Oxford & New York: Oxford University Press.

Lee, P. N. 2019. *Re-engineering Affordable Care in China.* London & New York: Routledge.

Sun, Z. 2013. Shishi daping baoxian shi jianqing renmin jiuyi fudang de guanjian (The key for lessening the burden for people in medical care is the implementation of major illness insurance). *Shehui baozhang zhidu.* (*Social Security System*). 3.

Wang, Y. 2008. *Zhongguo weisheng gaige yu fazhan shizheng yanjiu* (*Empirical Research on China's Health Care Reform and Development*). Beijing: Zhonguo laodong shehuibaoxian chubanshe.

Wang, Y., Liu, X. Cui, H., & Tang, J. 2007. Xinxing nongcun hezuo yiliao zhidu de jianli he fazhan (The establishment and development of new rural cooperative medical system). In Chen, J., & Wang. Y. (Eds.), *Zhuanxing Zhong de weisheng fuwu yu yiliao baozhang* (*The Health Care Reform and Medical Care*). Beijing: Shehui kexue wenxian chubanshe. 64–124.

Weishengbu, Caizhengbu & Nongyebu 2003. Guanyu jianli xinxing nongcun hezuo yiliao de yijian (Opinion concerning the establishment of the new rural cooperative medical care). www.gov.cn/zwgk/2005-08/12/content_21830.htm

Weishengbu, Caizhengbu & Nongyebu 2007. Guanyu jianli xinxing nongcun hezuo yiliao zhidu de yijian (Opinion concerning the establishment of a new rural cooperative medical care system). In Ge, Y., & Gong, S. (Eds.), *Zhongguo yigai: wenti, gengyuan, chulu (China's Medical Care Reform: Issues, Roots and Solutions)*. Beijing: Zhongguo fazhan chubanshe: 141–4.

Wu, R. 2013. Guanyu daping baoxian de sikao (Thoughts concerning the major illness insurance). *Shehui baozhang zhidu (Social Security System)*. 5.

Xiao, A. S. 2010. *Nongcun yiliao weisheng shiye de fazhan. (The Development of Enterprises of Rural Medical and Health Care)*. Zhengjiang: Jiangshu daxue chubanshe.

Xu, L., Zhou, L., & Rao, K. 2007. Xinxing nongcun hezuo yiliao guanli jigou diaocha fenxi (Analysis and investigation on managerial apparatus of new rural cooperative medical care) New rural cooperative medical care management). In Weishengbu tongji xinxi zhongxin (Ed.), *Zhongguo xinxing nongcun hezuo yiliao jinzhan jiqi xiaoguo yanjiu (The Progress of as well as the Research on the Effects of the New Rural Cooperative Medical Care in China)*. Beijing: Zhongguo xiehe yike daxue chubanshe. 9–19.

Zhongguo tongji nianjian (China Statistics Yearbook) 2007. Beijing: Zhongguo tongji chubanshe.

11 Packaging and Funding of NRCMCI

Further to the foregoing analysis on the policy initiation as well as institutional dimension concerning NRCMCI in the last chapter, the focus of the study will shift to the exercise of program specificity regarding the financial and managerial issues. In this chapter, here are some fundamental issues to be tackled: Namely, what kinds of products/services are provided? And how to find financing sources to cover the chosen types of products/services? These two issues fall into the arena of public financial management in NRCMCI, covering both funding and spending.

In the case of NRCMCI, the policymakers adopted a hybrid mode of governance that combined markets with hierarchy in handling all financial and managerial tasks to fulfill public policy purposes. The chapter will examine several salient aspects of financial management of NRCMCI. To begin with, an analysis will be devoted to the issue of how public financial management was restructured in the case of NRCMCI. To deal with the dynamic relations in the policymaking process, the study will then proceed to examine key policy actors in public finance pertaining to NRCMCI. Furthermore, discussion will be focused on the exercise of product/service. Finally, the study will make an assessment of implementation and policy outcomes.

Moreover, the study will try to make a comparative analysis of the differences and similarities between NRCMCI and URCMI. In policy evolution, NRCMCI is the predecessor of URCMI. Both were focused on HESI, but they each intended to address medical care demands of two entirely different sectors of the population in China, that is, the peasants and urban residents respectively. How do they differ from each other in the exercise of product/service specificity, financial management, and other operational issues? The study will try to tackle the above issues in the remaining passages in this chapter.

Remaking Public Financial Management

To analyze how public financial management was re-structured in the midst of marketization in the case of NRCMCI, it is necessary to examine not only the pure financial side of the case, but also the public policy implications. In the case of NRCMCI, policymakers adopted an amalgam of the inward-resource-flow (IRF) system with the outward-resource-flow (ORF) system in dealing with the matters of financial management, such as funding sources, fund management, and payment

DOI: 10.4324/9781003389934-14

schemes among others (Chapter 2). While the former played an important role in dealing with the pure financial side of NRCMCI, the latter addressed public policy issues such as externality. The study endeavors to demonstrate here how the two systems are functionally fused with each other in the hybrid mode of governance in NRCMCI from its policy-oriented formulation, highlighting public policy concerns.

Anchoring in the IRF system NRCMCI adopted the design of public insurance by working with the markets to ensure the matching of premium contributions with insurance payments and maintain a budgetary balance for the NRCMCI foundation, as it was in case of URMCI. NRCMCI operated with market mechanisms where both the government and the enrollee acted in their capacity as insurance payers in transactions with the insurer (i.e., represented by the executive agency), while installing transaction-centered management pertaining to the IRF system (Chapter 2). Like the case of URMCI, both the enrollee and the government assumed the role as purchasers, ensuring a rigorous calculation and accounting of each item of transaction with the insurer and thereby enhancing accountability in NRCMCI. The enrollee was given a pivotal part in the operation of market mechanisms in that the share of funding from the collective work unit and government could not procedurally enter NRCMCI unless the enrollee had already made a decision to subscribe to it. About managing NRCMCI financially, in other words, the government's funding role hinged on the peasant paying his own share of the premium contribution, albeit starting with a small share in the early phase of the institutional development. Also, the funding from the central government did not enter the account of the NRCMCI foundation unless the local governments had already submitted their share of contribution.

By design, NRCMCI was intended to provide funding in the delivery of a composite category of services (i.e., HESI cases) to the enrollee. NRCMCI operated with market transactions, dealing with both the buying side and selling side within the IRF system. On the one hand, the buying side embraced several actors: Enrollees, collective work units and echelons of government, who each contributed a share of the premium. On the other hand, the selling side was paid for providing insurance benefits, and it was represented by the insurer, namely, the executive agency, under the advice and instructions of the NRCMCI management committee, in accordance with the 2003 Opinion (Weishengbu, Caizhengbu & Nongyebu 2007).

Marking a further stage in the development of public policy in China, NRCMCI superseded RCMC not only in terms of novel types of services but also in new funding designs. In particular, the government played an entirely new funding role by subsidizing the demand side (or users/enrollees) in market transactions rather than merely the supply side as it used to when it only subsidized public providers. The collective work unit often was expected to subsidize the enrollee by paying premium contributions, albeit contributions considerably smaller than the days of RCMC. The relationship between the collective work unit and enrollees was not that of employer-employee relationship in business/industrial management, but based on a "cooperative" network as claimed in accordance with official policy line.

In the same process of marketization, the growth of hierarchies accompanied the ORF system in connection with product/service specificity. According to the government's formal policy intent, NRCMCI was designed to provide funding principally for the package of HESI (e.g., hospital care plus other exceedingly big expenditure cases). Accordingly, it was necessary for the government to intervene through the exercise of mandatory power on both the purchasing side (e.g., with premium contributions) and the spending side (e.g., for payment schemes, positive/negative listing of services etc.,) to provide medical care of HESI, together with quasi-collective goods to the members of the community at large. In the case of NRCMCI, the government acted as a "co-payer" for insurance. Like the case of URMCI, various echelons of the government directly subsidized the peasants through the channel of "direct subsidy" (or called "open subsidy", *mingbu* in Chinese expression) (Lee 2019: 75–97). The direct subsidy, namely, the subsidy to users, was taken as a managerial tool of transaction-centered management in the IRF system, as the user was granted a choice and a financial stake in transactions with the provider (Chapter 9). Through the direct subsidy, the government's share goes with the choice made by the user (or enrollee). As the user makes a choice as a buyer in a transaction, the insurer will benefit from the deal and thus be rewarded financially. Amounting to the idea of "every user as a manager," as a result, the user assumes a managerial role not only to gauge inwardly his/her own demand, but also assess his/her choice of services from a financial vantage point.[1]

According to Gu Xin, sovereign planners must face two optional schemes to address the issue of "reversal of choice," while maintaining a viable scale for funding the NRMCMI foundation.[2] The first scheme involves a mandatory plan, requiring all eligible members to subscribe to an insurance plan with common criteria, neither imposing pre-conditions of health, nor discriminating on the basis of income or other considerations. The second scheme makes use of community rates, requiring all enrollees from the same community to follow the common rates for premium contributions. Both options work against the reversal of choice and encourage the healthy and better income persons to stay on with the insurance plan, the effect of which is to sustain a viable scale for risk pooling.

It is evident that the first scheme was adopted for BMCI, while the second scheme applied to both NRCMCI and URMCI during the health care reforms in China. In the second scheme, community rates are based on one's residence and on a voluntary basis, allowing residents of a community freedom of choice. Moreover, the government addressed the issue of scale viability by providing subsidies to bolster enrollment in NRCMCI but refrained from exercising mandatory power to regulate the participation of peasants in the insurance plan.

From a comparative perspective, NRCMCI in China appears like the NHS in the UK in that both are marked by the significant role of the government in subsidizing health care. In the former case, the government injected considerable revenue to help the enrollee make premium contributions operating within the IRF system, albeit it was not part of the insurance plan. The latter case was characteristic of the ORF system. That is to say, the government commissioned the providers directly and picked up expenses on behalf of the patients, while the government was connected to providers through "service agreements," a non-contractual relationship, which, strictly speaking, did not constitute market transactions in terms of the quid pro quo exchange of values.

Key Actors in Financing NRCMCI

The NRCMCI funding scheme was transaction-oriented, as found in the operation of market mechanisms for collecting premium contributions, and it was also command-oriented, involving extensive, active state intervention through institution-building, policymaking, program and product/service specificity, regulatory control, and subsidies to users. Overall, sovereign planners assumed a significant role in designing and enforcing funding schemes pertaining to the adoption of market mechanisms relying on the IRF system. As a form of subsidy through the ORF system, they also use public revenue and resources to subsidize users while building NRCMCI.

What are the considerations behind the intervention of the government and other public organizations to take part in the payment of premium contributions to NRCMCI? In the interpretative frame of reference in the Chinese context, it appears that financial assistance from the government and from the collective work unit (e.g., production brigade at the township level or production team at the village level) may be better explained in terms of a version of the historically rooted obligation (taken as "historical debts"): The peasant shouldered a large burden for the financial accumulation at the collective work unit and the local government level under the CPE strategy during the pre-reform period. For instance, the peasants made considerable contributions to the growth of national wealth through taxation, retained revenue, and compulsory purchase rates of agricultural produce. Moreover, the peasants' contribution to the growth of public revenue and assets was enormous in terms of their sacrifice under the "scissor effect" during forced modernization under the CPE strategy: For example, the peasantry was burdened by the relatively high prices of not only consumers' goods but also industrial products (including modernizing input such as fertilizer, fuel, equipment, etc.). It is well argued, consequently, that peasants were left without adequate savings to pay for their retirement, health care and other social security demands, as funds had been converted into public revenue and assets, holders of which were and still are various echelons of government and collective work units (including collectively owned enterprises) (Wang 2003). This it is legitimate for peasants to lay claim to some kind of entitlement, for instance, a share of funds to make premium contributions to NRCMCI (Chapter 3).

How did the government and collective work units share their financial responsibility in funding NRCMCI exactly? In accordance with the 2003 Opinion, NRCMCI adopted funding mechanisms consisting of three components: The individual share, the assistance by the collective unit and the government's help (Weishengbu, Caizhengbu & Nongyebu 2007).

In principle, each share of an enrollee's premium contribution had to be matched by shares of subsidies provided by respective echelons of the government. In accordance with the 2003 Opinion, for example, the government needed to subsidize the enrollee (or the peasant) to make a premium contribution of 10 RMB each at a minimum starting in 2002. Subject to the decision of the local government concerned, however, the rate may be adjusted upward in an area enjoying better economic conditions. From 2003 to 2005, the minimum rate increased to 20 RMB. A further rise of the minimum rate to 40 RMB was introduced from 2006 onward (Gu 2008).

It appears that the government's share of subsidy adjusted over years considering economic growth, inflation and the increase of spending for medical care services. By 2009, for example, the central government's matching fund grew to a minimum of 40 RMB on average to each NRCMCI enrollee in the Central, Western, and the less developed part of the Eastern Region, while each enrollee needed to contribute 20 RMB at a minimum. In the less developed part of the Eastern Region, the premium contribution of the enrollee reached 100 RMB on average or more. Starting in 2010, there was still another raise of funding level to 150 RMB on average for each enrollee in NRCMCI, while the central government's share to the Central and Western Regions increased to 60 RMB, together with less developed part of the Eastern Region. Accordingly, the subsidy of local governments to NRCMCI increased further to 60 RMB, while each share of the enrollee was raised from 20 RMB to 30 RMB. As the provincial government was requested to shoulder the main portion of the increase in the subsidy, those local governments in financial hardship and difficulties were allowed a two-year grace period to meet the target of the increase in subsidy (Zheng 2011: 44–5).

Various echelons of the government were confronted with the scenario of chasing a moving financial target as there was a constant raise of subsidy over the years. Questions were raised about the sustainability of such a policy as well as the mechanisms adopted by sovereign planners to continue upward adjustments of the share of subsidy contributed by the echelons of the government, given the fluctuations in China's economy over a long period beyond the 2010s.

How did the echelons of government work out their division of shares of subsidy to enrollees? It is noteworthy that some interesting change took place between the central government and local governments in inaugurating NRCMCI. Not only did the central government take an active part in the funding, but it also tried to ensure that each echelon of the government would shoulder its share of financial responsibility to subsidize each enrollee's premium contributions to NRMCMI (Gu 2008: 188–203). While the central government made explicit that all funding responsibility had to rest squarely on provincial and local governments on top of the central government's share and had to avoid creating another form of tax burden on the peasantry. Meanwhile the central government would shoulder the initial financial appropriation to help meet the premium contribution of the peasants in the Central and Western Regions, together with selected counties in several provinces in the Eastern region (Wang et al. 2007: 70–6).

As given in Table 11.1, a compiled data set illustrates the division of the funding responsibility among echelons of governments, collective work units, enrollees and the central government covering the three regions (Eastern, Central and Western) in 2005. For the total funding of 754 million RMB in the country during 2005, the shares among contributors were as follows: Central government, 7.2 percent; provincial jurisdiction, 13.9; municipal jurisdiction, 7 percent; county government, 19 percent; township jurisdiction, 9.1 percent; peasant, 38.1 percent; other sources, 5.7 percent, as given in Table 11.1. In terms of the actual health care burden, the peasants' contribution is estimated at nearly 40 percent to pay for their NRCMCI insurance premium, in addition to their out-of-pocket payment (OPP) to the provider, often at 70 percent of the charges for services on average (Wang et al. 2007: 74).

There is no doubt that provincial and local governments were expected to shoulder large shares of funding to help the enrollee in premium contributions in view of the revenue reform of 1980 and 1994, as seen in the tendency taken as "load shedding": A smaller portion of revenue allocated to lower echelons of the government accompanying greater responsibility as demonstrated by a larger portion of expenditure in lower echelons.[3] It is new that the central government began to shoulder a share of the funding in health care, that is, 7.2 percent as noted in Table 11.1. However, the central government only helped the provincial/local jurisdictions selectively, normally concentrating on the Central and Western Regions, but not the Eastern region, for instance, 25.6 percent of funding for the Central Region and 21.8 percent for the Western Region.

The establishment of a minimum rate does not mean that all echelons of the government shoulder an equal share of the burden for funding of NRCMCI. Instead, it was up to the provincial and local jurisdictions to work out the proportions of financial responsibility for various echelons and enrollees. Consequently, the provincial/local governments adopted different schemes to divide up the shares among various echelons of government in the respective jurisdictions. According to Gu, there were three schemes to divide the sum of 10 RMB for each enrollee (to increase to 20 RMB within two years from 2006 onward) adopted among the provincial governments: The indiscriminate scheme (14 provincial jurisdictions), the discriminant scheme (13 jurisdictions), and the discretional-flexible scheme (2 jurisdictions) among the various echelons, attesting considerable variations in implementation across jurisdictions (Gu 2008: 234–49).

The foregoing analysis has so far shed light on the division of shares of funding among echelons of government, different roles in public policy, the legacy and system of finance, the actual operation at the provincial/local government level and the extent of help that the enrollee enjoyed to the funding of NRCMCI. Characteristic of one form of subsidy to users through the ORF system, various echelons of government worked closely to make funding to NRCMCI available and, accordingly, relieve the burden of the enrollee. With funding in place, it is germane to ask further what kind of medical care services are rendered and how they are delivered to the enrollee through NRCMCI.

Table 11.1 Financial Sources of NRCMCI Foundations (2005)

Nation & Region	Total Funding of the Year (100 Million)	Financial Sources of Foundation %							Average per Enrollee (RMB)	Central Funding (Average per Enrollee) (RMB)	Local Funding (Average per Enrollee) (RMB)
		Central Finance	Provincial Finance	Municipal Finance	County Finance	Township Finance	Individual's Finance	Other Sources			
Nation	7,540	7.2	13.9	7.0	19.0	9.1	38.1	5.7	42.2	3	20.7
Eastern Region	5,860	–	13.3	6.6	22.1	13.0	39.3	5.7	50.4	–	27.7
Central Region	1,190	25.6	14.4	8.8	12.9	0.1	37.8	0.3	28.0	7.4	10.5
Western Region	10.9	21.8	16.1	6.9	10.9	0.2	32.7	11.4	32.8	7.2	11.2

Source: Adapted from *Quanguo xinxing nongun hezou yiliao jiben xinxin baobiao 2005 (Basic statistical report of national NRCMCI)*, compiled by Ministry of Health, PRC. in Wang, Y., Liu, X. Cui, H., & Tang, J. 2007. Xinxing nongcun hezuo yiliao zhidu de jianli he fazhan (The establishment and development of a new rural cooperative medical system) in Chen, J. & Wang, Y. (Eds.), *Zhuanxing Zhong de weisheng fuwu yu yiliao baozhang (The Health Care Reform and Medical Care)*. Beijing: Shehui kexue wenxian chubanshe. 74.

The Exercise of Product/Service Specificity

Regarding the kinds of medical services covered and rendered, this study argues that program specificity, including product/service specificity, tended to foster both an evolution toward hierarchies in the process of the marketization of NRC-MCI. As a component of program specificity, product/services specificity involves the packaging of a composite category of medical care services, heavily relying on choices and preference mix, medical-technical decisions, financial and actuarial know-how, and designs and selections of managerial and institutional tools. According to Williamson, asset specificity is associated with the growth of hierarchy (Williamson 1996). By the same token, the exercise of program specificity requires additional resources and investment, most of which are command-centered types of decisions rather than market-centered types of choices.

In the case of NRCMCI, one needs to address the complex issues involving actors on the purchasing side as well as their divergent preferences. Often acting as a team, multiple actors, including echelons of government, collective work units, and enrollees, were responsible for the exercise of program specificity to enable NRCMCI to operate effectively as a public insurance plan. To focus on NRCMCI here, questions arise as to who the actors were and who decided directly and indirectly to buy insurance plans. Moreover, what kinds of preference mix lie behind enrollees' choices upon entering transactions? By what process and procedure do enrollees make their respective decisions? And finally, how is the market structured? To answer the above questions, it is evident, first, that by design, the enrollee plays a pivotal role by having the final say if (s)he wants to subscribe, by following the cardinal principle of voluntarism, to a given insurance plan pertaining to NRCMCI. In financial terms, several actors who represent various echelons of the government, together with the collective work unit, provide subsidies for the enrollee to make a larger portion of the premium payments to buy the insurance. Second, it is apparent that each enrollee's preference mix carries weight behind the decision to subscribe to a NRCMCI package. The enrollee, in the capacity of the insured, enters a transaction with the insurer for an insurance plan, and, subsequently, a transaction with the public providers for medical care services as chosen. Third, the kind of choice is personal, in part, regarding the sort of medical demands during illness, and it is internal concerning the enrollee's own preference mix to match payment, operating with the accounting procedures within the insurance plan. Fourth, as an integral part of the IRF system, the accounting procedures only calculate the costs and benefits for each item, incurred during transactions within the enclosed arena of a given transaction between the buyers and sellers without the involvement of third parties. Fifth, the government lends subsidies to the enrollee by helping a large share of premium contributions. The government is motivated by a mixture of policy considerations, including the policy concern of spill-over effects so generated (i.e., "positive externality") for example, protecting the community against high and ruinous expenditure due to illness among the residents and maintaining a healthy and productive labor force. Sixth, the residents in the community at large who benefit from positive externalities are not necessarily a party to the said market transaction pertaining to the insurance plan.

The government was confronted with a series of choices in the decision-making process in introducing NRCMCI in conjunction with the establishment of the hybrid mode of governance, making health care services available to the peasants through marketization. The government treated the package of public insurance over HESI cases as a topmost priority, but it was confronted with the scenario where the package was of low marketability among enrollees. Also, enrollees were caught in the conflict in their two-tier preference in the choice of NRCMCI packages (Gu, Gao & Yao 2006; Gu 2008: 195–7). The high-tier preference was concerned with large expenditure cases, often including hospital care and other HESI cases. The low-tier preference refers to less expensive clinical care that was tangible and attractive to many peasants.

In the exercise of product/service specificity, three possible options were entertained: First, only HESI including hospital care and other expensive services; second, clinical care plus HESI including hospital care and other expensive services; and third, the clinical care only. To implement NRCMCI, the peasants could only make choices between the first and second option in introducing NRCMCI, resulting in considerable policy disputes among policy actors concerned., The kind of medical care of RCMC was comparable with the third option, and it was not offered in NRCMCI. In a considerable number of cases, moreover, enrollees might be reluctant to subscribe to NRCMCI when *only* HESI cases (e.g., cases of the first option) were covered, because, in their narrow perception, these cases rarely occurred after all. The second option, appeared most acceptable to most of the peasants. For example, through the experience of pilot programs, there were cases where the NRCMCI package suffered somewhat from very low enrollment if *only* high expenditure cases were covered (e.g., cases of the first option) without including less expensive clinical cases (Gu, Gao & Yao 2006: 149–50).

As cited by Professor Hu Shanlian, for example, the survey of 1451 counties adopted three NRCMCI packages as given in Table 11.2, demonstrating the similar pattern of choices by the enrollees during of trial implementations and pilot programs across jurisdictions just noted above. Packages II and III were in common for both include clinical care and HESI cases (i.e. hospital care and other expensive items), except that Package III entertained a specially featured family clinical care.

- Package I, hospital care (plus other big expenditure cases) *only*;
- Package II, a combination of clinical care and hospital care (plus other expensive expenditure cases); and
- Package III, family clinical care and hospital care (plus other expenditure cases) (Hu 2008).

According to Hu, it is estimated overall that Package I and II consisted of 15.6 percent and 16.1 percent respectively in a sample of 1451 counties surveyed where NRCMCI plans were introduced as of 2006, and Package III covered 68.3 percent

Table 11.2 Package of NRCMCI (2006)

Nation & Region	Number of Counties	Package I, Hospital Care (%)	Package II, Hospital Care plus Clinical Care (%)	Package III, Family Clinical Care & Hospital Care (%)
Nation	1,451	15.6	16.1	68.3
Eastern Region	560	33.0	34.3	32.7
Central Region	378	9.0	1.3	89.7
Western Region	513	1.4	7.2	91.4

Source: Adapted from Hu, S. (2008). Woguo xinxing nongcun hezou yiliao zhidu de yunxing zhuang-kuan yu pingjia enfengxi (The operation and assessment of the new rural cooperative medical care system in China). *Zhongguo weisheng jingji* (*China's Medical Care Economics*). 27: 2.

of counties (see Table 11.2). In the Eastern Region, about 33 percent opted for Package I, 34.3 percent, for Package II, and 42.7 percent, for Package III. In the Central Region, 9 percent, 1.3 percent, and 89.7 percent chose Package I, II and III, respectively. And in the Western Region, 1.4 percent, 7.2 percent, and 91.4 percent matched with Package I, II and III, respectively as given in Table 11.2. Evidently Package I that only covered hospital care was least popular, while Package II & III that entertained clinical care fared much better. In fact, Package III with hospital care plus family clinical care plan was the most favorite choice among the three. Above all, any package that included clinical care with or without the require-ment of family membership tended to improve its marketability, promising better revenue to NRCMCI.

In another survey of expenditure for NRCMCI in 189 counties in 2006, making use of slightly different categories, and demonstrating the similar pattern of choice that lent weight to the package of combining hospital care with family clinical care, for example, 8.5 percent of the counties surveyed are counted for the hospital care package *only*, 8.5 percent for the package of hospital care plus high expenditure cases in clinical care, 24 percent for the package of hospital care plus special clini-cal care relying on risk-pooling, and 58.7 percent for the package of hospital care and the family clinical care account (Xu, Zhou & Rao 2007: 15).

Behavioral Adaptations in Implementation

In Williamson's formulation, once the decision-maker adopted a mode of govern-ance (either market, hybrid and hierarchy, it is expected at the phenomenal level that behavioral adaptation tends to take place in the direction of either Adaptation (A) or (C) (Williamson 1975, 1996; Chapter 2). In the case of NRCMCI as much as URCMI, it is interesting to monitor how policy actors concerned acted in the process of implementation of a chosen package of public insurance. It appeared that the package constituting (family clinical care plus hospital care and other ex-pensive services) was one of the most popular packages in NRCMCI, while the other two were discarded in a dynamic interaction among all involved. Overall, it is noteworthy that while Adaptation (A) enjoyed considerable saliency, Adaption (C) occurred too, in a context where both the markets and hierarchies grew further hand in hand).

There were pros and cons about the combination of the family clinical care account with hospital care (with other expensive services). In conflict with the government's original policy intent, proponents supported the family clinical care account in insurance plan for its merits in several important aspects. It is argued that the family clinical account represented an effective tool for fund-raising by relying on "social capital," taking advantage of voluntarism rooted in the community. And it came with its unique way of spending control, for example, the deposit in a family account constituted a natural spending ceiling. Besides, it enhanced awareness of the enrollee's personal need to seek a timely cure to prevent delays of treatment at an early stage (Gu, Gao & Yao 2006; Wang et al. 2007: 121–2; Gu 2008; Hu 2008).

Opponents argued against Package III, namely the incoperation of family clinical care account, with equal strength by pointing out that family account was superfluous after all for it hindered a better allocation of health care resources at the macro level. According to Hu, the high saving rates of the family clinical account in fact represented a poor option for making better use of health care resources (Hu 2008). It was argued, moreover, that the family clinical care account diverted funds from the unified funding account that operated with risk pooling mechanisms for really threatening risks to the health and economic well-being of the peasant family (Wang et al. 2007: 105–7). Regarding management at the micro level, it was strongly argued that the family clinical care account was never a better alternative to OPP, to deal with minor cases, with reference to prudent choices and cost consciousness. Some policy analysts raised another criticism against Package III, suggesting that in managerial terms, the family clinical care account did not offer desirable results for medical care, since the peasant family could always afford to take care of their clinical services though OPP. They went as far as to state that since enrollees could foot medical bills by themselves, it was better they paid directly to the provider, without an intermediary (Gu, Gao & Yao 2006).

It is claimed that in Package III, the family clinical care account was market-oriented and was dictated by narrow concerns at the micro level, lacking not only a public policy perspective, but also managerial concerns. After all, it was taken as a poor design for an insurance plan, failing to address even the requisites of resource management (e.g., three Es). In some cases, for example, enrollees were reluctant to claim reimbursement in view of its small and insignificant sum, and the excessive time and effort required to negotiate the difficult and tedious application. They even saved the unspent amount in the account and rolled it over to pay for premiums for the following year. It is also claimed that the sunk revenue in the family account tended to weaken the risk pooling mechanisms, to increase difficulties for fundraising and to create room for possible abuse at the local level. In addition, some analysts advanced the notion that the physical examination has only limited value in detecting potential illness and is actually unnecessary after all (Wang et al. 2007).

Like the case of URMCI, NRCMCI encountered the same policy dilemma in the exercise of product/services specificity, namely, mismatch between the government's policy priority and the enrollee's preference. As a matter of strategy for implementation, policymakers finally reached a consensus by opting for something like Package III just mentioned- a NRCMCI package that combined clinical care with hospital care (and/or HESI cases). On the one hand, it could fulfill the original policy intent to provide relief of the financial burden of HESI for enrollees, and meanwhile, enhance "positive externalities," for example, the protection of risks of HESI in the community at large. On the other hand, the clinical care component so included could attract a largest possible size of enrollment and thus maintain sufficient revenue stream to the NRCMCI foundation, meanwhile allowing hospital care (and/or HESI cases) to address the issue of HESI.

Clearly, in the subsidy scheme characterizing NRCMCI, actors on the selling side (the insurer) needed to work out a set of preference mixes to accommodate two divergent preferences (in both the high and low tier) of the insured. At the end of the day, family clinical care was finally accommodated in Package III noted above, a version of NRCMCI package to attract and maintain a sizable number of the enrollees who were motivated by a sense of "ownership" of the insurance plan of their own choice. Indicative of Adaptation (A), many jurisdictions added the physical examination to NRCMCI packages to enhance the marketability, for example, attractiveness to the enrollee upon the recommendation of the 2003 Opinion.

Like with other public insurances, furthermore, policy actors had to wrestle with the strain between the "spread of benefit" (*shuoyimian*) and the "amount of spending" *(shouyie)* in the markets during the implementation of NRCMCI. Here the term "spread of benefit" refers to the number of patients who benefit from health care services, while the "amount of spending" pertains to the absolute sum of expenditure in each case (Chapter 9; Lee 2019). As Hu observes, for example, the expenditure for hospital care ran as high as 67 percent to 79 percent of the total expenditure on average cases for medical care services in NRCMCI for the three years 2006 to 2008, albeit the "spread of benefit" was very narrow, for example, 3 percent to 4 percent of the total number of enrollees involved in the same case of hospital care (Hu 2008).

Indicative of Adaptation (A), overall, both NRCMCI and NRCMI moved to respond to market signals by accommodating the preference mix of enrollees, and thus ensure steady revenue stream to sustain the foundation. As a strategy of financial management, moreover, the name of the game in packaging both insurance plans appeared to be a combination of a relatively small number of big spenders with a largest possible size of small spenders.

Adaptation (A) and program specificity were found reinforcing with each other in the evolutionary adjustments of NRCMI in the process of implementation. This represented the growth of a financial cross-subsidization scheme, allowing a small number of enrollees who each involved big expenditure cases (including hospital care and HESI), meanwhile relying on the surplus of premium contributions generated from a sizable number of enrollees who only made use of clinical care and spent a much smaller portion of funds. In practice, the said design of financial cross-subsidization scheme was manifested in the existing pattern of financial performance. In the survey of the national total expenditure for NRCMCI conducted by MOH in 2005 as given in Table 11.3, for example, 74.2 percent was spent for hospital care, 20.4 percent for clinical care, 2.1 percent for physical examinations and 1.7 percent for high-risk cases (Wang et al. 2007: 75).

As given in Table 11.4, a data set prepared by MOH indicates that, as of 2005, only 3.3 percent of the total number of enrollees took advantage of hospital care, while 53.4 percent received compensation (i.e., co-payment) for clinical care from

Table 11.3 National Expenditure of NRCMCI Funds (2005)

Nation & Region	Total of Expenditure (Million)	Various Items of Expenditure				
		Hospital Care	Clinical Care	Physical Exam	Cases of Risk	Others
Nation	6175.004	74.2	20.4	2.1	1.7	1.6
Eastern Region	4053.318	75.1	18.7	2.0	2.3	1.9
Central Region	1036.031	76.8	18.5	2.8	0.3	1.6
Western Region	885.638	66.7	30.8	1.7	0.3	0.5

Source: Adapted from *Quanquo xinxing nongun hezou yiliao jiben xinxin baobiao 2005(Basic statistical report of national NRCMCI)*, compiled by Ministry of Health, PRC. in Wang, Y., Liu, X. Cui, H., & Tang, J. 2007. Xinxing nongcun hezuo yiliao zhidu de jianli he fazhan (The establishment and development of a new rural cooperative medical system) in Chen, J. & Wang. Y. (Eds.), *Zhuanxing Zhong de weisheng fuwu yu yiliao baozhang* (*The Health Care Reform and Medical Care*). Beijing: Shehui kexue wenxian chubanshe. 78.

Table 11.4 National NRCMCI: The Spread of Benefit (2004–2005) (Unit %)

Nation & Region	2004		2005	
	Hospital Care Compensation	Clinical Care Compensation	Hospital Care Compensation	Clinical Care Compensation
Nation	3.2	81.3	3.3	53.4
Eastern Region	3.0	59.2	3.0	55.7
Central Region	3.4	92.0	3.7	40.0
Western Region	3.1	105.5	3.6	62.7

Source: Adapted from *Quanquo xinxing nongun hezou yiliao jiben xinxin baobiao 2005(Basic statistical report of national NRCMCI)*, compiled by Ministry of Health, PRC. in Wang, Y., Liu, X. Cui, H., & Tang, J. 2007. Xinxing nongcun hezuo yiliao zhidu de jianli he fazhan (The establishment and development of a new rural cooperative medical system) in Chen, J. & Wang. Y. (Eds.), *Zhuanxing Zhong de weisheng fuwu yu yiliao baozhang* (*The Health Care Reform and Medical Care*). Beijing: Shehui kexue wenxian chubanshe. 90.

NRCMCI plans. The general pattern regarding the number of enrollees in various types of medical care services remained consistent throughout the three regions as of 2005: For hospital care only, 3 percent of enrollees in the Eastern Region, 3.7 percent in the Central Region, and 3.6 percent in the Western Region, while for clinical care, 55.7 percent in the Eastern Region, 40 percent for the Central Region and 62.7 percent for the Western Region (Wang et al. 2007: 90).

Further Growth of Hierarchies

The progress in the implementation of NRCMCI was impressive indeed, moving forward relatively fast within about six years from 2002 to 2008 while it was established in nearly 3,000 county jurisdictions throughout China. In each county jurisdiction, not only was a new organizational apparatus installed, but also the NRCMCI foundation was put in operation to cover a considerable portion of the medical care expenditure of enrollees. In such a rapid marketization process, however, some unanticipated policy outcomes (e.g., excessive saving) occurred, warranting to make Adaptation (C) relying on command-oriented management in hierarchies to enforce the public policy goal.

To begin with, overwhelming evidence indicates that in the process of inaugurating NRCMCI, excessive saving/deposit in the NRCMCI foundations was built up invariably in most of the pilot programs. Various policy analysts offer tentative explanations for this phenomenon from different angles. One explanation is concerns considerations of uncertainty inherent in the process of implementation itself. For example, it is suggested that policy actors in charge of introducing NRCMCI worried about possible shortfalls in collecting premiums, as they tried to avoid the risk of financial burden so created at the local government level. This often resulted in overly restrictive spending control measures, such as higher rates for deductible and co-payment, and high payment-ceiling at the expense of the patients. Also, excessive saving was attributable to the move taken by policy actors in low echelons to anticipate long delays for matching funds from higher levels (e.g., the central and provincial level) to enter the accounts in time (Gu, Gao, & Yao 2006; Wang et al. 2007).

In the NRCMCI foundation, excessive saving also resulted from managerial and institutional considerations. To begin with, one may treat excessive saving in the NRCMCI foundation as an unintended consequence stemming from overly restrictive spending control measures, such as deductibles, co-payments and payment-ceilings, similar to BMCI. A survey of 257 counties throughout the country indicates that the said spending control measures were introduced to varying degrees. For example, a spending ceiling was installed in nearly 90 percent of counties surveyed, suggesting that the issue of overspending was a serious concern of policymakers at the provincial/local level (Wang et al. 2007). It also became evident that as a matter of policy and managerial concerns, higher hurdles of deductible were adopted for hospitals in the higher echelons of the hierarchy in almost all cases in response to the excessive overconcentration of patients in high-grade hospitals as well as under-utilization of health facilities down below, characterized as a "reverse pyramid" shape (Lee 2019).

Second, it was argued in this study that the excessive savings built in the NRC-MCI foundation were the other side of the same coin regarding the dynamic of operation and management of funding within the IRF system, representing a key feature of transaction-centered management. On the one hand, it was desirable that the collection of premium payments was able to exceed insurance payment by a substantial safe margin to maintain an optimal scale of risk pooling and anticipate a sudden and unexpected increase in high expenditure cases, on top of regular funding requirements for the risk pooling reservoir. On the other hand, it was not deemed desirable to go beyond maintaining the safe margin of deposit but jeopardize the concern for better utilization of funds for the benefit of enrollees.

To remedy the "excessive" saving, yet maintain a safe margin of funds in the NRCMCI foundation, policy actors, including the county management committees and executive agencies, were expected to readjust the rates of deductibles, co-payments and payment-ceilings in timely fashion, and to find better ways to ensure that enrollees enjoy the benefits that they had paid for in the name of "value for money" (*wuyou shouzhi* in Chinese). Accordingly, policy actors often adjusted the spending control measures of pilot programs and to maintain a budgetary balance between the safety margin and appropriate utilization of funds. An official consensus was reached to control the safe deposit within the foundation at 15 percent of the annual average total of premium contributions (Xiao 2010: 226).

Last but not least, NRCMCI is concerned with how large the portion of financial burden is imposed on the enrollee in a fundamental sense. If NRCMCI cannot substantially provide relief to the enrollee, it defeats the rationale for its introduction. A sample of 27 county jurisdictions indicates that NRCMCI could only compensate 25.8 percent of hospital care expenditure by each enrollee in 2004, and 23.4 percent in 2005 (in the first six months). And in the same sample, it is found that NRCMCI was able to cover 27.9 percent of medical bills for clinical care in 2004 and 30.4 in 2005 (in the first six months) (Xu, Zhou & Yao 2007: 14–5).

According to Hu, it is estimated that for four years from 2003 to 2006, NRC-MCI was only able to shoulder about 30 percent of medical bills for hospital care for the enrollee, meaning that the enrollee concerned needed to be responsible for approximately 70 percent. Such a high percentage of OOP is considered burdensome to the peasants, as Hu claimed (Hu 2008). A set of statistics cited by Hu shows that enrollees were compensated 32.14 percent for their clinical care expenses and 31.31 percent for their hospital care expenses nationwide in 2004. And, indicative of Adaptation (C), the very low percentages of subsidy to medical care expenses through NRMCMI as cited above are attributable to overly restrictive spending control regarding deductibles, co-payments, and of payment-ceilings (Hu 2008: 199). This remains a crucial issue to be watched by policymakers, analysts and researchers for some time to come.

Concluding Remarks

In this chapter, the study argues that NRCMCI represents an innovative breakthrough in the public funding policy of medical care for the peasantry in China.

From a managerial and financial perspective, it is argued that NRCMCI relied on two funding sources: One derived from the enrollee's share of premium contributions, and other stemming from the government's subsidy to premium contributions. On the one hand, NRCMCI operates with the IRF system in that financial resources circulate within a closed arena, making sure that, in financial terms, input matches output in each item of transaction. On the other hand, one may characterize the financial relationship of the government to the enrollee in terms of the ORF system, through which the former directly subsidizes the latter in making premium contributions.

Notes

1 The direct subsidy addresses the matters of economy, efficiency, and effectiveness (the three Es) better by requiring more weighting and calculation regarding the services to be chosen in both qualitative and quantitative terms, and enhancing scrutiny over providers and accountability for their performance in the IRF system. By contrast, characteristic of the ORF system, the indirect subsidy allocates health care resources to the public providers who rely on public financial management, taking clues from authorities rather than the markets.

2 To be dealt with in the exercise of program specificity, "reversal of choice" refers to a process in the markets where, as a matter of calculating one's perceived self-interests, healthy and/or high-income users tend to refrain from subscribing to the plan, while less healthy and/or low-income users are more likely to stay with the plan, resulting in a shrinkage of enrollments to sustain the plan.

3 During the economic reform, provincial and local governments started to shoulder a heavy burden of expenditure, fluctuating in the region of 70 percent, and it increased visibly from 2003 onwards, for example, 69.9 percent from 2002 to 2003, 72.3 in 2004 and 74.1 percent in 2005. Besides, the share of revenue of provincial/local government shrank dramatically beginning from 1993 onwards, for instance, 78 percent in 1993 to 44.3 percent in 1994, 47.8 percent in 1995, 48.9 in 1996, and 45.4 in 2003, 45.1 in 2004 and 47.7 in 2005 (Gu 2008: 233).

References

Gu, X. 2008. *Zuoxian quanmin yibao: Zhongguo xinyigai de zhanlue yu zhanshu* (*The Strategy and Tactics of The New Medical Care Reform in China*). Beijing: Zhongguo laodong shehui baozhang chubanshe.

Gu, X., Gao, M., & Yao, Y. 2006. *Zhengduan yu chufang, zhimian Zhongguo yiliao tizhi gaige* (*Diagnosis and Prescription, Confronting China's Medical Care Reform*). Beijing: Shehui kexue wenxian chubanshe.

Hu, S. 2008. Woguo xinxing nongcun hezou yiliao zhidu de yunxing zhuangkuan yu pingjia enfengxi (The operation and assessment of the new rural cooperative medical care system in China). *Zhongguo weisheng jingji* (*China's Medical Care Economics*) 27: 2.

Lee, P. N. 2020. *Re-engineering Affordable Care in China*. London & New York: Routledge.

Wang, X. 2003. *Fenpei zhengyi yu shehui baozhang* (*Distributive Justice and Social Security*). Shanghai: Shanghai caijing daxue chubanshe.

Wang, Y., Liu, X., Cui, H., & Tang, J. 2007. Xinxing nongcun hezuo yiliao zhidu de jianli he fazhan (The establishment and development of a new rural cooperative medical system). In Chen, J., & Wang. Y. (Eds.), *Zhuanxing Zhong de weisheng fuwu yu yiliao baozhang*

(*The Health Care Reform and Medical Care*). Beijing: Shehui kexue wenxian chubanshe. 64–124.

Weishengbu, Caizhengbu & Nongyebu 2003. *Guanyu jianli xinxing nongcun hezuo yiliao de yijian* (Opinion concerning the establishment of a new rural cooperative medical care). www.gov.cn/zwgk/2005-08/12/content_21830.htm.

Weishengbu, Caizhengbu & Nongyebu 2007. Guanyu jianli xinxing nongcun hezuo yiliao zhidu de yijian (Opinion concerning the establishment of a new rural cooperative medical care system). In Ge, Y., & Gong, S. (Eds.), *Zhongguo yigai: wenti, gengyuan, chulu* (*China's Medical Care Reform: Issues, Origins and Solutions*). Beijing: Zhongguo fazhan chubanshe. 141–4.

Xiao, A. S. (Eds.) 2010. *Nongcun yiliao weisheng shiye de fazhan.* (*The Development of Rural Medical and Health Care Enterprises*). Zhengjiang: *Jiangshu daxue chubanshe*.

Xu, L., Zhou, L., & Rao, K. 2007. Xinxing nongcun hezuo yiliao guanli jigou diaocha fenxi jieguo (Investigation and analytical framework on new rural cooperative medical care management apparatus. In Weishengbu tongji xinxi zhongxin (Ed.), *Zhongguo xinxing nongcun hezuo yiliao jinzhan jiqi xiaoguo yanjiu* [The Progress as well as the Research on the Effects of the New Rural Cooperative Medical Care in China]. Beijing: Zhongguo xiehe yike daxue chubanshe. 9–19.

Zheng, G. 2011. *Zhongguo shehui baozhang gaige yu fazhan zhanlue* (China's Social Security Reform and Developmental Strategy). Beijing: *Renmin chubanshe*.

Part IV

Conclusion and Future Trend Analysis

12 Assessment and Discussion

The foregoing chapters have provided a portrait of healthcare insurance reforms in China, that built a network of three clusters of public medical care insurance, each centering on BMCI, NRCMCI, or URMCI respectively for more than three decades from the late 1980s. The BMCI programs formally commenced in 2001, involving a large scale of funding during a relatively long implementation time span from the early 1990s to the present. The NRCMCI was able to move faster, from 2003 to 2008, covering more than 90 percent of rural households and/or individuals enrolled in various packages. The URMCI began late in 2007 and was quickly extended to all residents who enjoyed household registration but were not employed or only employed part time in the public sector. Taken as a whole, these public medical care insurance packages were intended to cover the entire Chinese population.

Starting in 2016, the government decided to take further steps to merge the URMCI and NRCMCI into an urban & rural resident medical care insurance (URRMCI) as previously noted, but it appears that URRMCI is still at the early stage of implementation. And the National Healthcare Security Administration (NHSA), an entirely new ministerial ranking unit, was established in 2018. NHSA is supposed to oversee all functions under both the BMCI and URRMCI, among others. And in the latest policy paper on medical care insurance in 2020, the central government only urged the provincial/local government to promote territorial integration through strengthening "vertical management" and the command of municipal/prefectural jurisdiction. Meanwhile, the central government announced the commencement of pilot experiments of "unified funding" (*tongchou*) at the provincial level, and tried to take one step forward toward the national URRMCI (Zhonggong Zhongyang & Guowuyuan 2020). As China's healthcare reforms are taken as an on-going concern, the study here has been focused only on the BMCI, NRCMCI and URMCI, leaving URRMCI for further study till the dust becomes fully settled.

It is evident that the network of three clusters of public medical care insurance is intended to address the essential medical care demands of various sectors of the population, but they share some common features as well as similar issues of program specificity emerging from the dynamic of implementation. Arising from policy implementation, some of these issues merit further analysis in the remaining

DOI: 10.4324/9781003389934-16

passages as follows: the emerging trend, risk-pooling in operations, the product/services specificity concerning HESI, and the policy of integration.

The Emerging Trends

Representing a great leap forward in the realm of public policy in China, the government has built an entire network of public medical care insurances available to the population since the late 1980s. How to characterize the overall tendency of public policy that three programs represent? The study argues that the overall tendency of the network of public medical care insurances is marked by the rise of a hybrid mode of governance that features the application of markets, risk pooling design, and the concern of HESI cases in the realm of resource management. It is warranted here to examine what kinds of issues have emerged in conjunction with introducing the hybrid mode, and how the policymakers try to deal with them accordingly.

On the official records, the policymakers were able to install a network of public medical care insurances, covering nearly the entire population throughout China at the commencement of the new health care reform in 2009.[1] About one decade after, the NHSA announced statistics regarding enrollment in the major public medical care insurances in 2020, likely the most recent data available. As of 2020, the national total of enrollees in all public insurances for health care stood at 1,361,310,000, stably remaining at more than 95 percent of the population. The number of staff and workers subscribing to public insurance is 344,550,000 (including 254,290,000 currently employed and 90,260,000 retirees). For enrolled employees, the breakdown is as follows: 222,670,000 staff and workers in public enterprises, 62,320,000 public personnel in government and quasi-government units, and 44,260,000 flexibly employed personnel among others (Guojia yiliao baozhangju 2020). As of 2020, the total enrollment in URRMCI is 1,016,760,000 as given by NHSA without making any differentiation between NRCMCI and URMCI. As the research on URRMCI has yet to continue, nonetheless, NHSA provides breakdowns of URRMCI as follows: Adults, 750,100,000; students in primary and middle schools, 246,100,000, and college students, 20,560,000 (Guojia yiliao baozhangju 2020).

Mission is considered incomplete with regards to the reform of public medical care funding, however. The inauguration of public medical care insurances followed a sequential model of policymaking in the sense that it relied heavily on a series of the policy experimentations and pilot programs seemingly without a master plan to guide its path of development. According to Professor Zheng, three public medical care insurances each operated on their own and were isolated from one another in financial and managerial terms, as no functional linkage was installed to connect one with another at their early phase. Taken as a whole, he adds that the three programs were a kind of "patchwork" rather than a system holding all components together. In other words, the policymakers successfully installed BMCI, URMCI and NRCMCI in each of three clusters, albeit some gaps still have remained with regards to pockets of personnel who were left out of any medical care insurance plan.

The first cluster was concerned with the workforce in the urban area, some of whom were covered by BMCI in the planned sector, but others in the non-planned sector were not included in any insurance plan, for example, private enterprises and business of foreign investment, depending on the progress of economic reform. Among various public medical care funding programs, the BMCI was taken as the top priority, answering the funding demands of staff and workers in public enterprises. The BMCI was originally intended to replace the LIMC and PFMC. However, neither BMCI was able to achieve the integration between LIMC and PFMC by the new healthcare reform during 2009–2012, nor it succeeded to incorporate flexibly employed personnel and agricultural laborers owing to the narrowness of the BMCI design and slowness to catch up relatively fast industrial development and rapid social changes (Zheng 2011).

Taken as the topmost priority of the healthcare reforms, the BMCI was introduced earliest among various public medical care insurances. And it took the longest time span to install in the public sector in China, requiring considerable effort and injection of enormous funds from the provincial/local jurisdictions and public enterprises. For sure, the vested interests of the first several cohorts of the workforce who had worked under the CPE strategy during the pre-reform era carried weight in the making of BMCI. As indicated in Table 12.1, it took a lengthy period of nearly three decades for the echelons of government to expand enrollment of BMCI (including both employees and retirees) from 2,901,000 in the early 1990s and to 344,550,000 in 2020. And it is evident that BMCI is in operation despite gaps in implementation.

The study argues that the BMCI was introduced for two policy concerns. To deal with the issues arising from the forced modernization during the pre-reform era, first, it addressed the alienation of entitlement from funding that was responsible not only for the shortage of funding, but also for final breakdowns of conventional modes of funding of medical care. Second, it intended to provide public funding to basic medical care to the entire workforce, both senior and junior age groups, and in planned and non-planned sectors in the urban area. It appears that policymakers tried hard to fulfill both policy concerns, and a preliminary assessment based on various clusters and groups is overdue.

In the first cluster of public medical care insurances, there are four categories/ groups of people, and each faced with issues yet to be tackled. The first group was concerned with one of the most noted groups former enrollees of the conventional PFMC (i.e., those public personnel working for government and quasi-government units), estimated at 63,870,000 as of 2020 (Guojia yiliao baozhangju 2020), slightly less than one third of staff and workers in public enterprises. And they were supposed to join BMCI originally in accordance with the 1998 Decision, but they remained as a separate category enjoying different sets of medical care entitlements till the new healthcare reform in 2009 (Chapters 1 and 4). Some progress of integration between LIMC and PFMC has been registered for more than one decade since 2012. For example, some recent material indicates that in about

Table 12.1 Enrollment of Basic Medical Insurance 1993–2020 (Unit 10K)

Years	Total of Enrollees	Employees	Retirees
1993	290.1	267.6	22.5
1994	400.3	374.6	25.7
1995	745.9	702.6	43.3
1996	855.7	791.2	64.5
1997	1762.0	1588.9	173.1
1998	1877.7	1508.7	369.0
1999	2065.3	1509.4	555.9
2000	3787.0	2862.8	924.2
2001	7222.9	5407.7	1815.2
2002	9401.2	6925.8	2475.2
2003	10901.7	7974.9	2926.8
2004	12403.7	9044.5	3359.2
2005	13782.9	10021.7	3761.2
2006	15731.8	11580.3	4151.5
2007	18020.3	13420.3	4600.0
2008	19995.6	14987.7	5007.9
2009	21937.0	16410.0	5527.0
2010	-	-	-
2011	-	-	-
2012	26485.0	19861.0	6624.0
2013	27443.0	20501.0	6942.0
2014	28296.0	21041.0	7255.0
2015	28893.0	21362.0	7531.0
2016	29532.0	21720.0	7812.0
2017	30322.0	22288.0	8034.0
2018	31681.0	23308.0	8373.0
2019	32924.0	24224.0	8700.0
2020	34455.0	25429.0	9026.0

Sources: Gu 2010; Zheng 2011: 106–7; 115; NHSA 2021: 219.

25 out of 31 provincial units, PFMC was incorporated into LIMC, although a small pocket of enrollees still stay at the ministerial level and in provincial governments (https://baike.baidu.com/item/公费医疗/4897377).

The second group is concerned with the employed personnel of public enterprises, including retirees and former employees who had once been affiliated with work units, but did not enroll in BMCI for a variety of reasons, such as transfer to a new job, unemployment due to industrial reorganization (the policy of "transfer, closure, merging and stoppage") as well as bankruptcy and financial difficulties within the existing enterprises. In most cases, the work units were unable to find ways and means to make premium contributions for them to BMCI, where provincial/local jurisdictions could not afford to shoulder the financial responsibility to lend them needed help (Zheng 2011: 120–3).

The third group had to do with "flexibly employed personnel," estimated at 47,510,000 as of 2020, who remained active, being either self-employed or employed by non-public enterprises (Chapter 9; Guojia yiliao baozhangju, 2020).

Most flexibly employed personnel were not counted in the BMCI system. And, it became more difficult to incorporate them into the healthcare insurance as their size expanded further. The healthcare reform faced a dramatic increase of urban employees for a relatively short time of 15 years from 170,410,000 in 1990 to 283,000,000 in 2005, as the workers and staff employed by public enterprises under the conventional CPE framework remained stable for the same time period from 103,460,000 in 1990 to 111,610,000 as cited by Professor Gu (2008: 165). This means that sizable urban employees, an estimated additional 170,000,000 approximately, were still unaccounted for any healthcare insurance.

According to Professor Zheng, employees in public enterprises (SOEs and COEs combined) made up 12.1 percent of the total of registered industrial enterprises in 2008. The remaining, estimated at 87.9 percent, were non-public in nature, representing a new and thriving sector of China's reform economy (of which, 44.4 percent are private enterprises; 10.7 percent, Hong Kong/Taiwan investments; 11.7 percent, foreign investments; and 21.1 percent, other categories). And they were still not included in the network of healthcare insurance. Accordingly, the government tried to establish some form of public medical care insurance for staff and workers in "private enterprises" a selected sector of the flexibly employed personnel just noted, but the policy had been only partially implemented prior to the new healthcare reform in 2009, partly because of overloading caused by the rapid increase of flexibly employed personnel. Various jurisdictions were slow in catching up the task of providing insurance programs for them, and the situation turned worse. For example, as cited in a set of statistics, there witnessed a dramatic increase from 19.2 percent in 2003 to 28.9 percent in the total of enrolled employees in private enterprises in 2008 (Zheng 2011: 116–7).

The fourth group pertained to agricultural laborers, representing a substantial figure and on the rise as well, for example, 225,420,000 in 2008 and 229,780,000 in 2009 (Chapter 9; Zheng 2011: 118–20). Agricultural laborers working outside their home jurisdictions were counted as 140,410,000 (62.3 percent of the total of workforce) in 2008 and 145,330,000 (63.2 percent of the total of the workforce) in 2009. As a forerunner of medical care insurance reform in the case of Shenzhen, agricultural laborers were provided with medical care insurance in Scheme III and were "tied down" to some chosen clinics at the urban district level as previously noted (Chapter 9). The central government endeavored to incorporate agricultural laborers into some forms of medical care insurance. For example, the State Council promulgated the 2006 Several Opinions, urging the various municipal jurisdictions to introduce a kind of HESI insurance to cover agricultural laborers (Zheng 2011: 118–20) It appears that, in the long run, agricultural laborers need to find some form of essential medical care insurance in cities, for instance, either URCMI, NRCMCI, BMCI or some other insurance options, provided that various municipal jurisdictions could find ways to cross the hurdle of household registration as a restriction over eligibility to social security benefits (including medical care) in case of agricultural laborers (Zheng 2011). It is noteworthy, nevertheless, that the central policymakers did try to put the issue of public medical care insurance for the last three groups on the policy agenda starting amid the new healthcare reform in 2009–2011 (Guowuyuan Bangongting 2015).

The second cluster of public medical care insurances mainly covered urban residents, most of whom were family members of employees in the public sector, but they were left outside of the BMCI reform until 2007 (Chapter 9). In the designs of social security programs including LIMC and PFMC within the CPE framework, individual membership was adopted as a criterion for establishing eligibility for enrollment and as a result, family members were not able to be included into the said programs. As the former enrollees in LIMC and PFMC had to shift to BMCI formally in 2001, most urban residents were incorporated into URMCI instead. Meanwhile, there still existed pockets of residents who had to be accounted for in other options of public medical care insurances in view of their special status, demands, and funding requirements, for instance, the senior residents, primary and middle school pupils and college students among others (Chapter 9).

The third cluster embraced a vast group of peasants, many of whom had previously been covered by the RCMC before economic reform, but were brought into an entirely new public funding system of NRCMCI at the county level (Chapters 10 and 11). With exceptions, NRCMCI represented an institutional upgrade from the collective work unit (production brigade) to the party-state hierarchy, and it was county-centered in terms of managerial and financial function. Like URMCI, it relied upon risk pooling mechanisms and transaction-centered management run by the NDPE, a form of non-governmental body. Considering the funding design, the risk pooling scale was still limited as the policymakers considered options of an even larger scale of risk pooling to be managed at the prefectural/municipal level ore beyond. As portrayed above, the network of public medical care insurances represents an on-going policy trend of marketization, marking the beginning of a fresh cycle of policymaking, together with new sets of policy issues. However, the overall policy agenda is not immune from some limitations, for example, exceedingly heavy burden in repaying "historical debt," unanswered medical demands of fresh workforce released from rapid urbanization and new industries, fragmentation associated with many uncoordinated insurance plans, and privileges and distributive justice among strata of enrollees (Zheng 2011).

Risk-pooling Mechanisms in Operation

As the result of healthcare reforms, evidence indicates that public medical care insurances have operated as a novel system of public financial management on both the funding and the spending side in full swing. Among new financial issues of public medical care insurances, one of the principal concerns had to do with the holding and management of risk pooling on a considerable scale, in addition to the functions of input (i.e., funding) and output (i.e., spending). In all public medical care insurances, the hybrid mode of governance is characterized by transaction-centered management where the executive agency (a NDPE) plays the pivotal role as the insurer of the insurance foundation, as it is managerially connected with the enrollee (as the insured) and providers respectively through contractual relations.

All key services such as curative services, drug provision and medical devices are rendered and managed through negotiations in the markets (Guowuyuan Bangongting 2015).

However, not all public medical care insurances work managerially and institutionally in the same fashion. For example, BMCI differs significantly from NRCMCI and URMCI regarding a range of features such as legacy and policy evolutions, the designs of financial management, product/service specificity, risk pooling mechanisms, methods of funding and premium contribution, and spending and payments schemes. In BMCI, policymakers had to address the alienation of entitlements that was rooted in the conventional funding of medical care as well as the compensation policy under the CPE framework in the past (Chapter 4). To put it simply, the employees were given social security entitlements such as LIMC and PFMC during the forced modernization without a foundation to back up spending upon the due time (Chapters 6 and 7).

Once BMCI was put into operation, it started to work with a cycle of circulating funding and spending that operates with risk pooling mechanisms to meet the funding requirements of enrollees. To answer the funding demands incurred by LIMC and PFMC during the pre-reform period, it is warranted for BMCI to set aside a large sum of fund to sustain the risk pooling reservoir and provide a financial cushion for the spending in medical care for the future, especially among senior employees and retirees in the public sector. For instance, revenue of BMCI reached 1,573.2 billion RMB and expenditure 1286.7 billion RMB, resulting in a surplus of 246 billion, as of 2020. As 924.5 billion RMB was credited to the USFA accounts (including childbirth insurance) in 2020, the actual expenditure was 793.1 billion RMB, resulting in the annual saving of 131.4 billion RMB in USFA accounts (Guojia yiliao baozhangju 2020). While 658.7 billion was credited to PA accounts, expenditure came to 493.6 billion RMB in 2020, slightly less than equivalent to the annual revenue of PA account. However, for PA account, the accumulated saving was 1,009.6 billion RMB in 2020, indicative of its good financial health, but suggestive of needed improvements in effective use (Guojia yiliao baozhangju 2020).

It appears overall that BMCI enrollees' use of medical care services registered a visible increase slightly less than double over the decade of the 2010s and climaxed in 2019 when cases of treatment reached 21.2 billion in 2019 and 1.79 billion in 2020 respectively. However, regular clinical care and emergency cases were recorded as 1.5 billion in 2020, a reduction of 16.7 percent from 2019, and special clinical care cases for serious illness were 0.23 billion, about 8.8 percent less than 2019. Hospital care cases numbered 0.05 billion, or 12.3 percent less than that of 2019 (Guojia yiliao baozhangju, 2020).

As for the percentage of payment out of the total of the insurance fund, there was a steady improvement prior to the new healthcare reform in 2009. Several authors have tried to monitor the share contributed by public medical care insurances (including other forms of public funding) to alleviate a patient's medical care financial burden. Lee's study portrays the overall trend of improvement in payment out of public insurance funds from 24.1 percent at the lowest point in 2001 to 35.61 percent in 2012 (Lee 2019: 80). Gu Xin's statistical analysis confirms that in some visible way, there was an expanding share of public funding for medical care within the total expenditure for healthcare (including BMCI, URMCI, NRCMCI, and PFMC), from 28.9 percent in 2004, 32.3 percent in 2005, 34.8 percent in 2006, 32.7 percent in 2007 to the highest point, 38.2 percent in 2008 (Gu 2010a: 106).[2]

Given that variation among public medical care insurance packages, it appears that there will be much room on the part of policymakers to expand the share of public funding within the total expenditure for medical care, especially in both NRCMCI and URCMI that were far behind BMCI and even PFMC. According to the Fourth National Survey of Health Care Services conducted by MOH in 2008, insurance payments registered 63.2 percent on average in the total medical bill of BMCI, 49.3 percent in URMCI and 33.7 percent in NRCMCI (Gu 2010b: 60). Gu observes that in the said national survey, the proportion of self-payment (OPP) is highest in NRCMCI in the region of 60–70 percent and the lowest in BMCI in the range of 30–40 percent, while URMCI stands in between (Gu 2010b: 61). Parallel to Gu's study during the same period, Zheng's estimate in his study suggests that the reimbursement stands at approximately 30 percent in the case of NRCMCI (meaning 70 percent of OPP), while reimbursement for medical care reaches 50 percent (as expected) in the case of URMCI (about 50 percent of OPP) (Zheng 2011), attesting to the discrepancy between the two. The discrepancy between the two can be explained tentatively in terms of "half insurance" that enrollees enjoyed historically in case of URMCI (Chapters 4 and 9).

It appears that there is a considerable gap between the policy objective and the reality regarding the relatively low funding level in NRCMCI and URMCI. In accordance with the 2011 Major Tasks in Five Reforms of the Medical Care and Health Care, for example, it is suggested to raise the level of payments for hospital care to about 70 percentage of expenditure in URMCI and NRCMCI at the very end, coupled with a lift of payment-ceiling in the said two public insurances to six times of disposable income of urban residents or average net income of the peasant (Guowuyuan Bangongting 2015).

After one decade from 2011 to 2020, the NHSA's statistical bulletin indicates improvement in raising the level of payments in all three public medical care insurances. For example, insurance payments for hospital care were recorded at a national average of 85.2 percent for BMCI (i.e., 88.7 percent for 1st tier hospitals, 86.9 percent for 2nd tier hospitals and 84.3 percent for 3rd tier hospitals). In the case of URRMCI (i.e., the successor of NRCMCI plus URMCI), insurance payments for hospital care registered at a national average of 70 percent for hospital care (i.e., 79.8 percent for 1st tier hospitals, 73 percent for 2nd tier hospitals, and 65.1 percent for 3rd tier hospitals) (Guojia yiliao baozhangju 2020).

Attesting the risk pooling mechanism in operation, one of the most salient issues for the healthcare insurance reform among policymakers continues to be the rates of deposit. With reference to the rates of growth of savings, a set of data for BMCI indicates that the annual rates of saving within the total income ranged between 20 percent and 30 percent over one decade during 1999–2009 with the highest rate at 32.25 percent in 2002 and lowest at 24 percent in 1999 (Zheng 2011: 127). In 2009 the sum of accumulated deposits reached 405.5 billion RMB, including 266.1

billion RMB credited to USFA and 139.4 billion RMB to PA (Zheng 2011: 127, 129).

By the new healthcare reform during 2009–2011, policymakers were in the position to form an opinion on the issue of saving deposits.[3] The State Council urged various jurisdictions to strengthen the budgetary management of insurance foundations, establish the analysis and early warning system regarding the operation of foundation, and further improve control and efficient use of healthcare resources. It is advised that in some jurisdictions, the excessive saving of BMCI foundation needed to scale down gradually to a reasonable level, and the annual rate of saving of NRCMCI ought to observe the limit of 15 percent, and rate of accumulated saving to be controlled within 25 percent (Guowuyuan Bangongting 2015).

As no statistical data was available after launching the new healthcare reform in 2009, the latest and only set of statistics regarding public medical care insurances (including other forms of funding) for employees in the public sector indicates that in 2020 the annual savings for USFA was 121.4 billion RMB and the total of accumulated savings was 1,532.7 billion RMB (nearly equivalent to the annual income of 1,573.2 billion RMB) as just noted. In the same year, the annual savings to PA was 165 billion RMB, coupled with 1,009.6 billion RMB of accumulated deposits (amounting to about 1.6 times the annual income of 658.7 billion) (Guojia yiliao baozhangju 2020).

In addition, the revenue of the unified funding foundation of BMCI (including revenue sources other than premium contributions) was 914.5 billion RMB and expenditure was 793.1 billion RMB, generating a saving of 121.4 billion. The total accumulated savings of the foundation was 1,532.7 billion, nearly equivalent to the annual revenue (or 100 percent) of BMCI itself (Guojia yiliao baozhangju 2020). It is noteworthy that well within the policy intent in case of BMCI, overall, relatively high rates of saving tend to enhance its capacity to address the issue of alienation of entitlements from funding and strengthen its risk pooling mechanisms to cope with the arrival of large cohorts of employees with seniority and retirees in due course.

Based on integration between NRCMCI and URMCI formally commencing in 2016, the magnitude of URRMCI's financial foundation has grown considerably as well. As of 2020, the annual deposits stand at 9.49 billion RMB and accumulated deposits at 60.77 billion RMB (Guojia yiliao baozhangju 2020). Although other sources of statistical data are needed for double-checking and comparative analysis, it appears that the newly constructed health care insurance system has started to operate as a security net for people throughout the country for the first time in the history of PRC.

Debates on Product/Services Specificity

Representing a special concern of policymakers, the packaging of public medical care insurances is highlighted by emphasis on so-called high expenditure and serious illness (HESI) in the exercise of product/service specificity. However, it has been challenging for policy circles to come to a consensus on HESI at conceptual and definitional level. To begin with, the operational definition of "major illness" (*dabing*), together with its financial implications, persisted as a controversial policy issue, the resolution of which lent justification to interventions by the government. After all public medical care insurances were introduced, central policymakers did not take further initiatives until 2012 when the State Development and Reform Commission together with five ministerial units promulgated the 2012 Advisory Opinion spelling out for the first time the central government's new position regarding the key features of "major illness insurance" (Guojia fazhan gaigewei et al. 2012).

Conceptually speaking, one may define "major illness" (*dabing*) from two perspectives: It may be treated either as a serious illness from the pure consideration of medical science *or* from a financial point of view as a high expenditure case involving diagnosis, treatment, and recuperation. Of course, the two perspectives often overlap to a considerable extent. Major illness falls into a broad category of many types of medical care services, but only part of the services is considered serious enough to warrant funding through the public medical care insurance when the individual patient and/or work unit is not able to shoulder its financial burden. However, much ambiguity remains to be clarified in NRCMCI and URMCI, which are originally supposed to cover highly expensive medical care services.

Policymakers made it clear early on that NRCMCI was intended to help peasant families cope with impoverishment caused by serious illness (Chapters 10 and 11). In the process of implementation, moreover, NRCMCI and URMCI were focused mostly on HESI (by and large, including hospital care), while, by original policy intent, clinical care was supposed to be handled through OPP to be paid by the enrollees themselves. Nonetheless, many jurisdictions still incorporated clinical care in their insurance packages for enrollees to maintain a sense of "ownership" among enrollees and attractiveness of the said packages in the marketplace (Chapters 9–11).

The 2012 Advisory Opinion represented the first attempt for central policymakers to work on operational definitions, producing a set of classifications for "major illness." From considerations of product/service specificity, "major illness" embraces three types of medical care: (1) regular hospital care to be covered by payments under the payment-ceiling; (2) high expenditure and serious illness (*gaoe zhongbing* or HESI), namely, treatment normally involving payments above the payment-ceiling but less than payments for catastrophic illness; and (3) types of catastrophic medical care events that are often listed and treated as a separate category of extremely high and uncontrollable expenditure, to be handled through specially designed funding programs (Guojia fazhan gaigewei et al. 2012; Guowuyuan Bangongting 2015). Accordingly, the 2012 Advisory Opinion recommends lending priority to HESI in all public medical care insurance programs, making it the core feature of NRCMCI and URMCI (Sun 2013).

In the exercise of product/service specificity, for instance, preference mix carried weight in the market transaction between the insured (i.e., the enrollee) and insurer (i.e., the insurance foundation). On the one hand, the enrollee dictated, in full and in part, the preferred package. On the other hand, command was relevant to the extent that hierarchy (i.e., government) impacts the pattern of market choices through subsidizing a certain desirable preference mix lending priority to "major illness," the operational definition of which was constructed through actuarial science and financial analysis in line with the government's policy requirements (Zhu, Song & Wang 2013; Xu & Li 2015; Xu & Du 2016).

In the policy evolution of public medical care insurance, ironically, neither at the central nor at the provincial/local level did policymakers maintain sequential consistency for funding major illness in two policymaking episodes, where the central government and provincial/local jurisdictions each reversed their respective positions. As the study examined the first episode in case of BMCI (Chapter 8), the second episode has to do with URMCI and NRCMCI that was quite complex and difficult to handle in theoretical terms (Chapters 9–11).[4]

In fact, HESI created tensions in the "marketizing" process of URMCI and NRCMCI, which raised the question whether, in market transactions, the parties involved were necessarily motivated by "preference", a notion yet to be defined and operationalized. Theoretically speaking, as one party in each transaction, the enrollee is *not* dictated by one preference alone, but by a cluster of preferences (or called preference mix) with varying weight in his or her behavior of choice in the market, as demonstrated during the implementation of URMCI and NRCMCI (Chapters 9 and 11). That is to say, the enrollee needed to deal with more than a preference—one set of preferences (e.g., between serious illness versus common and frequent disease, and between HESI versus clinical care, etc.) when entering transactions within the insurance market. In theoretical terms, moreover, it is not expected that all enrollees will act with the same preference mix, given the relative weight of preference mix in market transactions. For instance, depending on the enrollees concerned, clinical care might carry more weight than HESI (mostly hospital care), or vice versa. In the case of NRCMCI and URMCI, most enrollees expected regular clinical care to be covered with a sense of "ownership" of the insurance packages that they subscribed to (Chapters 9 and 11). In a subjective sense, the insurance plan that enrollees could not enjoy often enough in daily life is taken as too remote and therefore not relevant to themselves. A considerable number of enrollees would rather take a chance by not including HESI and other expensive items such as hospital care into their insurance package because these cases rarely take place anyway (Gu 2008).

Further tension arises due to HESI involving a relationship between the government and the enrollee. From the public policy perspective, the government tended to regard highly expensive and uncontrollable costs of those items of service (including hospital care and HESI) as top policy priority, although it was not a party to the transaction as shown in case of NRCMCI and URMCI (Chapters 9–11). In both NRCMCI and URMCI, nevertheless, the government wielded financial power to subsidize enrollees, nudging them to focus on expensive items of services in the insurance plan they subscribed to. By doing so, the government pushed for a different agenda for public policy purposes (e.g., provision of positive externalities), the enforcement of which relied on public finance and the exercise of authority (Chapters 9–11).

As the dust settled after the implementation of NRCMCI and URMCI during the early 2010s, the central policymakers became aware that the said two insurance packages fell short of the earlier expectation of maintaining an adequate level of funding for HESI, and tried to upgrade the two packages through a number of adjustments in the managerial and financial realm. As claimed in the 2012 Advisory Opinion, the funding level for HESI cases was too low, and enrollees registered a strong desire for alleviating the financial burden of HESI in the respective insurance packages. Accordingly, not only did the 2012 Advisory Opinion recommend making better use of actuarial and scientific methods, but also it explored answers to the question of feasibility either by using the savings of the insurance funds or by adjusting the rates of premium contributions to finance HESI (Guojia fazhan gaigewei et al. 2012).

How is medical care under HESI to be funded? It is proposed in the 2012 Advisory Opinion that the medical care insurance plans under HESI ought to be funded principally through existing insurance plans such as URMCI and NRCMCI by setting aside one portion of the fund from existing savings derived from premium contributions, and/or by raising additional percentage of premium contributions if existing savings are found inadequate, as this had been put into practices in some jurisdictions. Based on policy experiments and pilot programs at the early phases of healthcare reform, it was well taken that in the designs of public medical care insurances, there existed feasible and effective options to deal with HESI within the available funding sources so prescribed. The issue of HESI could be resolved through simple actuarial and financial exercises on a limited scale without resorting to major program restructuring.[5]

The 2012 Advisory Opinion urges provincial/local jurisdictions to aim high at the expenditure level for catastrophic illness whenever feasible by devising new funding alternatives for HESI. Also, it suggests adopting either the annual average disposable income of urban residents or the annual average income of peasants as a concrete criterion for calculating a reasonable funding level for medical care. To strengthen the funding for HESI, it further suggests that each insurance package sets minimum requirements for the insurance foundation to cover at least 50 percent of a payment in case of HESI. From a long-term policy perspective, it urges expanding the scale of economy for risk pooling by upgrading the jurisdiction of the insurance plan from the county level to the municipal level (conventionally, prefectural level) (Guojia fazhan gaigewei et al. 2012; Guowuyuan Bangongting 2015).

Furthermore, according to the 2012 Advisory Opinion, the role of the commercial insurance company needs to play a principal role in order to manage HESI, and the government ought to organize the bidding by making a selection among commercial insurance corporations and adopt contractual mechanisms to shoulder the financial burden of HESI insurance. Also, in a concrete form of management, the government recommended the experimental program of Chongqing Municipality, as put forth in 2001 (Guojia fazhan gaigewei et al. 2012). The design of Chongqing's insurance program was market-oriented, as funding for high expenditure cases mainly was entrusted to a commercial insurance company, relying on a funding source from co-insurance by the work unit and enrollees, and operating with risk-pooling mechanisms (Congqingshi laodong he shehui baozhangju & Congqingshi caizhengju 2001).

The 2012 Advisory Opinion was slow to make any fundamental change in conceptual terms, treating HESI as a "supplement, extension and expansion of basic medical care." Wu Mutu takes exception to this while arguing that HESI ought to be treated instead as an inalienable part of basic medical care from considerations of maintaining life from a medical standpoint. Even though it is difficult to predict and estimate the costs of any given HESI event, it is nonetheless necessary despite the unpredictability to cover such costs for the sake of maintaining good health and saving lives. In Wu's view, therefore, public medical care insurance ought to incorporate HESI regardless of its cost, even if exceedingly high.[6] He argues, furthermore, that although major illness is expensive, many clinical care items are, in some cases, equally expensive, such as items treating chronic illnesses, expenses for which can accumulate to a small fortune over time (Wu 2013). As the argumentation goes on, it appears that consensus has yet to be forged on the operational dimension of HESI.

Policy of Integration

As public funding packages for health care became prolific in China, there witnessed considerable institutional fragmentation, inadequacy of coordination, an inefficient use of healthcare resources as well as in absence of distributive justice (Zheng 2011). For several unsolved issues as noted, it was well warranted for sovereign planners to move forward, introducing a policy of integration to improve the performance of public medical care insurances, better serve the basic medical care demands of the people, and alleviate the existing disparities among various sectors of population, among others.

The notion of integration (or *zhenghe* in Chinese) is multi-dimensional. And, in operational terms, it may entertain three senses: Territorial integration, program integration and functional integration. In practice, one kind of integration might overlap with another, and often be supplemented with one another. The first refers to the combination among small territorial jurisdictions at the lower level of the jurisdiction into the large one at the higher level, for example, from the county level to municipal/prefectural level or even provincial level. In the design of public medical care insurance, territorial integration concerns itself with maximizing the scale of risk pooling to absorb costs of each episode of HESI. The second is program-centered, meaning an endeavor of merging similar programs into one under one singular command within the same jurisdiction, ensuring that a given sector/group of enrollees is treated in a common and standard fashion, for example, URCMI with NRCMCI. The third is concerned with functional linkages. Examples include referral between hospitals of various specialties or of different classes of hospitals for medical treatments; portability of insurance plans across regions, and coordination at the managerial and financial level, such as sharing of operational information and data on medical care insurance through the internet, etc. In light of Zheng' analysis, functional integration is built on connectivity in several functional realms: Funding, spending, management, service delivery, information and computer services, and institution and environment (Zheng 2011).

The policy of integration was articulated with regards to two sets of integration among several public medical care insurances from the late 1980s to the 2010s. One set was concerned with fusing PFMC and LIMC into BMCI, and the other set pertained to combining NRCMCI and URMCI into urban/rural resident insurance (abbreviated as URRMCI; i.e., *chengxiang jumin baoxian* in Chinese). As noted in Figure 12.1, policymakers tried to take steps to achieve program integration of all four public medical care insurances, and eventually build a national health care insurance system, interfaced with intermediary stages of combining smaller territorial jurisdictions into larger ones at the territorial level (e.g., from county level, to municipal/prefectural level and provincial level).

As originally recommended in the 1998 Decision, the first set of program integration was intended to merge PFMC and LIMC into one program (namely BMCI), embracing all employed personnel in the public sector (both public personnel of the government and quasi-government units and staff and workers of

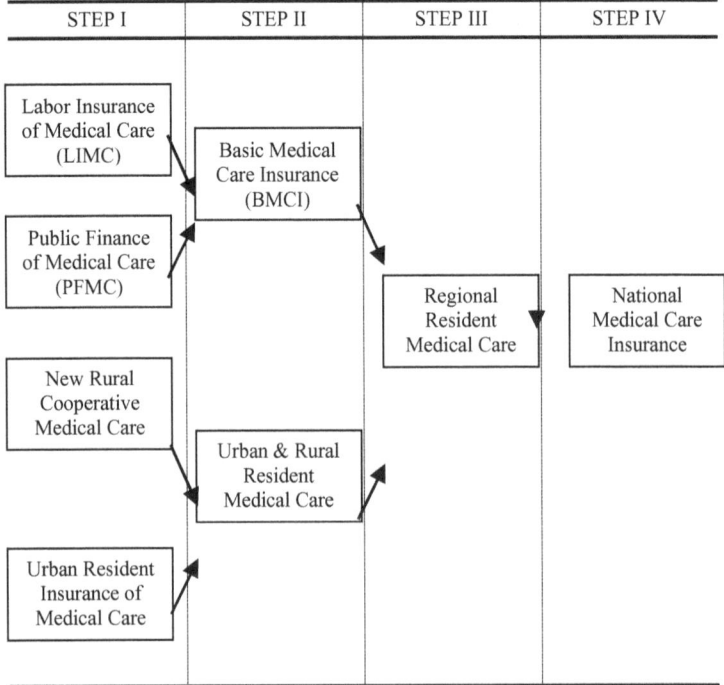

Figure 12.1 The Proposed Policy Agenda of Integration of Public Medical Care Insurances.

Source: Adapted and translated with minor revisions from: Zheng, G. 2011. *Zhongguo shehui fazhan zhanlue* (*Social Security Reform and Strategy for Development*). Beijing: Renmin chubanshe. 135

public enterprises) as noted in Figure 12.1. On the surface, there existed considerable homogeneity between the said two programs with reference to the types of entitlements and the standards of funding. Neither PFMC nor LIMC was financed through an institutionalized funding approach during the pre-reform period, however, as they each were taken as "work-unit centered," in a managerial or even financial sense and in fact, funded through their respective channels of financial source in common with other budgeted items in the social security system (Chapter 4).

It is noteworthy that even in the transition to BMCI reform, sovereign planners endeavored to maintain some measure of comparability between PFMC and LIMC. For example, the top policymakers found it necessary to remedy the thrifty version of BMCI by installing SMCI during the early phase of policy experiments, adding still another layer of insurance entitlement through SMCI during the late 1990s and, similarly, PFMC was given the comparable layer of SMCI (Chapter 8). From 2001 onwards, the funding for PFMC maintained considerable continuity except that it involved a change of title in that state budget (listed instead as "*xingzhen jiguo he shiye danwei jingfei,*" "current expenses for medical care for the administrative apparatus and service work units"), still representing a different public funding channel for medical care running parallel to BMCI for the time being (Chapter 4).

Evidence suggests that the PFMC enrollees enjoyed better medical care entitlements than that of BMCI enrollees, attesting the perpetuation of substantial vested interests among government officials and party cadres in retaining PFMC (Huang 2020: 129–33). As of 2002, for instance, the total expenditure for PFMC stood at 25.17 billion RMB, compared with 60.78 billion RMB for staff and workers (about 41.4 percent), while the size of PFMC enrollees was less than one third of that of BMCI (Zheng 2011: 121–2). Overall, the funding for PFMC enrollees registered an upward trend from 21.1 billion RMB in 2000 to 47.1 billion RMB in 2008 (Zheng 2011: 121). Despite inertia and resistance, the central policymakers did try to take a gradual and soft approach to enforce the policy of integration of PFMC with BMCI in accordance with the 1998 Decision. As early as 2009, a pilot program on such integration was first introduced to Pingu county in Beijing, and the policy formally commenced there in 2012. Other provinces joined the implementation of the integration policy from 2012 to 2002, and, at the end of day, 24 out of 31 provincial units adopted the integration policy of PFMC with BMCI for public personnel affiliated with echelons of the provincial/local government and service work units at the provincial/local level. As the central policymakers to push the said integration policy, only a small pocket of public personnel still stays with PFMC, embracing the officials and cadres directly affiliated with ministerial units and provincial governments as of today (https://baike.baidu.com/item/公费医疗/4897377).

As indicated in Figure 12.1, furthermore, central policymakers seized the opportunity to merge URMCI and NRCMCI into one singular urban/rural resident insurance (abbreviated as URRMCI, or *chengxiang jumin baoxian* in Chinese) in 2016, representing a significant landmark of healthcare reform since 2009. The State Council put forth its 2016 Opinion, urging respective provincial/local jurisdictions to plan and make arrangements for integration between the said two before the end of June, 2016 and prepare to implement the proposals concretely by the end of the same year. Intending to merge NRCMCI and URMCI in URRMCI, the 2016 Opinion requires provincial/local jurisdictions to achieve "unity" (*tongyi*) in several functional areas at the municipal level: The coverage of enrollees (all residents within the jurisdiction except for enrollees in BMCI and PFMC), the same funding policy, common entitlements, standard insurance catalogs for services and drugs, the common list of designated providers, and a similar insurance foundation management (Guowuyuan 2016).

With regards to product/service specificity, both NRCMCI and URMCI were focused on insurance packages for so-called "major illness," covering relatively expensive types of services, from hospital care to the illnesses above the payment-ceiling (e.g., HESI and catastrophic medical care events). According to Cong, major illness insurance is a distinctive design focusing on healthcare risks involving much uncertainty and unpredictability, and it differs from retirement security in that it represents an income redistribution policy and a compulsory saving system. In addition, the funding of major illness insurance needs to be independent of the financial management of CPE and operate with risk-pooling mechanisms relying on a sizable scale of economy beyond the work unit (Cong 2006). From a public policy perspective, policymakers at both the central and provincial/local level intended to prevent or, at least, control impoverishment caused by HESI at the individual/family level (especially in case of NRCMCI), and to alleviate the financial burden of the work units (in case of URMCI).

Among policy analysts in China, Professor Zheng took pains to demonstrate the homogeneity between URMCI and NRCMCI to show feasibility of the program integration (Zheng, 2011). For instance, enrollees in both programs were required to subscribe to insurance plans as family members, albeit they were not employed in the public sector (i.e., neither staff and workers of public enterprises, nor public personnel of government and quasi-government units). For both programs as of 2010, the government set up a subsidy of 120 RMB for each enrollee. And while both were focused on "unified social funding" (or risk pooling) for "major illness" (including hospital care), they were allowed flexibility in extending gradually to clinical care over time. They were comparable in their payment schemes, for example, deductible, co-payments and payment-ceiling although URMCI was offered slightly favorable terms for funding. In addition, both adopted standard forms of spending control measures.

The prospect of integration is often associated with some challenges, for instance, potential rivalry between departments. Conceivably, the policy of integration between URCMI and NRCMCI needed to address their existing difference of institutional affiliation that entails considerable tension between the labor and social security bureau and healthcare bureau at the provincial/local level (Qian 2021: 81–99). They each had been under a different command system for coordination and management of public funding/insurance for residents in respective jurisdictions. For example, the healthcare bureau oversaw NRCMCI, while the labor and security bureau assumed main responsibility for URMCI. On a vertical level, meanwhile, each bureau was under the command of its ministerial unit, that is, either the Ministry of Labor and Social Security (MLSS) or Ministry of Health (MOH) respectively. Integration means that two programs need to be assigned to one ministry rather than two, tending to engender debates on pros and cons.[7] To circumscribe the potential conflicts between two ministries, together with possible frictions between their local counterparts down below, it appeared as a better option to establish an entirely new ministerial ranking unit—National Healthcare Security Administration (NHSA) to be in charge of URRMCI that combines both URMCI and NRCMCI. And it did happen in 2018.

According to Zheng, URRMCI stood as a favorable option to take advantage of an effective managerial apparatus and an expanded scale of risk pooling for the URRMCI foundation at the municipal/prefectural level. Moreover, the municipal government was endowed with financial resources and found itself in a better position to attract previous NRCMCI or URMCI enrollees at the county/urban district level to join URRMCI. In the case of a great disparity of economic development and income levels, however, it was challenging indeed to work with unified and standard premium schemes for different brackets of enrollees. In the pilot program in Xian municipality, for instance, the program integration entertained several brackets of premium contribution, coupled with various types of entitlements and funding levels commensurate with the classes of enrollees (Zheng 2011). Nevertheless, one ought not to under-estimate the complexity and difficulty regarding the undertaking of URRMCI, given that the echelons of the provincial/local jurisdiction to shoulder financial burden of subsidy to the enrollee's premium contribution and administrative and managerial workload in supervisory and managerial tasks with or without in the URRMCI program. What would then be new funding sources for the newly established URRMCI? As URRMCI marks the latest healthcare reform effort in China, one has to wait till the dust is settled, and an assessment of its progress will be warranted in due course.

Concluding Remarks

This study has dwelled on the discussion over and assessment of the gigantic undertaking of making public medical care insurances during economic reform in China, coupled with an analysis of recent developments, to conclude this book.

Overall, there are some questions left to be tackled, for instance, sustainability of the new system considering the contionus income growth and economic development, spread of rule of law and legal culture, and further consolidation of mixed economy, among others. Regarding the achievements. As argued, the network of three clusters of public medical care insurance was not only indigenous but innovative since it first emerged from policy experimentations and pilot programs in various provincial/local jurisdictions starting in the late 1980s and was subsequently adopted throughout the country. All three major programs of public medical care insurances relied not only on the use of risking-pooling schemes but also on market mechanisms, despite differences in terms of the enrollees covered, types of services offered, levels of funding, jurisdictions and scale of economy, policy legacies and vested interests among others. After the policymakers' attempt to fine-tune public medical care insurances by strengthening the financial management of HESI, especially in NRCMCI and URMCI, another major restructuring was soon made in 2016 to enforce the integration of NRCMCI and URMCI in URRMCI, marking a further step toward a prospective national health care insurance, a new policy agenda for the future.

Notes

1 For instance, it has been indicated in one of the latest sets of analysis available that the national total of enrollees in public medical care insurances reached an estimated 1,231,470,000, as of 2009. As for the breakdown of the national total, the enrollment figure in BMCI reached 219,370,000; that of URCMI was recorded at 182,100,000 while those enrolled in NRCMCI were counted to be 833,000,000 in 2009 (Zheng 2011: 46–7).

2 It is noted that Gu Xin in his previous analysis on the same subject-matter (Gu 2010a: 106) registers a slight discrepancy from the statistical data cited here (Gu 2010b: 60). This study adopts the latter in view of the greater detailed references provided.

3 For example, the Ministry of Human Resources and Social Security put forth the circular concerning full extension of the work of urban resident basic medical care insurance (abbreviated as the 2009 Circular) in 2009, advising various jurisdiction to maintain the appropriate balance of insurance fund, avoid excessive saving and ensure that more enrollees to benefit from the insurance plans (Renshebu 2009).

4 In the first policy episode involving the thrifty version of BMCI, the central government insisted to incorporate clinical care, in the mix of HESI (including hospital care) and regular clinical care, while the provincial/local jurisdictions were inclined to include HESI cases only for many employees and enterprise units suffering ruinous consequences during the early phase of economic reform (Chapter 5; Lee 2019). The issue of HESI was not handled seriously until the introduction of supplementary medical care insurance (SMCI), as evident in the drafting of the 1998 Decision (Chapter 7; Lee 2019). In the second episode pertaining to NRCMCI and URMCI, the central government shifted its priority as it determined to install HESI mainly for public policy considerations, as the provincial/local jurisdictions endeavored to answer the enrollees' demands for clinical care, and meanwhile, to protect and maintain a revenue source from premiums contributed by a sufficiently large number of enrollees through market mechanisms (Chapters 8–10).

5 For instance, in Shenzhen, the executive agency would handle HESI within 0.4 percent of expenditure of the SMI plan it had implemented. And as for the SMCI plan administered by the Labor and Social Insurance Administration in Guangzhou, enrollees needed to contribute a premium of 0.29 percent of the average monthly wage in order to cover up to 95 percent of payment for major illnesses in the above-ceiling payment category (i.e., critical hospital care and designated clinical care). As an option to commercial medical care insurance plans, the Shanghai Federation of Labor Unions, offered a medical care mutual security plan (*yiliao huzu baozhang jihua*), embracing four schemes: Scheme 1 for seven types of "particularly serious illness" (catastrophic illnesses); Scheme II for major illness involving above-ceiling payments by staff and workers in order to cover hospital care, specially defined clinical care, family care services, and emergency observation; Scheme III for retirees; and Scheme IV for special cases for women (breast and ovarian cancers). For all four schemes, enrollees have an option to pay either as a monthly fee (without refund) or as a lump sum (with refund) (Chapter 8).

6 Wu states that basic medical care ought to maintain the minimal requirement for ensuring the continuity of life and the biggest threat to life is major illness, not minor ailments

such as common and frequent illnesses. He adds that medical care entitlements differ from other types of social security entitlements in that the former are contingent upon risk factors whose costs cannot be defined, calculated and even fixed in quantitative terms like retirement pension or housing benefits (Wu 2013).

7 It is argued that the division of labor was better delineated in the case of URMCI, if it was to be assigned to the labor insurance bureau at the local level. To put it in another way, while the labor insurance bureau could perform an impartial role regulating and supervising the medical care insurance, and maintaining its institutional integrity on the funding side, the health care bureau could be held responsible for supervising providers on the spending side. In the case of NRCMCI, by contrast, one singular set of organizations, namely, the health care bureau, was in command of both the insurance funding apparatus (such as the executive agency of the insurance foundation) and providers and public health care facilities. And, this was likely to produce policy distortion in the sense that the health care bureau might be given discretion to distort its role of supervising spending at the expense of maintaining integrity of control and financial discipline in performing its funding role (Zheng 2011).

References

Cong, S. 2006. Lun guojian yi dabing baozhang wei hexin de yiliao baozhang zhidu (On the medical care security system focusing on major illness insurance). *Shehui baozhang zhidu (Social Security System)* 6, 45–50.

Congqingshi laodong he shehui baozhangju & Congqingshi caizhengju. 2001. Congqing-shi chengzhen zhigong jiben yiliao baoxian shiji tongcuo dae yiliao fuzu jijin zanxin banfa (The provisional measures of municipal-wide unified high expenditure medical care mutual help foundation for medical care insurance for staff and workers in cities and towns of Congqing municipality). http://www.rongchang.gov.cn/zwgk.264/zcjd/201912/PO20191220436982021987.docx November 20, 2021. 6:50pm, 1–3.

Gu, X. 2008. *Zuoxian quanmin yigai, zhongguo xinyigai de zhanlue yu zhanshu (Towards Universal Coverage of Healthcare Insurance, the Strategical Choices and Institutional Frameworks of the New Health Care Reform)*. Beijing: Zhongguo laodong shehui baozhang chubanshe.

Gu, X. 2010a. Xinyigai weijinlu (The unfinished journey to new medical care reform). *Tizhi gaige (System Reform)* from Zhonggo renmin daxue shubao zhiliao zhongxin. (originally from Caijing 2010. 6, 28–32).

Gu, X. 2010b. *Quanmin yibao de xintansuo (New Exploration for the National Medical Care Insurance)*. Beijing: Shehui kexue wenxian chubanshe.

Guojia fazhan gaigewei et al. (2012). Guanyu kaizhan chengxiang jumin dabing baoxiang gongzou de zhidao yijian (The advisory opinion regarding the launching of the task of major illness insurance for residents in cities and countryside). In Guojia weisheng jishen-wei (Eds.) *2012 nian shenhua yigai wenjian huibian (The 2012 Collected Documents of Further Health Care Reform)*. Beijing: Guojia weisheng jishenwei.

Guojia yiliao baozhangju (Eds.) (2020). 2020 nian quanguo yiliao baozhang shiye fazhan tongji 20/21. 6:50pm gongbao (*Statistical Communique of National Medical Care Security*). http:www.nhsa.gov.cn/art/2021_7_5232.htm 12/2/21. 9:35am, 1–8.

Guowuyuan. 2016. Guowuyuan guanyu zhenghe chengxiang jumin jiben yiliao baoxian zhidu de yijian (The opinion of the state council regarding the integration of basic medical care in-surance for urban and rural residents). http://baike.baidu.com/reference/4277454/1873Urw zYuLMHXs…IGXsOc388e3krl_Ao2rhdf6MFcp65MFcp65Hs8woThXBrYgRSi1-PJjw

Guowuyuan Bangongting 2015. Yiyao weisheng tizhi wuxiang zhongdian gaige 2011 niandu zhuyao gongzuo anpai (The 2011 major task schedule of five key reforms in the system of medical care and health care). in Guojia weisheng jishenwei (Eds.), *2011 nian shenhua yigai wenjian huibian* (*The 2011 Collected Documents of Further Medical Care Reforms*) 29–39. Beijing: Guojia weisheng shengjiwei.

Huang, X. 2020. *Social Protection under Authoritarianism, Health Politics and Policy in China.* New York: Oxford University Press.

Lee, P. N. 2019. *Re-engineering Affordable Care Policy in China, Is Marketization A Solution?* London & New York: Routledge.

Qian, J. 2021. *The Political Economy of Making and Implementing Social Policy in China.* Singapore: Palgrave Macmillian.

Renshebu 2009. Guanyu quanmian kaizhan chengzhen jumin jiben yiliao baoxian gongzuo de tongzhi (The Circular concerning the task of full extension of urban resident basic medical care insurance) in Guojia weisheng jishen wei (Eds.), *2009 nian Shenhua yigai wenjian huibian* (*The 2009 Collected Documents of Further Medical Care Reforms*). 43–5. Beijing: Guojia weisheng jishengwei.

Sun, Z. 2013. Shishi dabing baoxian shi jianqin renmin jiuyifudan de guanjian (The key link to lessening the people's burden is through big expenditure insurance). *Shehui baozhang zhidu* (*Social Security System*) 3: 49–52.

Wu, R. 2013. Guanyu dabing baoxian de sikao (Considerations on the reform of major illness insurance). *Shehui baozhang zhidu* (*Social Security System*) 5: 59–62.

Xu, W. & Du, Z. 2016. Dabing baoxian shishi xiaoguo pinjia (Assessment of the results of implementing major illness insurance). *Weisheng jingji yanjiu* (*Research of Health Care Economics*) 9.353: 54–7.

Xu, W. & Li, M. 2015. Jiben yiliao baoxiang dui zhongda de baozhang xiaoying yanjiu (The impact of basic medical care insurance on major illness security). *Weisheng jingji yanjiu* (*Research on Health Economics*) 8.340: 36–9.

Zheng, G. 2011. *Zhongguo shehui baozhang gaige yu fazhan zhanlue* (*The Reform and Strategy of Development of Social Security in China*). Beijing: Remin chubanshe.

Zhonggong Zhongyang & Guowuyuan 2020. "Guanyu Shenhua yiliao baozhang zhidu gaige de yijian" (Opinion regarding the further reform of medical care insurance system) (abbreviated as the 2020 Opinion). Retrieved from http://www.gov.cn/zhengce/2020-03/05/content_5487407.htm 12/9/21, 11.23 AM. 1–5

Zhu, M., Song, Z. & Wang, Y. 2013. Dabing baoxian puchan moshi de sikao (Considerations regarding the compensation model for major illness insurance). *Shehui baoxian zhidu* (*Social Security System*) 5: 63–71.

Index